Athletic Injuries of the Hip

Editors

DUSTIN L. RICHTER
F. WINSTON GWATHMEY

CLINICS IN
SPORTS MEDICINE

www.sportsmed.theclinics.com

Consulting Editor
MARK D. MILLER

April 2021 • Volume 40 • Number 2

ELSEVIER

1600 John F. Kennedy Boulevard • Suite 1800 • Philadelphia, Pennsylvania, 19103-2899

http://www.theclinics.com

CLINICS IN SPORTS MEDICINE Volume 40, Number 2
April 2021 ISSN 0278-5919, ISBN-13: 978-0-323-77842-8

Editor: Lauren Boyle
Developmental Editor: Donald Mumford

Clinics in Sports Medicine (ISSN 0278-5919) is published quarterly by Elsevier Inc., 360 Park Avenue South, New York, NY 10010-1710. Months of issue are January, April, July, and October. Business and Editorial Offices: 1600 John F. Kennedy Blvd., Ste. 1800, Philadelphia, PA 19103-2899. Customer Service Office: 3251 Riverport Lane, Maryland Heights, MO 63043. Periodicals postage paid at New York, NY and additional mailing offices. Subscription prices are $364.00 per year (US individuals), $931.00 per year (US institutions), $100.00 per year (US students), $405.00 per year (Canadian individuals), $964.00 per year (Canadian institutions), $100.00 (Canadian students), $475.00 per year (foreign individuals), $964.00 per year (foreign institutions), and $235.00 per year (foreign students). Foreign air speed delivery is included in all *Clinics* subscription prices. All prices are subject to change without notice. **POSTMASTER:** Send address changes to *Clinics in Sports Medicine*, Elsevier Health Sciences Division, Subscription Customer Service, 3251 Riverport Lane, Maryland Heights, MO 63043. Customer Service (orders, claims, online, change of address): Elsevier Health Sciences Division, Subscription Customer Service, 3251 Riverport Lane, Maryland Heights, MO 63043. **Tel: 1-800-654-2452 (U.S. and Canada); 314-447-8871 (outside U.S. and Canada). Fax: 314-447-8029. E-mail: journalscustomerservice-usa@elsevier.com (for print support); journalsonlinesupport-usa@elsevier.com (for online support).**

Reprints. For copies of 100 or more of articles in this publication, please contact the Commercial Reprints Department, Elsevier Inc., 360 Park Avenue South, New York, NY 10010-1710. Tel.: 212-633-3874; Fax: 212-633-3820; E-mail: reprints@elsevier.com.

Clinics in Sports Medicine is covered in *MEDLINE/PubMed (Index Medicus) Current Contents/Clinical Medicine, Excerpta Medica,* and *ISI/Biomed.*

Contributors

CONSULTING EDITOR

MARK D. MILLER, MD
S. Ward Casscells Professor, Head, Department of Orthopaedic Surgery, Division of Sports Medicine, University of Virginia, Charlottesville, Virginia; Team Physician, Miller Review Course, Harrisonburg, Virginia

EDITORS

DUSTIN L. RICHTER, MD
Assistant Professor, Sports Medicine, Director, Sports Medicine Fellowship Program, Department of Orthopaedic Surgery, University of New Mexico Health Sciences Center, University of New Mexico, Albuquerque, New Mexico

F. WINSTON GWATHMEY, MD
Associate Professor, Sports Medicine, Director, UVA Residency Program, Department of Orthopaedic Surgery, University of Virginia School of Medicine, University of Virginia Medical Center, Charlottesville, Virginia

AUTHORS

MATTHEW B. ANASTASI, MD
Mayo Clinic, Orthopedics, Sports Medicine Department, Phoenix, Arizona

ERIC AZUA, BS
Division of Sports Medicine, Department of Orthopedic Surgery, Section of Young Adult Hip Surgery, Rush Medical College of Rush University, Rush University Medical Center, Chicago, Illinois

JENNIFER A. BELL, MD
Orthopaedic Surgery Resident, USC Epstein Family for Sports Medicine at Keck Medicine of USC, Los Angeles, California

IOANNA K. BOLIA, MD, MS, PhD
Research Associate, USC Epstein Family for Sports Medicine at Keck Medicine of USC, Los Angeles, California

BRIAN D. BUSCONI, MD
Orthopedic Sports Medicine Surgeon, Department of Orthopedics and Physical Rehabilitation, University of Massachusetts Medical School, Worcester, Massachusetts

JACOB G. CALCEI, MD
Department of Orthopaedic Surgery, University Hospitals of Cleveland, Case Western Reserve University, Cleveland, Ohio

JONATHAN W. CHEAH, MD
Department of Orthopaedic Surgery, Orthopedic Surgeon, Sports Medicine Specialist, Santa Clara Valley Medical Center, San Jose, California

ZACHARY K. CHRISTOPHER, MD
Mayo Clinic, Orthopedics, Sports Medicine Department, Phoenix, Arizona

CHRISTOPHER C. CHUNG, BS
Medical Student, Department of Orthopaedic Surgery, University of Virginia Medical Center, Charlottesville, Virginia

PETE CICINELLI, PT, DPT
Major League Head Physical Therapist, Atlanta Braves, Truist Park, Southeast, Atlanta, Georgia

REBECCA A. DUTTON, MD
Assistant Professor, Department of Orthopaedics and Rehabilitation, University of New Mexico, Albuquerque, New Mexico

KOSTAS J. ECONOMOPOULOS, MD
Mayo Clinic, Orthopedics, Sports Medicine Department, Phoenix, Arizona

AMANDA N. FLETCHER, MD, MS
Department of Orthopaedic Surgery, Orthopaedic Surgery Resident, Duke University Medical Center, Durham, North Carolina

F. WINSTON GWATHMEY, MD
Associate Professor, Sports Medicine, Director, UVA Residency Program, Department of Orthopaedic Surgery, University of Virginia School of Medicine, University of Virginia Medical Center, Charlottesville, Virginia

ARIANNA L. GIANAKOS, DO
Orthopaedic Surgeon, Department of Orthopaedic Surgery, Robert Wood Johnson Barnabas Health – Jersey City Medical Center, Jersey City, New Jersey

KYLE E. HAMMOND, MD
Assistant Professor of Orthopaedic Surgery, Emory University Sports Medicine Center, Atlanta, Georgia

DAVID A. HANKINS, MD
Lexington Orthopaedics, West Columbia, South Carolina

JOSHUA D. HARRIS, MD
The Houston Methodist Hip Preservation Program, Houston Methodist Orthopedics and Sports Medicine, Associate Professor, Houston Methodist Academic Institute, Houston, Texas; Associate Professor of Orthopedic Surgery, Weill Cornell Medical College, New York, New York; Adjunct Assistant Professor, Texas A&M University, College Station, Texas

JEFFREY D. HASSEBROCK, MD
Mayo Clinic, Orthopedics, Sports Medicine Department, Phoenix, Arizona

LEE KNEER, MD
Assistant Professor of Physical Medicine and Rehabilitation, Assistant Professor of Orthopaedics, Emory University Sports Medicine Center, Atlanta, Georgia

LUCAS KORCEK, MD
Slocum Center for Orthopaedics and Sports Medicine, Eugene, Oregon

TIMOTHY P. LANCASTER, MD
Resident Physician, Department of Orthopaedic Surgery, University of Virginia Medical Center, Charlottesville, Virginia

BRIAN D. LEWIS, MD
Department of Orthopedics, Duke University Medical Center, Durham, North Carolina

RICHARD C. MATHER III, MD, MBA
Department of Orthopaedic Surgery, Associate Professor of Orthopaedic Surgery, Orthopaedic Surgeon, Sports Medicine Specialist, Duke University Medical Center, Duke Sports Science Institute, Durham, North Carolina

MARY K. MULCAHEY, MD
Orthopaedic Surgeon, Department of Orthopaedic Surgery, Tulane University School of Medicine, New Orleans, Louisiana

TIMOTHY J. MULRY, DO
Orthopedic Sports Medicine Fellow, Department of Orthopedics and Physical Rehabilitation, University of Massachusetts Medicine School, Worcester, Massachusetts

SHANE J. NHO, MD, MS
Department of Orthopaedic Surgery, Associate Professor of Orthopaedic Surgery, Orthopaedic Surgeon, Sports Medicine Specialist, Midwest Orthopaedics at Rush, Section of Young Adult Hip Surgery, Rush Medical College of Rush University, Rush University Medical Center, Chicago, Illinois

MARC A. NICHOLES, BA
Medical Student, School of Osteopathic Medicine, University of the Incarnate Word, San Antonio, Texas

KWAN J. PARK, MD
The Houston Methodist Hip Preservation Program, Houston Methodist Orthopedics and Sports Medicine, Houston, Texas

KEVIN C. PARVARESH, MD
Division of Sports Medicine, Department of Orthopedic Surgery, Section of Young Adult Hip Surgery, Rush Medical College of Rush University, Rush University Medical Center, Chicago, Illinois

JONATHAN RASIO, BS
Division of Sports Medicine, Department of Orthopedic Surgery, Section of Young Adult Hip Surgery, Rush Medical College of Rush University, Rush University Medical Center, Chicago, Illinois, USA

DUSTIN L. RICHTER, MD
Assistant Professor, Sports Medicine, Director, Sports Medicine Fellowship Program, Department of Orthopaedic Surgery, University of New Mexico Health Sciences Center, University of New Mexico, Albuquerque, New Mexico

PAUL E. RODENHOUSE, DO
Orthopedic Sports Medicine Fellow, Department of Orthopedics and Physical Rehabilitation, University of Massachusetts Medicine School, Worcester, Massachusetts

MARC R. SAFRAN, MD
Department of Orthopaedic Surgery, Stanford University Medical Center, Palo Alto, California

MATTHEW R. SCHMITZ, MD
Chair, Department of Orthopaedics, San Antonio Military Medical Center, Fort Sam Houston, Texas

PAUL B. SCHROEDER, MD
Resident, Department of Orthopaedics, San Antonio Military Medical Center, Fort Sam Houston, Texas

SELINA R. SILVA, MD
Department of Orthopaedic Surgery, University of New Mexico, Albuquerque, New Mexico

ALEXANDER E. WEBER, MD
Assistant Professor of Orthopaedics, USC Epstein Family for Sports Medicine at Keck Medicine of USC, Los Angeles, California

KATHRYN C. YEAGER, MD
Department of Orthopaedic Surgery, University of New Mexico, Albuquerque, New Mexico

JOHN W. YUREK, DO
Orthopaedic Surgeon, Department of Orthopaedic Surgery, Robert Wood Johnson Barnabas Health – Jersey City Medical Center, Jersey City, New Jersey

Contents

Hip pain is a common complaint in athletes and can result in a significant amount of time lost from sport. Diagnosis of the source of hip pain can be a clinical challenge because of the deep location of the hip and the extensive surrounding soft tissue envelope. Establishing whether the source of hip pain is intra-articular or extra-articular is the first step in the process. A thorough history and a consistent and comprehensive physical examination are the foundation for the proper management of athletes with hip pain.

Athletic injuries of the hip often require radiographs and advanced imaging for diagnosis. Plain radiographs evaluate for osseous injury, provide a structural context behind an athlete's symptoms and examination, and offer a backdrop for interpretation of advanced imaging. An understanding of normal anatomy, imaging findings, and radiographic measurements allows for recognition of pathoanatomy and ability to diagnose accurately. Advanced imaging modalities, including magnetic resonance imaging, computed tomography, and ultrasonography, each play a role in evaluation of the athlete's hip. Although MRI and CT provide high-resolution imaging of the hip, ultrasonography offers the unique ability to perform dynamic imaging and guided injections.

Femoroacetabular impingement and associated labral tearing is a common source of hip pain in athletes. This article reviews the hip joint anatomy and complex interplay between alterations on the femoral and acetabular sides, in addition to evaluation of soft tissue stabilizers and spinopelvic parameters. Symptom management with a focus on arthroscopic treatment of abnormal bony morphology and labral repair or reconstruction is discussed. In select patients with persistent pain who have failed conservative measures, hip arthroscopy with correction of bony impingement and labral repair or reconstruction has yielded good to excellent results in recreational and professional athletes.

Acetabular dysplasia represents a structural pathomorphology associated with hip pain, instability, and osteoarthritis. The wide spectrum of dysplasia anatomically refers to a 3-dimensional volumetric- and surface area-based insufficiency in coverage and is classified based on the magnitude and location of undercoverage. Borderline dysplasia has been variably defined and leads to management challenges. In symptomatic dysplasia, treatment addresses coverage with periacetabular osteotomy. Concomitant simultaneous or staged hip arthroscopy has significant advantages to address intra-articular pathology. In nonarthritic individuals, there is evidence PAO alters the natural history of dysplasia and decreases the risk of hip arthritis and total hip arthroplasty.

In this review, the recent literature evaluating the anatomic considerations, etiology, and management options for athletes with hip instability are investigated. Studies on the osseous, chondrolabral capsuloligamentous, and dynamic muscular contributions to hip stability are highlighted. Microinstability, iatrogenic instability, and femoroacetabular impingement-induced instability are discussed with a focus on demographic and outcomes research in athletes. Surgical techniques including both open and arthroscopic approaches are additionally evaluated.

Athletic injuries to the hip flexors and iliopsoas have been described in populations across all levels of competitive sports. Overall estimates of hip flexor pathology have ranged from 5% to 28% of injuries among high-risk sport specific groups. Although most of these injuries are successfully treated with conservative management, and high rates of return to play are observed, significant rehabilitation time can be involved. As the understanding of hip pathology with imaging modalities such as MRI has advanced, greater importance has been placed on accurately diagnosing hip flexor injuries and initiating rehabilitation protocols early to minimize time loss from sport.

The hip trochanteric bursa, tendinous insertions of the gluteal muscles, and the origin vastus lateralis make up the main structures of the peritrochanteric space. Greater trochanteric pain syndrome (GTPS) refers to pain generated by one or multiple disorders of the peritrochanteric space, such as trochanteric bursitis, gluteus medius and minimus tendinopathy or tear, and disorders of the proximal iliotibial band. Patients with GTPS might present with associated intra-articular hip pathology, which requires further investigation and appropriate management. Successful midterm outcomes have been reported in patients undergoing surgical treatment of GTPS using an open or endoscopic approach.

CLINICS IN SPORTS MEDICINE

SERIES OF RELATED INTERESTED

Orthopedic Clinics
https://www.orthopedic.theclinics.com/
Foot and Ankle Clinics
https://www.foot.theclinics.com/
Hand Clinics
https://www.hand.theclinics.com/
Physical Medicine and Rehabilitation Clinics
https://www.pmr.theclinics.com/

THE CLINICS ARE AVAILABLE ONLINE!
Access your subscription at:
www.theclinics.com

Foreword
Hip, Hip, Hurrah!

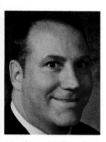

Mark D. Miller, MD
Consulting Editor

In the sports medicine world, you are either a "hipster" or you are not. If you are not, you need to have one (or more) of them on your team, and you need to know enough about the hip to know who to refer. This issue of *Clinics in Sports Medicine* is primarily focused on us "nonhipsters," and it is hoped, will make us just a little bit smarter in the eyes of the true "hipsters." It is also an update and treatise on athletic hip injuries for those of us who take care of these problems, and all aspiring "hipsters" out there.

This issue includes articles on evaluation and workup, treatment of many hip conditions, with a focus well beyond arthroscopy, and addresses many special situations, such as the adolescent hip, gender differences, and rehabilitation. I am proud of my partner at University of Virginia, Dr Winston Gwathmey, and former University of Virginia fellow, Dr Dustin Richter, for putting together such an outstanding issue—Go 'Hoos!

Mark D. Miller, MD
Division of Sports Medicine
Department of Orthopaedic Surgery
University of Virginia
Charlottesville, VA, USA

Miller Review Course
Harrisonburg, VA, USA

513 Half Mile Branch Road
Crozet, VA 22932, USA

E-mail address:
MDM3P@hscmail.mcc.virginia.edu

Clin Sports Med 40 (2021) xiii
https://doi.org/10.1016/j.csm.2021.02.001
0278-5919/21/© 2021 Published by Elsevier Inc.

sportsmed.theclinics.com

Preface

Hip Pain in the Athlete: The Source is Key

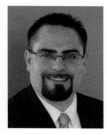 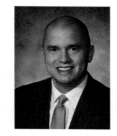

Dustin L. Richter, MD   F. Winston Gwathmey, MD
Editors

Compared with the diagnosis and management of pain in the knee and shoulder, diagnosis and management of hip pain in the adolescent and young adult population had been relatively neglected until the twenty-first century. During the past 2 decades, there has been an explosion in the understanding of hip pathologic condition and management of hip conditions in the younger population without arthritis. Improved indications and modern techniques have been developed that make the field of hip arthroscopy relatively safe with a low complication rate.

Examining a patient with hip pain can seem quite daunting, because of more than 20 muscles that cross the hip joint and because of both intraarticular and extraarticular sources of pain. Thankfully, we've compiled a group of experts in the field to shed some light on how to work up and treat these patients to achieve optimal outcomes. We would like to thank our friends and colleagues who have given their time and talent to contribute to this issue of *Clinics in Sports Medicine*. They are leaders in their field, many of whom serve as team physicians with a vested interest in returning athletes to their prior level of competition. All our contributors are dedicated to advancing the understanding and management of hip pain in the athlete through surgeon, physician, trainer, and patient education. In this issue of *Clinics in Sports Medicine*, you will learn to properly evaluate and image patients with pain in the hip region. The diagnosis and management of both intraarticular and extraarticular hip issues are reviewed. Additional excellent articles on special topics, including the adolescent athlete and sex-based differences in injury rates, help round out the current issue.

Enjoy perusing articles to learn about what radiographs and advanced imaging are necessary to make an accurate diagnosis? If a patient has hip dysplasia: Who can safely be treated with an arthroscopic approach and who may require an acetabular osteotomy? What are the indications for doing a labral reconstruction versus a labral repair? How do you manage stress fractures in elite athletes or pelvic avulsion injuries

Clin Sports Med 40 (2021) xv–xvi
https://doi.org/10.1016/j.csm.2021.01.004
0278-5919/21/© 2021 Published by Elsevier Inc.   **sportsmed.theclinics.com**

in the adolescent athlete? These are just some of the topics we hope to provide guidance on by sharing our knowledge through practice and evidence-based medicine.

Dustin L. Richter, MD
Department of Orthopaedic Surgery
University of New Mexico Health Sciences Center
MSC 10 5600
Albuquerque, NM 87131, USA

F. Winston Gwathmey, MD
Department of Orthopaedic Surgery
University of Virginia School of Medicine
PO Box 800159
Charlottesville, VA 22908, USA

E-mail addresses:
Dustin.richter1818@gmail.com (D.L. Richter)
FWG7D@hscmail.mcc.virginia.edu (F.W. Gwathmey)

Evaluation of Athletes with Hip Pain

Jacob G. Calcei, MD[a], Marc R. Safran, MD[b],*

KEYWORDS

- Hip pain • Femoroacetabular impingement • Labral tear • Instability
- Musculotendinous strain

KEY POINTS

- Determining the source of athletic hip pain can be a clinical challenge.
- Obtaining a thorough history and performing a consistent, comprehensive physical examination are the vital initial steps in the proper management of athletes with hip pain.
- The first delineation is whether the source of hip pain is intra-articular or extra-articular.
- Intra-articular sources of pain are generally not tender to palpation, or exacerbated with resisted muscle testing.
- Common sources of hip pain in athletes include impingement and labral tears, hip microinstability, hip flexor and adductor muscle strains, and core muscle injuries.
- Other causes of nonmusculoskeletal hip-related pain, such as hernias, intra-abdominal and genitourinary disorders, or lumbar radiculopathy, should be identified and evaluated when present.

INTRODUCTION

Athletes are constantly subjecting their hip joints to high forces, large ranges of motion (ROMs), and compromising positions as they run, jump, cut, pivot, and kick. A 3-year study at Stanford University found that nearly 10% of all musculoskeletal complaints to athletic trainers by athletes involved the hip (Safran, unpublished data, 2013). Thus, hip pain is a common complaint in athletes and can lead to a significant amount of time lost from sport.[1–10] In recent years, the identification of hip injuries and appreciation for hip-related disorders has increased among team physicians and other clinicians caring for athletes.[11–13] Whether the evaluation of an athlete with hip pain starts on the field, in the training room, or in the office, the clinician must obtain a reliable history

a Department of Orthopaedic Surgery, University Hospitals of Cleveland, Case Western Reserve University, 11100 Euclid Avenue, Cleveland, OH 44106, USA; b Department of Orthopaedic Surgery, Stanford University Medical Center, Palo Alto, CA, USA
* Corresponding author. 450 Broadway, M/C 6342, Redwood City, CA 94063.
E-mail address: MSafran@Stanford.edu
Twitter: @drcalcei (J.G.C.)

Clin Sports Med 40 (2021) 221–240
https://doi.org/10.1016/j.csm.2020.11.001
0278-5919/21/© 2020 Elsevier Inc. All rights reserved.

and perform a consistent and comprehensive physical examination to provide an accurate and timely diagnosis.

Correct diagnosis can lead to efficient and effective treatment of hip pain; however, making the correct diagnosis about the hip has traditionally been thought to be difficult because of the difficulty of examining this deep structure, as well as the broad differential diagnosis of hip pain resulting from many surrounding structures and pain that may radiate to the hip joint (**Table 1**). However, with a thorough history and physical examination, clinicians can narrow down the diagnoses and, combined with appropriate imaging, can identify the true source of hip pain and formulate a treatment plan to get the athletes back to their sports.

DISCUSSION
History of Hip Pain

Initial evaluation of an athlete with hip pain should include a thorough history of the patient's hip pain. The clinician should start with the athlete's sport and level of play, and the presence of a specific inciting event or injury that caused the pain. Onset, duration, and aggravating and relieving maneuvers or positions should be elicited. Any history of hip-related disorders and/or treatment should be noted. Patients with a history of acetabular dysplasia or femoral-sided disorders such as slipped capital femoral epiphysis or Legg-Calve-Perthes syndrome may be predisposed to developing hip pain, particularly in athletes.

The location of the athlete's pain can help to differentiate between an intra-articular and extra-articular source of the pain. Importantly, clinicians must differentiate between groin, lateral hip, and low back pain, while ruling out referred and radiating intra-abdominal disorders, hernias, and other nonmusculoskeletal causes of pain around the hip. Pain within the hip joint typically manifests as anterior groin pain, along the inguinal crease. However, referred pain to the thigh or even down to the knee can be a finding in patients with intra-articular hip disorders. Patients with intra-articular

---

Table 1
Common sources of hip pain in athletes

Intra-articular	Referred
• Femoroacetabular impingement	• Lumbar spine disorders
• Labral tear	○ Radiculopathy
• Chondral injury	○ Pars injuries
• Ligamentum teres tear	○ Facet arthropathy
• Loose body	○ Disc degeneration
• Hip dysplasia	○ Disc herniation
• Hip microinstability	•Abdomen: gastrointestinal
• Hip dislocation	• Pelvis: genitourinary
Extra-articular	• Abdominal muscle strains
• Iliopsoas strain and tendinopathy	• Hernia (inguinal)
• Adductor strain and tendinopathy	
• Greater trochanteric bursitis	
• Gluteus medius strain and tendinopathy	
• External snapping hip syndrome	
• Internal snapping hip syndrome	
• Hamstring strain and tendinopathy	
• Piriformis syndrome	
• Core muscle injury/athletic pubalgia/sports hernia	
• Osteitis pubis	
• Sacroiliac joint dysfunction	

pain often form what is called the C sign with their hands when asked to show the location of their pain, noting that the pain is deep, between the 2 fingers forming the C[14,15] (**Fig. 1**).

Pain localized posteriorly in the buttocks or that radiates to the posterior or lateral thigh or distally past the knee is concerning for a lumbar spine origin, although piriformis syndrome, sacroiliac (SI) joint dysfunction, and hamstring disorders may also be the cause of buttock pain. Pain localized to the adductor tubercle or the lower abdominal muscles at the pubic tubercle are more consistent with a proximal adductor strain or core muscle injury/athletic pubalgia. Lateral hip pain at the greater trochanter may be the result of a several sources, now grouped as greater trochanteric pain syndrome, including trochanteric bursitis and gluteus medius strain or syndrome, and can coincide with iliotibial band tightness and snapping that is pathognomonic for external snapping hip syndrome. Posterolateral hip pain may be more consistent with piriformis syndrome, whereas pain just proximal to the greater trochanter may be caused by a gluteus medius strain. Pain and snapping anteriorly in the groin are often secondary to iliopsoas inflammation and internal snapping hip syndrome.

Clinicians should ask the patients to qualitatively describe their symptoms. The presence of mechanical symptoms, such as locking, clicking, or catching in the hip, is concerning for intra-articular disorders, specifically a labral tear or chondral flap. Duration and frequency of pain, as well as certain motions, movements, or activities that aggravate or relieve the symptoms, should be documented.

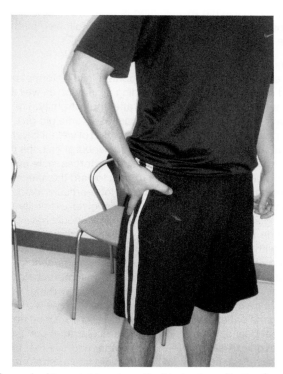

Fig. 1. C sign. When asked to point to where the hip hurts, patients often grab the hip and state that the hip hurts deep, at the junction between the thumb and long finger. (© 2020 Marc R. Safran.)

The initial history can provide the clinician with a short list of preliminary diagnoses and allow a more focused physical examination of the athlete with hip pain. An extensive list of physical examination maneuvers of the hip to be combined with the thorough history outlined earlier are presented here.

Physical Examination of the Hip

The hip can be a challenging joint to examine because of the deep location and extensive surrounding soft tissue envelope. However, if approached in a focused and stepwise manner based on the patient's complaints and injury history, clinicians can begin to narrow down the potential causes of hip pain and formulate an accurate diagnosis. The patient should be in clothing that allows unrestricted hip motion, usually short pants or possibly leggings.

The first step is determining whether pain is coming from the hip, thus ruling out a remote source of radiating pain such as hernias, intra-abdominal and genitourinary pain, or lumbar spine pain. It is then important to delineate whether the pain is originating from an intra-articular or extra-articular source with reference to the femoroacetabular joint. Although intra-articular disorders are typically exacerbated by passive motion of the hip, extra-articular disorders often become more painful with palpation or resisted active motion. It is important that examiners approach the examination of athletes with hip pain in a comprehensive and stepwise manner. The examination begins when the patient enters the office, because the clinician should observe the patient's gait, how the patient is sitting, and how the patient transitions between positions. A comprehensive hip examination is described later, organized by patient positioning, beginning with the standing examination, followed by the seated, supine, lateral, and prone examinations[14,16,17] (**Table 2**).

Standing examination

A basic standing examination can provide important initial information, such as height, body habitus, and gross lower extremity standing alignment, as well as whether the patient does not want to fully bear weight on the affected extremity. The patient should be asked to walk down the hall to observe the gait. In an antalgic gait, the patient has a shortened stance phase to attempt to limit the duration of weight bearing on the affected side, whereas, in a coxalgic (also known as Trendelenburg) gait, the patient lurches the center of gravity toward the affected side to distribute forces more evenly across the hip joint. A pelvic wink is seen when the patient rotates toward the affected side to allow full terminal hip extension and may be a sign of hip intra-articular disorders, ligamentous laxity, or abnormal femoral version.[18] Any obvious lower extremity malalignment and foot progression angle should be noted. The examiner should have the patient perform short and long stride walking as well as internal and external foot progression angle walking. Patients with instability or ischiofemoral impingement have pain in terminal extension with long stride walking.[19] Ischiofemoral impingement in particular is more painful in extension and external rotation. Patients with femoroacetabular impingement (FAI) have more pain with internal foot progression angle walking, whereas those with instability have more pain with external foot progression angle walking.[20]

Simply observing the patients walk into the office and transition from sit to stand can often provide a great deal of information, with particular attention paid to the patients compensating or favoring 1 side more than the other and whether they use their arms to get out of the chair. Patients with FAI often avoid sitting straight up in the chair to decrease hip flexion and impingement, and they also do not like to sit in low chairs, like a low couch. Patients with piriformis syndrome often lean toward the contralateral hip to avoid putting pressure on the affected side.

Table 2
Summary of the basic hip examination in athletes organized by patient positioning

Standing examination	Supine examination
Gait	Range of motion
Trendelenburg/abductor strength	• Flexion
Leg length assessment	• Internal and external rotation
Sitting examination	• Abduction and adduction
Internal and external rotation	Thomas test
Iliopsoas strength	Adductor strength
Neurovascular examination	Hamstring tightness
• Pulses (DP and PT)	Straight leg raise
• Sensation	Scour/labral stress test
• Motor strength	FADIR/impingement test
• Deep tendon reflexes	Stinchfield test
	McCarthy test
	Patrick FABER test
	Log roll
	Axial loading and foveal distraction test
	Hyperextension external rotation test
	Beighton score
	Palpation
	• Abdomen
	• Pubic symphysis
	• Adductor and Iliopsoas
	Hesselbach test
Lateral examination	Prone examination
Palpation	Range of motion
• Trochanteric bursa	• Internal rotation
• Gluteus medius muscle	• External rotation
• Piriformis tendon	Domb instability test
Ober test	Glute-hamstring dominance
Guanche instability test	

Abbreviations: DP, dorsalis pedis; FABER, flexion, abduction, external rotation; FADIR, flexion, adduction, internal rotation; PT, posterior tibialis.

A Trendelenburg gait is where the patient's contralateral hip drops toward the floor during the stance phase of gait because of abductor weakness of the standing leg. Patients may compensate by doing an abductor lurch, leaning toward the weight-bearing side. Abductor weakness can also be identified using a single-leg stand, or Trendelenburg sign. With the clinician assessing from posterior and visualizing the posterior ilium, the clinician's hands are placed on the athlete's iliac crests (**Fig. 2**A), and the athlete lifts 1 leg off the ground. If the pelvis on the side that is lifted rises up (**Fig. 2**B), the Trendelenburg sign is negative, signaling good gluteus medius strength. If the ipsilateral pelvis drops or the athlete shifts the upper body away from the lifted side, the test is considered positive (**Fig. 2**C), suggesting abductor weakness.[17,21] In conjunction with the Trendelenburg sign, the clinician can assess for pelvic tilt and any gross leg length discrepancies. A quantification of leg length discrepancy can be performed by using wooden blocks under the shorter side until the pelvis is level.[14]

Seated examination
The patient moves to the seated position with the legs hanging over the side of the examination table and knees bent 90°. In the seated position, the examiner can obtain an initial assessment of hip ROM and iliopsoas strength testing as well as perform a complete bilateral lower extremity neurovascular examination.

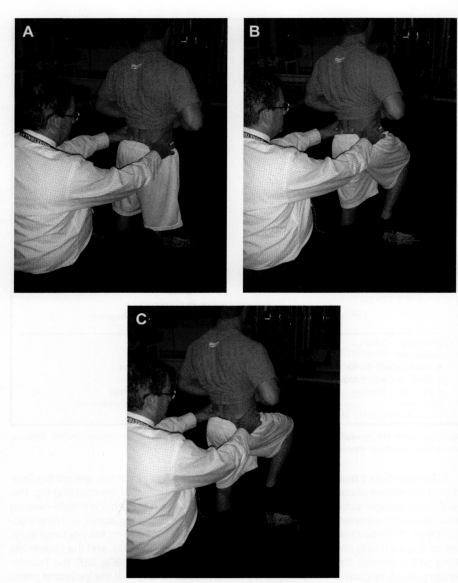

Fig. 2. Trendelenburg sign. The examiner sits behind the standing patient and observes the posterior pelvis (*A*). The examiner's fingers are then placed on the iliac wings and the thumbs by the posterior superior iliac spine. The patient lifts 1 leg/knee. If the ipsilateral pelvis goes up (*B*), the Trendelenburg sign is negative, suggestive of good gluteus medius strength. If the ipsilateral pelvis (seen by the examiner's thumb) drops (*C*), the Trendelenburg sign is positive, consistent with gluteus medius weakness. (© 2020 Marc R. Safran.)

Range of motion and strength Hip internal and external rotation should be tested in the seated position and documented compared with ROM in the supine and prone positions (**Table 3**). In the seated position, the pelvis is grounded on the table with the hip flexed at 90°, so the examiner is able to obtain an accurate measurement of actual hip motion while avoiding side-to-side rocking of the pelvis.

Examiners can best assess iliopsoas strength in the seated position. This examination is performed as the athlete flexes the hip and holds against resistance as the examiner tries to pull the knee down toward the floor (**Fig. 3**). The iliopsoas is a powerful hip flexor; thus, it is important that the athletes stabilize themselves by holding the edge of the bed so that the iliopsoas strength can be accurately assessed.[18] Even a small amount of iliopsoas weakness compared with the contralateral side can serve as a cause of anterior groin pain. Pain with iliopsoas testing is concerning for iliopsoas tendinopathy. In general, strength testing is documented on a standard 0 to 5 scale, and pain is noted when present.

When indicated, internal and external hip rotation strength can also be assessed with the patient seated on the table and the hips and knees flexed at 90°.

Neurovascular assessment Importantly, the clinician should always perform a neurovascular assessment of the lower extremities, which can be done with the patient in the seated position. This assessment includes bilateral lower extremity pulses, sensation, motor strength, and deep tendon reflexes.[22] Side-to-side variations in the neurovascular assessment should be documented and further work-up pursued, as indicated.

Supine examination

A large portion of the hip examination is performed with the patient in the supine position. With the athlete supine on the examination table, the clinician can best delineate between intra-articular and extra-articular causes of the hip pain. The supine hip examination starts with palpation, hip ROM, identification of flexion contractures with the Thomas test, and strength testing, followed by special tests for labral disorders, FAI, SI joint disorders, and hip instability. These special tests help the examiner differentiate between intra-articular versus extra-articular causes of hip pain, thus narrowing the differential diagnosis. In addition, other causes of hip and groin pain can be ruled out by palpation of the abdomen, pubic symphysis, adductor, and iliopsoas.

Range of motion and strength The hip is taken through full passive ROM testing, including hip flexion, internal and external rotation with the hip flexed at 90°, and abduction and adduction with the hip extended. During ROM testing, the examiner should place 1 hand on the pelvis to avoid compensatory pelvic motion. If there is

| Table 3 | |
Range of normal active hip range of motion	
Flexion	110°–120°
Extension	10°–15°
Abduction in extension	30°–50°
Adduction in extension	30°
External rotation in flexion	40°–60°
Internal rotation in flexion	30°–40°

Adapted from: Safran MR. Evaluation of the painful hip in tennis players. *Aspetar Sport Med J*. 2014;3:516-525; with permission.

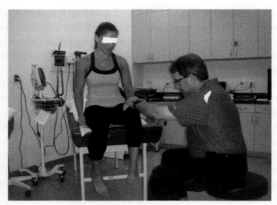

Fig. 3. Iliopsoas strength test. Because the iliopsoas provides most of the strength at greater than 90° of hip flexion, the patient's hip flexion is tested, seated at the end of a table. The patient then flexes the hip and the examiner attempts to push down toward the table to determine strength. (© 2020 Marc R. Safran.)

concern for a flexion contracture of the hip, this can be assessed and quantified using the Thomas test. In the Thomas test, the athlete flexes up the contralateral hip and holds the knee while the leg being examined is allowed to passively extend; the angle between the thigh and table is then measured (**Fig. 4**).

Pain at extremes of motion can be particularly concerning for intra-articular disorders, specifically a labral tear or chondral flap. In addition, this may result in a decrease in ROM over time as the patient avoids painful positions and movements. A loss of internal rotation is commonly seen in FAI. The impingement test, which is not pathognomonic for FAI, is performed with the patient supine, hip flexed to 90°, adducted, and then internally rotated, causing pain. In addition, patients with FAI may have obligatory abduction and external rotation with flexion often seen in patients with slipped capital femoral

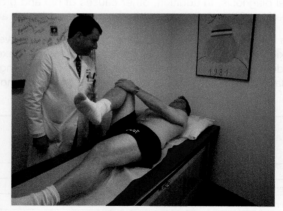

Fig. 4. Thomas test. The athlete flexes up the contralateral hip and holds the knee to stabilize the pelvis. The lower spine should be in neutral, and can be checked by the clinician with the hand at the lower back while the positioning the contralateral hip. The leg being examined is allowed to passively extend; the angle between the thigh and table is then measured. (© 2020 Marc R. Safran.)

epiphysis, known as the Drehmann sign.[23] Pain with full passive flexion may be seen with FAI, anterior inferior iliac spine subspinous impingement, and iliopsoas tendinitis. Limited internal and external rotation of the hip in the context of radiographs that do not show arthritis is consistent with an idiopathic stiff hip (also known as frozen hip).

Adductor strength can be tested in the supine position, both with the hips in full extension and flexed so that the athlete's feet are flat on the examination table (**Fig. 5**). Pain with resisted adduction can be concerning for adductor strain or core muscle injury, which typically are accompanied by localized tenderness to palpation, as described later.

Hamstring muscle tightness should be quantified by measuring the popliteal angle on each side. Tightness of the hamstring muscle group can cause a flexion-extension muscular imbalance leading to relative weakness and hip pain and should be addressed through physical therapy and a home stretching program.

A straight leg raise test to rule out lumbar disc herniation and radiculopathy can be performed with the patient supine or sitting. In the supine examination, the patient lies flat while the examiner puts the sciatic nerve on stretch by passively flexing the patient's hip with the knee in full extension. The examiner then dorsiflexes the foot. Pain in the posterior hip and thigh and/or paresthesias down the posterior leg and into the foot are a positive result and concerning for lumbar spine disorders as a potential cause of the athlete's hip pain.

Special tests

Labral tears of the hip are a common cause of intra-articular hip pain in athletes. The labral stress test, also known as the scour maneuver, is performed with the patient supine starting with the affected hip in abduction and external rotation. The hip is then adducted and internally rotated while being moved into extension (**Fig. 6**). This provocative movement stresses the labrum and is likely to cause pain in the presence of a labral tear.

Internal impingement of the hip can be examined by putting the hip into flexion, adduction, and internal rotation (FADIR), also known as the impingement test. The hip is flexed to 90°, then brought into adduction and internal rotation (**Fig. 7**). Pain with FADIR is considered a positive test and, although not specific for hip impingement or labral tear, the test is sensitive for intra-articular disorders in general.[24]

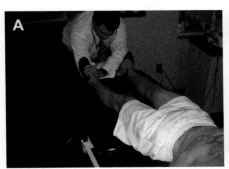 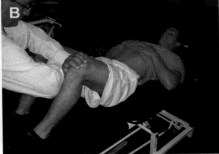

Fig. 5. Adductor strength testing. With the patient supine, adductor strength testing is performed with the hips in extension (*A*) and 45° of flexion (*B*) to assess different parts of the adductors. The authors have found that having examiners cross their arms to test adductor strength is easier and less strenuous, and can help less muscular examiners resist the powerful adductor muscles. (© 2020 Marc R. Safran.)

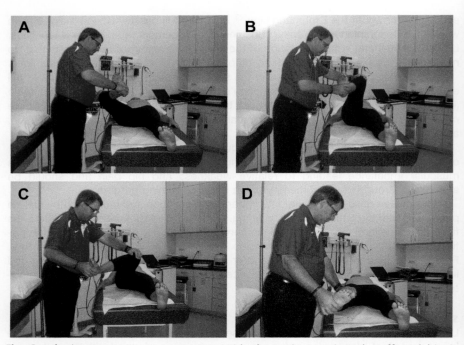

Fig. 6. Labral stress test/scour maneuver. With the patient supine, the affected hip is brought into flexion, abduction, and external rotation (*A*). The hip is then adducted and internally rotated (*B* & *C*)), while being moved into extension (*C* & *D*). (© 2020 Marc R. Safran.)

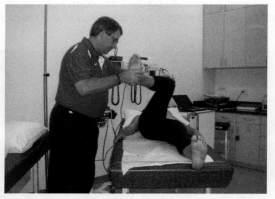

Fig. 7. Impingement test/FADIR maneuver. With the patient supine, the hip is flexed to 90°, then adducted and internally rotated. This test should produce pain, which may be intra-articular. Although the name suggests it is to diagnose hip impingement (FAI), it is not pathognomonic for FAI/hip impingement, because other hip disorders (intra-articular and some extra-articular, such as iliopsoas tendinitis) may cause pain with this maneuver. (© 2020 Marc R. Safran.)

Other dynamic tests that can point toward an intra-articular cause for the athlete's groin pain include the Stinchfield and McCarthy tests. In the Stinchfield test, the athlete performs a straight leg raise against resistance (**Fig. 8**). The Stinchfield test can serve as a quick screening maneuver for intra-articular disorders or hip flexor tendinitis. The McCarthy test consists of the athlete starting with the hip in a maximally flexed, adducted, and internally rotated position, then moving to an abducted and externally rotated position on the way to full extension. The wide arc of motion in the McCarthy test allows the examiner to find a specific site of impingement.[22] Pain and clicking with the McCarthy test indicates intra-articular disorder, such as a labral tear.

In the Patrick test, the athlete is positioned with half the buttock off the side of the table. The athlete puts the ipsilateral extremity in a figure-4 position with the ankle resting just above the contralateral knee and downward pressure is placed on the affected knee. This position puts the hip in a flexed, abducted, and externally rotated (FABER) position (**Fig. 9**). Pain posteriorly in the pelvis is consistent with SI joint disorder. Pain anteriorly in the groin points toward iliopsoas inflammation or osteitis pubis, whereas lateral pain is seen in FAI, gluteus medius tendinopathy, and/or trochanteric impingement. General hip stiffness can be assessed with the supine athlete having the leg in a figure-4 position and the distance between the lateral joint line and examination table measured (**Fig. 10**).

Patients with more acute intra-articular disorders often have pain with a simple log-rolling maneuver and gentle passive motion of the hip point. In contrast, patients with extra-articular disorders typically do not have pain with log rolling. In addition, the modified log roll test, which includes passive external rotation of the hip in extension noting the angle of the foot, followed by passive internal rotation and then letting the foot fall back into external rotation, can assess for iliofemoral ligament laxity or anterior hip instability.

Pain with axial loading of the hip also points toward intra-articular disorder or fracture. The foveal distraction test is the opposite of axial loading because the examiner brings the athlete's hip into 30° of abduction and applies axial traction on the hip. Relief with this maneuver points toward an intra-articular cause of the patient's pain because it decreases the load experienced by the femoroacetabular joint.

Microinstability of the hip is an underdiagnosed cause of anterior groin pain and is common in athletes because of the amount of force that is often placed on the hip joint

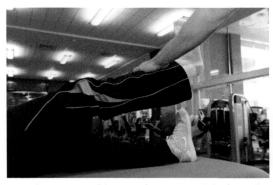

Fig. 8. Stinchfield test. The supine athlete performs a straight leg raise against resistance. Pain in the hip may be caused by hip flexor strain or potentially anterior labral tear. (© 2020 Marc R. Safran.)

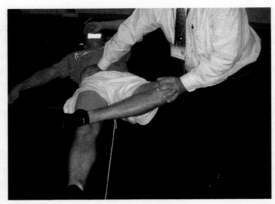

Fig. 9. Patrick test. The athlete is positioned with half the buttock off the side of the table. The athlete puts the ipsilateral extremity in a figure-4 position with the ankle resting just above the contralateral knee and downward pressure is placed on the affected knee. This position puts the hip in a FABER position. Pain anteriorly is consistent with labral tear, osteitis pubis, or iliopsoas tendinitis. Pain posteriorly is the result of posterior greater trochanteric impingement or sacroiliac joint pain. (© 2020 Marc R. Safran.)

and hip capsule in different twisting and turning motions. The hyperextension external rotation test is performed with the patient supine and can identify anterior labral disorders or anterior instability of the hip. In this maneuver, the patient moves to the edge of the table and stabilizes the pelvis by holding the contralateral knee to the chest. The affected extremity hangs off the edge of the bed and the hip is placed in a hyperextended and externally rotated position, putting stress onto the anterior labrum and capsule (**Fig. 11**). Anterior hip pain may result from hip microinstability, although anterior labral tear may also produce pain in this position. Posterior hip pain with the hyperextension external rotation test may be the result of posterior hip impingement. Other tests for microinstability are performed in the lateral and prone positions.

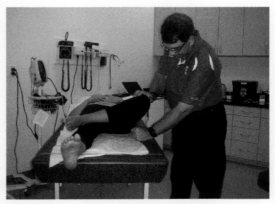

Fig. 10. FABER test. General hip stiffness can be assessed with the supine athlete having the leg in a figure-4 position and the distance between the lateral joint line and examination table is measured. (© 2020 Marc R. Safran.)

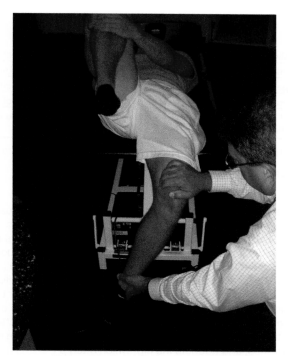

Fig. 11. Hyperextension–external rotation test for microinstability. The hyperextension external rotation test is performed with the patient supine and the patient's buttocks at the very edge of the examination table. The athlete then holds 1 leg near the chest to stabilize the pelvis. The other (affected) extremity hangs off the edge of the bed and should be in a hyperextended position. The examiner then grabs the lower leg/ankle and externally rotates the lower extremity. Pain anteriorly may be the result of anterior microinstability or anterior labral tear. Pain posteriorly may be the result of posterior hip impingement. (© 2020 Marc R. Safran.)

Generalized ligamentous laxity may be of concern in patients that have increased ROM testing throughout. In that case, the clinician can calculate a Beighton score to quantify the patient's general ligamentous laxity[25,26] (**Table 4**). Patients with a score of 4 or greater are considered hypermobile with generalized ligamentous laxity.

Palpation

Several structures can be palpated with the athlete in the supine position. A basic palpation of the 4 quadrants of the abdomen can help the clinician to rule out any intra-abdominal cause of pain about the hip joint. Next, the examiner can palpate the symphysis pubis to rule out osteitis pubis or other pubic symphysis–related sources of pain.

Adductor strains are a common source of proximal thigh and groin pain, particularly in soccer, hockey, and track and field athletes.[4] Adductor injuries commonly lead to weakness in hip adduction as well as point tenderness to palpation at the site of adductor strain. More significant strains can result in ecchymosis along the proximal inner thigh.

Despite being a deep structure that lies directly anterior to the hip capsule, the iliopsoas tendon can be palpated. The iliopsoas is found by having the patient externally

Table 4 Beighton score	
Small finger passive extension at MCP joint past 90°	1 point for each side
Thumb passively flexed to touch the volar forearm	1 point for each side
10° of elbow hyperextension	1 point for each side
10° of knee hyperextension	1 point for each side
Standing forward bend with knees locked in extension and palms flat on the floor	1 point total

Maximum score of 9 points; patients with a score of 4 or greater are considered to have generalized joint hypermobility.
Abbreviation: MCP, metacarpophalangeal.

rotate and flex the hip about 30°: the sartorius will be evident, because it is the most superficial anterior hip muscle stressed by this position. The iliopsoas is just medial to the sartorius and distal to the inguinal crease. The examiner's fingers are kept on the iliopsoas, and the patient brings the extremity back to a resting position on the examination table. The patient then lifts the leg from the examination table (doing a straight leg raise of only 30°) and the examiner can feel the contraction of the iliopsoas tendon. Pain with this maneuver is consistent with iliopsoas tendinopathy or bursitis.

Internal snapping hip can be elicited by having the patient do one of several active maneuvers that result in an audible snap or clunk. One test has the patient lying supine and starting with the hip flexed, abducted, and externally rotated. The patient then extends, internally rotates, and adducts the hip, which often produces the clunk that patients feel and may cause discomfort or pain; frequently, the examiner can hear the clunk. Another provocative test has the supine patient flex the hip, then abduct and externally rotate, and move into extension and back to midline. A final physical examination maneuver to reproduce snapping from the iliopsoas is having the patient do a straight leg raise, elevating the leg to 60 cm (2 feet) above the examination table. The patient then moves from abduction with external rotation to adduction with internal rotation.

Core muscle injury, formerly known as sports hernia or athletic pubalgia, can be another cause of extra-articular hip pain. Core muscle injury or athletic pubalgia is an injury to the soft tissues of the lower abdominal or posterior inguinal wall.[27,28] Core muscle injury is a common cause of chronic groin pain in athletes and typically manifests as pain in the lower abdomen or proximal adductors with activity, exacerbated by contraction of the abdominal musculature in a resisted sit-up or with Valsalva maneuvers.[29,30] The examiner must be sure to rule out an inguinal hernia when there is concern.[31] Although more of a diagnosis of exclusion, sports hernia evaluation can be performed with the Hesselbach test (**Fig. 12**). In this examination maneuver, the clinician palpates the edge of the rectus abdominus muscle near its insertion on the pubis while the athlete attempts to perform a sit-up. Pain with this maneuver is consistent with core muscle injury or athletic pubalgia, and the diagnosis should be supported by properly protocoled MRI.[32,33] Another test for core muscle injury includes pain with a simple resisted sit-up.

Lateral Examination

Palpation

Once completed with the supine examination, the athlete is asked to roll onto one side into the lateral decubitus position. The examiner starts by palpating important

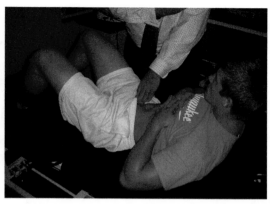

Fig. 12. Hesselbach test. With the athlete supine, the clinician palpates the lateral edge of the rectus abdominus muscle near its insertion on the pubis while the athlete attempts to perform a sit-up. Pain with this maneuver is consistent with core muscle injury or athletic pubalgia. (© 2020 Marc R. Safran.)

potential pain generators in the lateral hip. The first location of palpation is the trochanteric bursa, which is at the most prominent aspect of the lateral hip along the greater trochanter but also along its borders, especially proximally and posteriorly. Pain at the trochanteric bursa can be related to inflammation and irritation of the bursa or a sequela of a tight iliotibial band.

The next site of palpation is the gluteus medius, which is a fan-shaped muscle that originates along the ilium and inserts onto the proximal aspect of the greater trochanter. Tenderness along the gluteus medius insertion is consistent with gluteus medius tendinopathy, whereas tenderness 2 cm or more proximal to its insertion may be consistent with gluteus medius syndrome.

Third is the piriformis tendon. Athletes with piriformis syndrome complain of deep posterolateral hip or buttock pain with associated tenderness along the piriformis tendon. The piriformis is best palpated with the patient in the lateral position with the hip flexed and adducted so that the knee on the side being examined is resting on the examination table. This position helps to expose the piriformis tendon, which is palpated between the ischial tuberosity and greater trochanter. In addition, piriformis strength can be tested by starting in this flexed and adducted position while the patient lifts the knee off the table against resistance. This test may cause pain if the patient has piriformis syndrome.

Special tests

The Ober test is also performed in the lateral position and assesses for hip abductor tightness and iliotibial band contracture.[34] The hip and knee are first flexed, then the hip is abducted, followed by extending of the hip to neutral while letting the hip fall into adduction (**Fig. 13**). The test is positive when the knee is unable to drop below neutral, signaling iliotibial band tightness. Gluteus maximus contracture can be tested by having the patient start in the same position with the hip and knee flexed, then the hip is abducted, followed by some extension (but not quite to midline) and then letting the hip fall into adduction. If the hip does not drop below neutral, then gluteus maximus contracture is present.

The presence of anterior hip instability can be identified using the abduction-hyperextension external rotation test.[35] With the patient in the lateral position, the affected hip is abducted, extended, and externally rotated while the examiner places

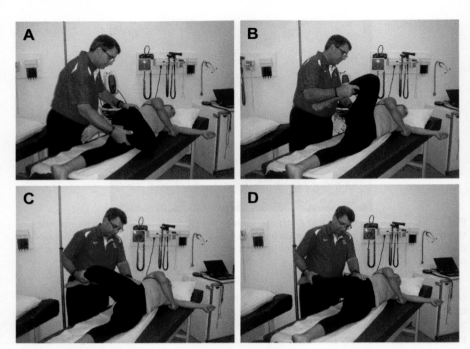

Fig. 13. Ober test. This test for iliotibial band contracture or tightness is performed in the lateral position. The hip and knee away from the examination table are first flexed (*A*). The hip is then abducted (*B*), and then extended (*C*) while the knee is maintained in flexion. The knee and thigh are allowed to drop toward the table, falling into adduction (*D*). If the knee does not adduct past midline/parallel to the table, then the hip abductors/iliotibial band are tight. If a similar maneuver is performed but the hip is not extended past neutral and the thigh allowed to adduct, gluteus maximus is assessed for tightness and contracture. (© 2020 Marc R. Safran.)

an anteriorly directed force on the posterior greater trochanter (**Fig. 14**). This provocative maneuver stresses the anterior hip, and athletes with anterior microinstability complain of pain anteriorly.

Prone Examination

In addition, the athlete is asked to move to the prone position on the examination table. While in the prone position, the examiner can again test ROM, perform a special test for instability, and assess gluteus-hamstring firing pattern. Hamstring tendinopathy and ischial bursitis may be identified by tenderness to palpation of the ischial tuberosity in the prone position.

Range of motion

A third data point for hip internal and external rotation can be collected with the patient in the prone position, avoiding any rocking of the pelvis. These ROM values should be noted and compared with the internal and external rotation values collected with the patient in the seated and supine positions.

Special tests

The prone instability test described by Domb and colleagues[36] is performed by the examiner externally rotating the hip while putting an anteriorly directed force on the

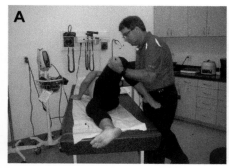 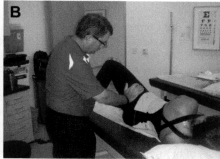

Fig. 14. Abduction-extension–external rotation test. This test for hip anterior microinstability is performed with the athlete in the lateral position. The affected hip is abducted, extended, and externally rotated while the examiner places an anteriorly directed force on the posterior greater trochanter (*A, B*). Anterior pain is seen with hip microinstability but may also cause discomfort with iliopsoas tendinitis. (© 2020 Marc R. Safran.)

posterior greater trochanter (**Fig. 15**). Patients with instability of the hip complain of anterior groin pain with this maneuver.

Improper muscular activation and firing pattern of the gluteus maximus and hamstring muscles during hip extension can lead to muscle imbalances around the hip and resultant pain. Firing pattern is tested with the athlete in the prone position with the knees flexed at 90°. The examiner puts 1 index finger on the gluteus maximus muscle and the other index finger on the hamstring muscles to detect the sequence of muscle activation as the athlete actively extends the hip. A normal firing pattern is gluteal dominant, with the gluteus maximus firing first followed by the hamstrings. A hamstring-dominant firing pattern, with the hamstrings activating first, is abnormal and should be addressed by a referral to physical therapy for neuromuscular reeducation to establish a proper activation sequence of gluteus maximus followed by hamstrings.[18]

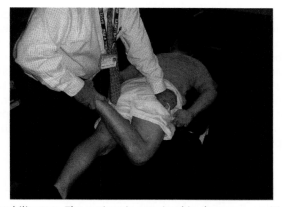

Fig. 15. Prone instability test. The patient is examined in the prone position. The extremity being tested is externally rotated and the examiner applies an anteriorly directed force on the posterior greater trochanter. Patients with instability of the hip complain of anterior groin pain with this maneuver. (© 2020 Marc R. Safran.)

SUMMARY

Hip pain is a common complaint in athletes and has garnered increasing interest from clinicians and team physicians in recent years. Determination of the source of athletic hip pain can be a clinical challenge, but, by using a stepwise approach starting with a thorough history and a consistent and comprehensive physical examination, clinicians can start to narrow down the differential diagnosis. Clinicians should first establish whether the source of hip pain is intra-articular or extra-articular and, because of its location, must rule out any nonmusculoskeletal causes of hip-related pain. Ultimately, clinicians can combine their history and clinical examination findings with appropriate imaging studies and other diagnostic tools to formulate an accurate and timely diagnosis of hip pain to guide treatment of these athletes.

CLINICS CARE POINTS

- Determining the source of athletic hip pain can be a clinical challenge and clinicians should combine a thorough history and comprehensive physical examination with appropriate imaging and other diagnostic mediums to establish an accurate and timely diagnosis.
- Differentiating between an intra-articular and extra-articular source of pain is the first major delineation in the diagnosis of athletic hip pain.
- Common intra-articular causes of athletic hip pain include FAI, labral tears, and microinstability, whereas common extra-articular causes include hip flexor and adductor muscle strains, and core muscle injuries/athletic pubalgia.
- Clinicians must identify nonmusculoskeletal causes of hip pain, such as hernias, intra-abdominal and genitourinary disorders, or lumbar radiculopathy.

DISCLOSURE

J.G. Calcei declares no potential conflicts of interest with respect to the research, authorship, and/or publication of this article. M.R. Safran has the following disclosures: *American Journal of Sports Medicine*, editorial or governing board; Biomimedica, stock or stock options; unpaid consultant; DJ Orthopaedics, IP royalties; International Society for Hip Arthroscopy, board or committee member; International Society of Arthroscopy, Knee Surgery, and Orthopedic Sports Medicine, board or committee member; AAOS, board or committee member; American Orthopaedic Society for Sports Medicine, board or committee member; *JISAKOS*, editorial or governing board; *Journal of Hip Preservation Surgery*, editorial or governing board; Medacta, paid consultant, paid presenter or speaker; Saunders/Mosby-Elsevier, publishing royalties, financial or material support; Smith and Nephew, IP royalties; paid presenter or speaker, research support; Stryker, IP royalties; Wolters Kluwer Health, Lippincott Williams & Wilkins, publishing royalties, financial or material support.

REFERENCES

1. Abrams GD, Renstrom PA, Safran MR. Epidemiology of musculoskeletal injury in the tennis player. Br J Sports Med 2012;46(7):492–8.
2. Coleman SH, Mayer SW, Tyson JJ, et al. The epidemiology of hip and groin injuries in professional baseball players. Am J Orthop (Belle Mead NJ) 2016; 45(3):168–75.

3. Dalton SL, Zupon AB, Gardner EC, et al. The epidemiology of hip/groin injuries in National Collegiate Athletic Association Men's and Women's Ice Hockey: 2009-2010 through 2014-2015 academic years. Orthop J Sport Med 2016;4(3). https://doi.org/10.1177/2325967116632692.

4. Eckard TG, Padua DA, Dompier TP, et al. Epidemiology of hip flexor and hip adductor strains in National Collegiate Athletic Association Athletes, 2009/2010-2014/2015. Am J Sports Med 2017;45(12):2713–22.

5. Epstein DM, McHugh M, Yorio M, et al. Intra-articular hip injuries in national hockey league players: A descriptive epidemiological study. Am J Sports Med 2013; 41(2):343–8.

6. Feeley BT, Powell JW, Muller MS, et al. Hip injuries and labral tears in the national football league. Am J Sports Med 2008;36(11):2187–95.

7. Jackson TJ, Starkey C, McElhiney D, et al. Epidemiology of hip injuries in the national basketball association: A 24-year overview. Orthop J Sport Med 2013;1(3). https://doi.org/10.1177/2325967113499130.

8. Kantrowitz DE, Trofa DP, Woode DR, et al. Athletic hip injuries in major league baseball pitchers associated with ulnar collateral ligament tears. Orthop J Sport Med 2018;6(10). https://doi.org/10.1177/2325967118800704.

9. Kerbel YE, Smith CM, Prodromo JP, et al. Epidemiology of hip and groin injuries in collegiate athletes in the United States. Orthop J Sport Med 2018;6(5). https://doi.org/10.1177/2325967118771676.

10. Kerr ZY, Kroshus E, Grant J, et al. Epidemiology of national collegiate athletic association men's and women's cross-country injuries, 2009-2010 through 2013-2014. J Athl Train 2016;51(1):57–64.

11. Lynch TS, Bedi A, Larson CM. Athletic hip injuries. J Am Acad Orthop Surg 2017; 25(4):269–79.

12. Frank JS, Gambacorta PL, Eisner EA. Hip pathology in the adolescent athlete. J Am Acad Orthop Surg 2013;21(11):665–74.

13. Frank RM, Walker G, Hellman MD, et al. Evaluation of hip pain in young adults. Phys Sportsmed 2014;42(2):38–47.

14. Martin HD, Shears SA, Palmer IJ. Evaluation of the Hip. Sports Med Arthrosc 2010;18(2):63–75.

15. Nepple JJ, Carlisle JC, Nunley RM, et al. Clinical and radiographic predictors of intra-articular hip disease in arthroscopy. Am J Sports Med 2011;39(2):296–303.

16. Safran MR. Evaluation of the hip: History, physical examination, and imaging. Oper Tech Sports Med 2005;13(1):2–12.

17. Safran MR. Evaluation of the painful hip in tennis players. Aspetar Sport Med J 2014;3:516–25.

18. Herickhoff PK, Safran MR. Physical evaluation of the hip. In: DiGiacomo G, Ellenbecker TS, Kibler WB, editors. Tennis medicine. A complete guide to evaluation, treatment and rehabilitation. Switzerland: Springer Nature Publishers; 2018. p. 101–10.

19. Martin HD, Reddy M, Gómez-Hoyos J. Deep gluteal syndrome. J Hip Preserv Surg 2015;2(2):99.

20. Ranawat AS, Gaudiani MA, Slullitel PA, et al. Foot progression angle walking test: a dynamic diagnostic assessment for femoroacetabular impingement and hip instability. Orthop J Sport Med 2017;5(1). https://doi.org/10.1177/2325967116679641.

21. Trendelenburg F. Trendelenburg's test: 1895. Clin Orthop Relat Res 1998;(355):3–7.

22. Braly BA, Beall DP, Martin HD. Clinical examination of the athletic hip. Clin Sports Med 2006;25(2):199–210.

23. Kamegaya M, Saisu T, Nakamura J, et al. Drehmann sign and femoro-acetabular impingement in SCFE. J Pediatr Orthop 2011;31(8):853–7.

24. Reiman MP, Mather RC, Hash TW, et al. Examination of acetabular labral tear: A continued diagnostic challenge. Br J Sports Med 2014;48(4):311–9.

25. Beighton P. Hypermobility scoring. Br J Rheumatol 1988;27(2):163. Available at: http://www.ncbi.nlm.nih.gov/pubmed/3365538.

26. Shu B, Safran MR. Hip instability: anatomic and clinical considerations of traumatic and atraumatic instability. Clin Sports Med 2011;30(2):349–67.

27. Trofa DP, Mayeux SE, Parisien RL, et al. Mastering the physical examination of the athlete's hip. Am J Orthop (Belle Mead NJ) 2017;46(1):10–6.

28. Elattar O, Choi HR, Dills VD, et al. Groin injuries (Athletic Pubalgia) and return to play. Sports Health 2016;8(4):313–23.

29. Ross JR, Stone RM, Larson CM. Core muscle injury/sports hernia/athletic pubalgia, and femoroacetabular impingement. Sports Med Arthrosc 2015;23(4):213–20.

30. De Paulis F, Cacchio A, Michelini O, et al. Sports injuries in the pelvis and hip: diagnostic imaging. Eur J Radiol 1998;27. https://doi.org/10.1016/S0720-048X(98)00043-6. Elsevier Sci Ireland Ltd.

31. Taylor DC, Meyers WC, Moylan JA, et al. Abdominal musculature abnormalities as a cause of groin pain in athletes: Inguinal hernias and pubalgia. Am J Sports Med 1991;19(3):239–42.

32. Mullens FE, Zoga AC, Morrison WB, et al. Review of MRI Technique and imaging findings in athletic pubalgia and the "sports hernia. Eur J Radiol 2012;81(12):3780–92.

33. Zoga AC, Kavanagh EC, Omar IM, et al. Athletic pubalgia and the "sports hernia": MR imaging findings. Radiology 2008;247(3):797–807.

34. Martin HD, Kelly BT, Leunig M, et al. The pattern and technique in the clinical evaluation of the adult hip: the common physical examination tests of hip specialists. Arthroscopy 2010;26(2):161–72.

35. Domb B, Brooks A, Guanche C. Physical examination of the hip. In: Guanche C, editor. Hip and pelvis injuries in sports medicine. Philadelphia: Wolters Kluwer/Lippincott Williams and Wilkins; 2010. p. 62–70.

36. Domb BG, Stake CE, Lindner D, et al. Arthroscopic capsular plication and labral preservation in borderline hip dysplasia: Two-year clinical outcomes of a surgical approach to a challenging problem. Am J Sports Med 2013;41(11):2591–8.

Hip Imaging and Injections

Timothy P. Lancaster, MD, Christopher C. Chung, BS,
Winston F. Gwathmey, MD*

KEYWORDS

- Hip • Imaging • Pelvis • X-ray • Radiograph • Ultrasound • MRI • CT

KEY POINTS

- The ability to critically interpret plain radiographs is essential in the evaluation of the athlete's hip. Radiographs augment physical examination findings and provide context for advanced imaging.
- An understanding of normal anatomy, imaging findings, and radiographic measurements allows for the recognition of pathoanatomy and the ability to diagnose accurately.
- A thorough understanding of the strengths and limitations of various advanced imaging modalities helps guide imaging choice.
- Magnetic resonance imaging and computed tomography provide high-resolution imaging of the hip, whereas ultrasonography offers the unique ability to perform dynamic imaging and guided injections.

INTRODUCTION

Initial assessment of an athlete's hip involves a thorough physical examination and detailed history, which should allow for formation of a differential diagnosis and guide next steps in obtaining imaging studies. Radiographic imaging of the pelvis provides structural context, which augments clinical examination findings and can provide insight into disruptions in normal hip function. Radiographs help to establish baseline anatomy and provide a necessary backdrop for interpretation of advanced imaging. Advanced imaging with computed tomography (CT), magnetic resonance imaging (MRI), and ultrasonography (US) provides high-resolution characterization of a patient's anatomy, allowing for accurate diagnosis and surgical planning.

RADIOGRAPHS

Radiographs are indicated in most, if not all, patients with athletic injuries of the hip to evaluate for acute osseous injury in addition to gaining insight into the underlying structural morphology. A standard series, including anteroposterior (AP) pelvis,

Department of Orthopaedic Surgery, University of Virginia Medical Center, PO Box 800159, Charlottesville, VA 22908, USA
* Corresponding author.
E-mail address: fwg7d@virginia.edu

Clin Sports Med 40 (2021) 241–258
https://doi.org/10.1016/j.csm.2020.11.002
0278-5919/21/© 2020 Elsevier Inc. All rights reserved.

sportsmed.theclinics.com

Dunn lateral, and false-profile views, provides an excellent overview of hip anatomy from which an abundance of information can be gathered. The following sections detail techniques for obtaining various pelvic radiographic views and descriptions of key measurements, which have important clinical implications.

Anteroposterior Pelvic Radiograph

The AP radiograph can be obtained with a patient standing or supine. Bilateral lower extremities should be internally rotated 15°, which maximizes the length of the femoral neck by offsetting for normal anteversion (**Fig. 1**). The optimal x-ray tube-to-film distance is 120 cm, with the tube oriented perpendicular to the film. The coccyx should be centered in line with the pubic symphysis, and the radiation beam should be centered between the 2 horizontal lines connecting anterior superior iliac spines (ASISs) bilaterally and superior aspects of the pubic symphysis, respectively.[1] Some providers prefer standing AP images, asserting that weight bearing may affect joint positioning and certain hip angles for evaluation.

A well-centered, well-tilted, and well-rotated image is essential for the interpretation of apparent abnormalities. A well-centered AP image aligns, along a vertical axis, the pubic symphysis with the midline of the sacral vertebrae. Offset of the symphysis from the sacral midline suggests a rotated image, which also may be indicated by asymmetry in the appearance of obturator foramina, ischial spines, and radiographic teardrops. The pubic symphysis and tail of the coccyx should be approximately 1 cm to 3 cm in distance for an appropriately inclined hip image.[1] These markers of image quality should be screened routinely prior to more in-depth evaluation and interpretation of hip radiographs.

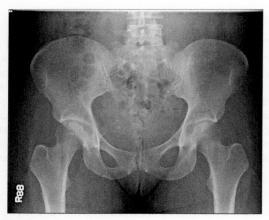

Fig. 1. AP radiograph of pelvis.

Frog-Leg Lateral View

The frog-leg lateral view is obtained with the patient placed supine, the hip of interest abducted to 45°, and the ipsilateral knee flexed to 30° to 40° (**Fig. 2**). The ipsilateral heel should rest comfortably against the opposite knee. The cassette is placed with the superior edge of the film aligning with the ASIS and the beam aimed at the midway point between the ASIS and pubic symphysis. The tube-to-film distance should be approximately 40 in (102 cm).[1]

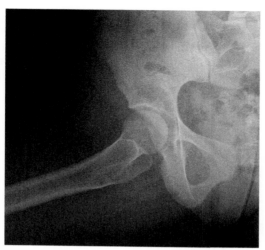

Fig. 2. Frog-leg lateral view.

Dunn Lateral View, 90° or 45°

The Dunn lateral radiograph is obtained with the patient supine and hips flexed to 90° (for 90° Dunn) or 45° (for 45° or modified Dunn). The Dunn radiograph provides a view of the elongated neck for better characterization of proximal femoral morphology. For both the 90° and 45° Dunn views, the hip is abducted 15° to 20°, with the pelvis and tibia aligned in neutral rotation, parallel to the long axis of the body (**Fig. 3**). The tube-to-film distance is approximately 40 in (102 cm) from the table, with the tube perpendicular to the table and the x-ray beam centered at the midpoint of the ASIS and pubic symphysis.[1] An AP radiograph of the pelvis with both hips positioned for the Dunn Lateral view provides a comparison of the proximal femoral anatomy of each hip.

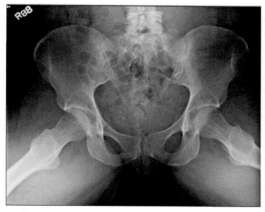

Fig. 3. 45° Dunn lateral view.

False-Profile View

The false-profile view is obtained from the standing patient, with the hip of interest placed closest to the cassette film. The ipsilateral foot should run parallel with the plane of the cassette, and the pelvis is angled 65° from the plane of the cassette (**Fig. 4**). The x-ray beam is centered on the femoral head, perpendicular to the film, with a tube-to-film distance of approximately 40 in (102 cm).[1]

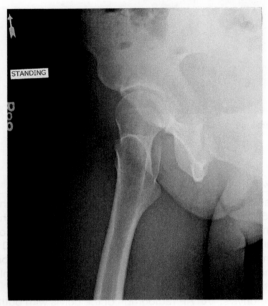

Fig. 4. False-profile view.

Acetabular Version

Acetabular version describes the AP orientation of the acetabulum in the horizontal plane. Normal version is considered to be 15° to 20° anteversion. It is essential to evaluate acetabular anatomy on an AP pelvis radiograph so that pelvic tilt and rotation can be taken into account. On the AP pelvis film, version can be assessed by evaluation of the relative positions of the anterior and posterior walls. To assess version, outline the anterior and posterior acetabular rims extending to the lateral sourcil. In the anteverted acetabulum, the anterior and posterior rim lines do not cross when traced to the lateral sourcil. If the outline of the posterior rim crosses with the anterior rim before either extends to the lateral sourcil, this is known as the *crossover sign*, and may signify retroversion of the acetabulum (**Fig. 5**).[1] Specifically, crossover sign on AP radiograph represents focal retroversion, or anterior overcoverage. By comparison, global retroversion is demonstrated by presence of the posterior wall sign, in which the center of the femoral head is lateral to the posterior wall.[1] Also associated with retroversion is the presence of a prominently visible ischial spine on AP film. It is important to consider that inappropriately tilted hips can introduce artificial crossover signs bilaterally, and a rotated pelvis can induce a unilateral crossover sign with an excessively anteverted appearance of the contralateral side.

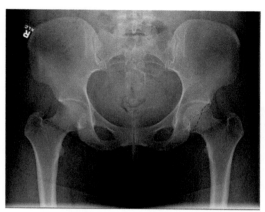

Fig. 5. Crossover sign. The anterior (*red*) and posterior (*blue*) rim lines cross, signifying focal retroversion of the acetabulum.

Acetabular Depth

Acetabular depth is delineated in reference to the ilioischial line. Normal depth on AP pelvic radiograph demonstrates the medial aspect of the femoral head positioned lateral to the ilioischial line. If an aspect of the acetabular fossa is touching or crossing medial to the ilioischial line, it is considered coxa profunda. If the medial aspect of the femoral head crosses medial to the ilioischial line, this is termed, protrusio acetabuli (**Fig. 6**).[1]

Acetabular Angles

Acetabular angles are useful metrics for assessing structural stability. In determining these angles, it is helpful to establish the center of the femoral head and demarcate the horizontal pelvic plane, which in a well-positioned AP pelvis radiograph can be obtained by drawing a line between the 2 teardrops.

The lateral center-edge angle (angle of Wiberg) describes superolateral coverage of the femoral head. The angle is created by drawing 2 lines: (1) a vertical line through the femoral head center, perpendicular to the horizontal pelvic plane, and (2) a line connecting the femoral head center to the lateral sourcil (**Fig. 7**). The normal range is between 25° and 40°. An angle greater than 40° is overcovered whereas an angle less than 20° is considered dysplastic; an angle 20° to 25° is considered borderline dysplasia.[1]

Acetabular inclination, measured by the Sharp angle, is determined by the following 2 lines: (1) the horizontal pelvic plane drawn between the teardrops and (2) the line connecting the teardrop to the lateral sourcil (**Fig. 8**). The normal range is 40° to 45°, with angles greater than 45° suggesting dysplasia.[1]

Acetabular index, or Tonnis angle, is another measure of acetabular coverage. It is defined as the angle between a horizontal line through the medial sourcil and a line that connects the medial sourcil to the lateral edge of the sourcil (**Fig. 9**). A normal Tonnis angle is between 0° and 10°.[1] An upsloping Tonnis angle greater than 10° may be structurally unstable, whereas a downsloping angle (less than 0°) increases the risk for femoroacetabular impingement (FAI) by creating pincer deformity.

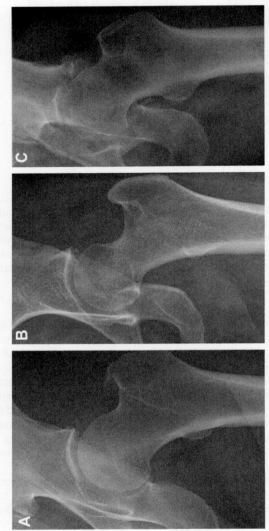

Fig. 6. (A) Normal depth: the acetabular fossa is lateral to the ilioischial line. (B) Coxa profunda: the acetabular fossa is medial to the ilioischial line. (C) Protrusio acetabuli: the medial aspect of the femoral head is medial to the ilioischial line.

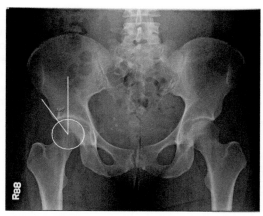

Fig. 7. Lateral center-edge angle (angle of Wiberg). Normal range is 25° to 40°.

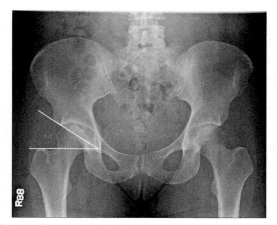

Fig. 8. Sharp angle (acetabular inclination).

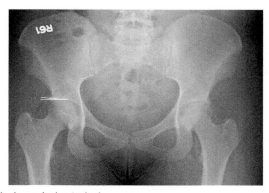

Fig. 9. Tonnis angle (acetabular index).

Extrusion Index

The extrusion index describes the percentage of femoral head that is uncovered by the acetabulum on AP imaging. Two distances are identified: (1) the horizontal distance between the lateral-most aspect of the femoral head and the lateral-most aspect of the acetabulum and (2) the total head diameter (**Fig. 10**). The first distance is taken as a percentage of the second to determine the extrusion index. An index less than 25% is normal, whereas a hip with greater than 25% is undercovered.[1]

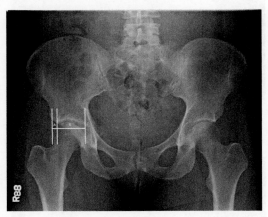

Fig. 10. Extrusion index, calculated by dividing distance A by distance B.

Alpha Angle

The alpha angle, originally described on MRI, can be extrapolated from lateral radiographs of the hip. The angle is created by 2 lines: (1) a line from the center of the femoral head drawn through the middle of the femoral neck and (2) a line drawn from the center of the femoral head to the point at which the femoral neck exits the circular profile of the head (the point at which the femoral head is noted to lose its sphericity) (**Fig. 11**).[1] It is important to recognize the position of the hip when measuring the alpha angle on a plain radiograph. The 45° Dunn lateral radiograph characterizes an anterlateral cam deformity whereas a 90° Dunn lateral radiograph characterizes deformities more anteriorly based. Values greater than 55° are associated with cam deformity.

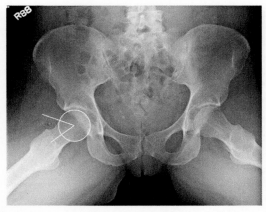

Fig. 11. Alpha angle. Values greater than 55° are associated with cam deformity.

Femoral Head-Neck Offset and Offset Ratio

Femoral head-neck offset provides another metric for assessing morphology at the head-neck junction. With the Dunn lateral radiograph, head-neck offset is calculated as the distance between the following 2 lines drawn parallel to the femoral neck axis: (1) a line tangent to the anterior-most aspect of the femoral head and (2) a line tangent to the anterior-most aspect of the femoral neck (potential area of impingement) (**Fig. 12**).[1] Normal offset is greater than 9 mm, whereas offset less than 9 mm suggests cam deformity. The offset ratio is calculated as a ratio of head-neck offset to the diameter of the femoral head. Offset ratio less than 0.18 is suggestive of cam deformity.[1]

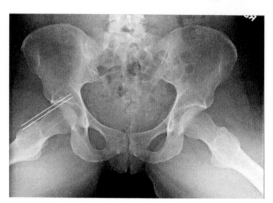

Fig. 12. Femoral head-neck offset. Offset less than 9 mm suggests cam deformity.

Anterior Center-Edge Angle

The anterior center-edge angle, or angle of Lequesne, is obtained from the false-profile radiograph and assesses anterior femoral coverage (**Fig. 13**). The angle is created by the intersection of 2 lines: (1) a vertical line through the center of the femoral head and (2) a line connecting the center of the femoral head to the anterior-most aspect of the acetabular sourcil.[1] Normal values for anterior center-edge angle range between 25° and 40°. An angle between 20° and 25° is borderline dysplastic, whereas angles less than 20° suggest instability and dysplasia. Angles greater than 40° indicate anterior overcoverage.[1]

Anterior Inferior Iliac Spine/Subspine Morphology

Anterior inferior iliac spine (AIIS) morphology has been described as a contributor to hip impingement. Originally described by Hetsroni and colleagues via CT imaging, the AIIS can be classified into 3 types from a false-profile radiograph: (I) upsloping AIIS from the acetabular sourcil, (2) AIIS at the level of the sourcil, and (3) downsloping AIIS from the acetabular sourcil. Types II and III AIIS morphology are associated with decreased hip flexion and internal rotation at 90° flexion, with the AIIS causing impingement at terminal positions. There is growing evidence for consideration of operative decompression of severe AIIS dysmorphology to treat subspine impingement.[2]

Osteoarthritis

Arthritic changes in the hip are assessed easily from the AP pelvis film. The joint space should be assessed for narrowing, with attention specifically directed toward the superior, superolateral, and superomedial aspects of the joint. False-profile view is

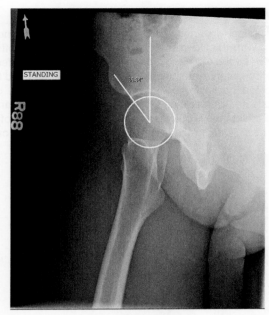

Fig. 13. Anterior center-edge angle (angle of Lequesne). Normal range is 25° to 40°.

useful for evaluation of the anterior joint space. Joint space measurement less than 2 mm at any position is associated with poor outcomes following arthroscopic debridement and indicates a high risk for conversion total hip arthroplasty.[3] Other markers of osteoarthritis include the presence of osteophytes, subchondral cysts, and subchondral sclerosis; these findings are incorporated into the Tonnis classification for hip osteoarthritis (**Table 1**), with higher grades indicating increasing severity of degenerative changes.[4]

Table 1
Tonnis classification for hip osteoarthritis

Grade	Radiographic Features
0	No signs of osteoarthritis
1	Mild joint space narrowing Mild sclerosis
2	Moderate joint space narrowing Moderate sclerosis Subchondral cysts
3	Severe joint space narrowing Osteophytes Large subchondral cysts

Higher Tonnis grades indicate increasing severity of osteoarthritis.

Os Acetabuli

Os acetabuli refers to the presence of ossicles, or bony fragments, along the acetabular rim (**Fig. 14**). These rim fragments arise from various etiologies, including unfused secondary ossification centers or stress fractures from repetitive loading.[5] They have

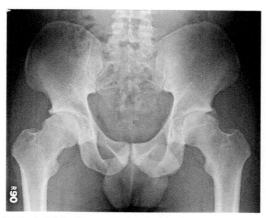

Fig. 14. Os acetabuli. The left hip demonstrates the characteristic bony fragment seen along the acetabular rim.

been associated with hip dysplasia and with FAI. In cases of hip dysplasia, overloading of the lateral acetabulum due to undercoverage of the femoral head is thought to contribute to fatigue fractures of the lateral rim. FAI contributes to the development of rim fragments through repetitive impingement of the femoral neck on the acetabular rim, resulting in ongoing microtrauma and eventual fracture.[6] Other proposed etiologies include avulsion sequelae or soft tissue calcification/ossification.[5]

MAGNETIC RESONANCE IMAGING

MRI is an invaluable imaging modality in evaluation of the athlete's hip. After initial patient assessment with a focused physical examination and plain radiographs, MRI is the preferred modality for evaluation of the labrum, articular cartilage, bone marrow, and soft tissues around the hip.[7] A fluid-sensitive fat-suppressed imaging sequence with a large field of view to include the pubic symphysis provides an overview of the patient's anatomy and pathology. This should be followed by focused hip imaging with a small field of view, with the affected hip centered in the field and use of surface coils to improve image quality.[8] Axial images should be oriented perpendicular to the axis of the femoral neck. If there is suspicion for intra-articular pathology, the diagnostic value of MRI can be enhanced by the use of arthrography with gadolinium contrast. MRI arthrogram of the hip has been shown to have increased sensitivity for detection of labral tears and acetabular cartilage lesions compared with standard MRI.[9] Arthrography often is combined with an intra-articular anesthetic injection, which may provide additional diagnostic and therapeutic value. A physical examination performed before and after anesthetic injection can shed light on the origin of hip pain; intra-articular pathology typically improves after injection, whereas extra-articular pathology likely remains unchanged.[10]

Accurate diagnosis of common hip pathologies requires an understanding of normal hip anatomy and familiarity with characteristic MRI findings. In the evaluation of the athlete's hip, MRI may reveal femoral stress fracture, FAI, labral tear, cartilage injury, and muscle or tendon injury, among other conditions.

Femoral stress fractures occur most commonly at the medial femoral neck and are represented by bone marrow edema on fluid-sensitive sequences (**Fig. 15**). Plain

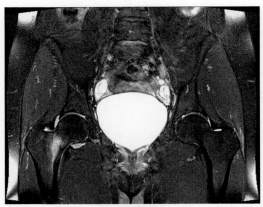

Fig. 15. Femoral neck stress fracture. T2-weighted coronal plane imaging reveals medial (compression-sided) stress fracture with edema and a dark linear fracture line.

radiographs often are negative, especially early in the course of the injury, or may demonstrate a lucent fracture line and sclerosis. Suspicion for stress injury in the setting of normal radiographs should be investigated with MRI in order to prevent delay or missed diagnosis.

FAI is a condition in which there is abnormal contact between the femoral head/neck and the acetabular rim, resulting in repetitive impingement and microtrauma during normal range of motion. This causes injury to the anterosuperior labrum and adjacent cartilage and is associated with characteristic MRI findings.[10] Labral tear is demonstrated as a linearly increased signal intensity on fluid-sensitive imaging, or on arthrogram is seen as contrast extending into the tear in the substance of the labrum. Superior labral tears may be evaluated on coronal images, whereas anterior superior tears are best identified on sagittal or axial imaging (**Fig. 16**).[10]

Articular cartilage consists of 4 distinct layers, including superficial, transitional, deep, and calcified. On fluid-sensitive MRI sequences, the superficial layer is low signal, transitional layer is high signal, and deep and calcified layers are low signal. Cartilage defects re evidenced by focal signal change, thinning, or abnormal cartilage contour; these findings are exemplified by gadolinium contrast which outlines cartilage margins.[10]

MRI also is useful for evaluation of the surrounding extra-articular ligaments and musculotendinous structures of the hip. It permits detailed evaluation of muscle, tendon, and soft tissues for diagnosis of tears, tendinitis, and avulsion injuries.

COMPUTED TOMOGRAPHY

CT of the hip is most useful in the setting of acute trauma and has a limited role in the evaluation of sports-related hip injuries. CT provides excellent bony anatomy and high spatial resolution and can be used for 3-dimensional reconstruction of complex femoral neck anatomy for surgical planning.[11] CT may be useful in characterizing osseous deformities implicated in FAI or in visualizing acetabular rim fragments. MRI, however, provides an adequate view of bony anatomy in addition to the adjacent soft tissue structures, such that the risks associated with radiation exposure often obviate CT evaluation, particularly in younger patients.

CT arthrography with multidetector CT, however, may provide an alternative for patients with contraindications to MRI or prior surgical patients in whom MRI imaging

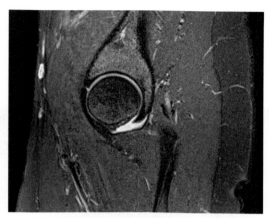

Fig. 16. Anterior superior labral tear. T2-weighted sagittal plane imaging reveals contrast extending into the substance of the labrum, seen as a linear disruption of the anterior labrum.

may be difficult to interpret. There is of interest in the use of CT arthrography for evaluation of subtle labral pathology and chondral injury.[12]

CT may be used to assess femoral version accurately. Femoral version is defined as the angle in the axial plane created between the long axis of the femoral neck and the posterior condylar axis of the knee. Normal femoral anteversion is approximately 8° to 15°, although there is significant variation across the population. Femoral version plays a role in FAI symptomatology; for example, femoral retroversion exacerbates the functional impact of an anterior cam deformity, because it positions the femoral neck into closer proximity with the anterior rim of the acetabulum. In a retrospective study by Lerch and colleagues,[13] 52% of patients with symptomatic FAI or hip dysplasia were found to have abnormal femoral version. A CT scanogram is useful for making this measurement: this low-dose noncontrast study is obtained using thick cuts through the trochanteric region and the distal femur in order to define the angular relationship between the femoral neck and posterior condyles (**Fig. 17**). The McKibbin index combines the values of acetabular version and femoral version to predict instability or impingement at the hip.[14] An index between 30° and 60° is considered normal. Values less than 30° are suggestive of impingement pathology, whereas values greater than 60° may indicate hip instability.

ULTRASONOGRAPHY

With advances in resolution and accessibility of US, it is becoming a widely utilized imaging modality for assessment of the athlete's hip. Its advantages include point-of-care real-time imaging, no exposure to radiation, relatively low cost, and ability to perform dynamic imaging.[15] It also allows for simultaneous diagnostic imaging and therapeutic intervention in the form of injection or aspiration. For these reasons, a thorough understanding of hip US is a vital asset in evaluation of sports injuries to the hip.

Although US does provide limited information regarding intra-articular pathology, its primary application is in the assessment of extra-articular pathology, including evaluation of muscle, tendon, and soft tissue injuries. Abnormalities in anatomic relationships and changes in echogenicity may suggest soft tissue injury or tendon tears.[16] Hypoechogenicity or heterogenous echogenicity with enlargement of tendon fibers

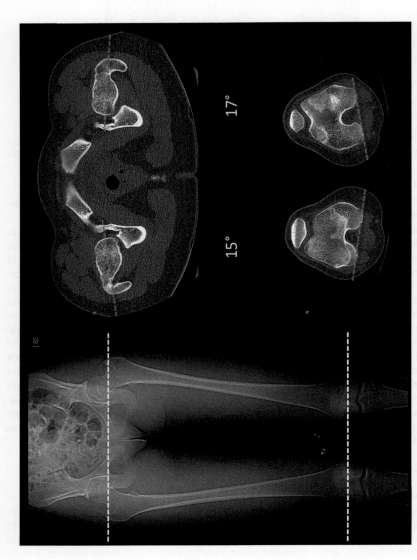

Fig. 17. CT scanogram. White lines indicate the level of the axial CT cuts. Red lines delineate the orientation of the femoral necks and posterior condyles in the axial plane. Femoral version is the angle created between the long axis of the femoral neck and the posterior condylar axis of the knee.

may represent tendinosis. Anechoic clefts represent areas of torn tendon. Complete disruption with intervening heterogenous hematoma may be seen with complete tendon tear.[15] In assessment of tendon tears, US has an advantage over MRI in that a dynamic assessment may be conducted. Active muscle contraction under US visualization may demonstrate gapping at the site of the tear, indicating complete disruption of fibers and distinguishing from a partial tear.[17]

Dynamic Imaging and Snapping Hip

Unique to US is the ability to perform dynamic imaging examinations. This may be employed in the diagnosis of snapping hip syndrome. This condition is categorized further into external and internal snapping hip.

External snapping hip syndrome refers to the abnormal transient catching of the gluteus maximus and iliotibial (IT) band over the greater trochanter during hip flexion, leading to painful popping and snapping over the lateral hip. Although typically a clinical diagnosis, US may provide additional diagnostic value through a dynamic assessment of the IT band and gluteus maximus during hip flexion and extension. With the patient in lateral decubitus position, the hip is moved from extension into flexion. A US probe positioned over the greater trochanter may visualize a sudden release of the IT band from posterior to anterior as the hip is flexed.

Internal snapping hip syndrome describes a similar snapping sensation in the anterior hip due to abrupt movement of the iliopsoas tendon. The mechanism of internal snapping hip is thought to involve abnormal motion of the iliopsoas tendon relative to the iliac muscle and the superior pubic ramus.[18] With the US probe placed in the transverse plane just proximal to the hip joint and parallel to the pubic bone, the hip is placed in the position of flexion, abduction, and external rotation. In this position, a portion of the iliacus muscle becomes interposed between the superior pubic ramus and iliopsoas tendon. As the hip is returned to neutral position, the iliopsoas muscle suddenly shifts laterally, allowing the tendon to abruptly snap back into contact with the pubic bone.[18] In certain cases, US-guided injections into the iliopsoas bursa may be appropriate for pain relief or diagnostic purposes.[19]

Trochanteric Pain and Bursa Injections

The greater trochanteric bursa, also called the subgluteus maximus bursa, is a common source of painful inflammation termed, trochanteric bursitis. It often is targeted for therapeutic relief through corticosteroid injections.[16] The greater trochanter is best viewed with the patient in lateral decubitus position. Placing the US probe in the transverse plane between the anterior and lateral facets of the greater trochanter should bring into view the short axis of the gluteus minimus and medius inserting onto the greater trochanter.[20] With rotation of the probe to the long-axis view of the gluteus muscles, the lateral trochanteric attachment of the gluteus medius and the anterior attachment of the gluteus minimus can be traced back to their muscular origins to identify any tendon tears or disruptions.[21] Returning to the short-axis view over the lateral facet, the greater trochanteric bursa can be identified as the plane between the gluteus medius and the overlying gluteus maximus.[21] Posteriorly, the greater trochanteric bursa continues deep to the gluteus maximus over the posterior facet.[22] Greater trochanteric bursitis may be identified by a hypoechoic fluid collection in these potential spaces or by bursal wall thickening.[16]

Injections of the greater trochanteric bursa are best done with needle-in-plane technique, with a well-positioned fluid injection in the bursal plane verified by hypoechoic expansion between the gluteus medius and maximus muscle layers.

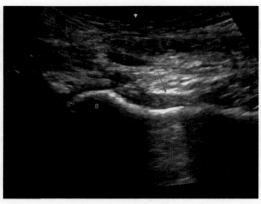

Fig. 18. Intra-articular injection of the femoroacetabular joint. In the oblique position, oriented along the long axis of the femoral neck, the acetabulum (A), femoral head (B), and joint capsule (C) can be visualized. Injected fluid (D) can be seen within the joint capsule.

Intra-articular Assessment and Injections

US evaluation of the femoroacetabular joint typically begins by placing the patient supine with the hip slightly abducted. The probe is placed obliquely along the long axis of the femoral neck, in order to visualize the acetabulum, femoral head, and head-neck junction in the same plane. From the oblique view, the iliopsoas muscle can be identified as a marbled appearing structure above the hyperechoic joint capsule. A cross-section of the lateral circumflex femoral neurovascular bundle also should be identified and followed proximally and distally. If the probe is turned 90° to view the short-axis of the psoas tendon, the femoral vein, femoral artery, and femoral nerve can be seen medial to the tendon. Doppler color visualization can help identify these landmarks. An intra-articular effusion can be detected by assessing capsular distention: 7 mm of total capsular distention as measured from the femoral neck to the outer margin of the capsule is suggestive of joint effusion.[17] Paralabral cysts also may be identified from this view and are suggestive of a labral tear, although sensitivity is not sufficient for the use of US as a rule-out test for labral pathology.[17]

In order to perform an injection or aspiration, the probe is placed in the oblique (femoral neck long axis) position, and the needle-in-plane technique is used to guide the needle toward the head-neck junction. Once the tip of the needle is placed within the joint capsule, fluid can be injected and should cause distension of the joint capsule visible under US (**Fig. 18**).

US has several limitations in its use. Its resolution diminishes with increasing depth of tissue, and thus is primarily effective for superficial structures. The bony anatomy of the hip joint limits use of US in evaluation of intra-articular pathology. Lastly, US is distinctly operator -dependent, and high-quality imaging requires an experienced and skilled ultrasonographer.

SUMMARY

A variety of imaging modalities are available for evaluation of the athlete's hip. The treating physician must keep in mind the various strengths and limitations of each modality when determining the most appropriate imaging for each patient. In general, plain radiographs and physical examination provide an excellent foundation on which to build a differential diagnosis and act as a backdrop for interpretation of advanced imaging. Familiarity with normal anatomy and characteristic imaging findings allow for recognition of pathoanatomy and accurate diagnosis of injuries to the athlete's hip.

CLINICS CARE POINTS

- Plain radiographs provide the structural context behind an athlete's symptoms and physical examination. They act as a backdrop for interpretation of advanced imaging.

- It is essential to confirm that plain radiographs are well centered, well tilted, and well rotated prior to evaluation. Poor-quality imaging can lead to inaccurate measurements and flawed diagnoses.

- Imaging findings always must be correlated with a patient's history and physical examination. Abnormal imaging findings may be incidental and asymptomatic.

- It is important to screen for and recognize osteoarthritis in patients with sports injuries of the hip, because this strongly impacts outcomes and treatment options.

- MRI arthrography provides excellent intra-articular imaging of the hip and allows for simultaneous diagnostic or therapeutic injection.

- US increasingly is utilized in evaluation of the athlete's hip because it is uniquely capable of providing real-time dynamic imaging.

DISCLOSURE

The authors have nothing to disclose.

REFERENCES

1. Clohisy JC, Carlisle JC, Beaulé PE, et al. A systematic approach to the plain radiographic evaluation of the young adult hip. In: Journal of Bone and Joint Surgery - Series A. J Bone Joint Surg Am 2008;90:47–66.
2. Hetsroni I, Poultsides L, Bedi A, et al. Anterior inferior iliac spine morphology correlates with hip range of motion: a classification system and dynamic model hip. Clin Orthop Relat Res 2013;471:2497–503. Springer New York LLC.
3. Skendzel JG, Philippon MJ, Briggs KK, et al. The effect of joint space on midterm outcomes after arthroscopic hip surgery for femoroacetabular impingement. Am J Sports Med 2014;42:1127–33. SAGE Publications Inc.
4. Kovalenko B, Bremjit P, Fernando N. Classifications in brief: tonnis classification of hip osteoarthritis. Clin Orthop Relat Res 2018;476(8):1680–4.
5. Martinez AE, Li SM, Ganz R, et al. Os acetabuli in femoro-acetabular impingement: stress fracture or unfused secondary ossification centre of the acetabular rim? HIP Int 2006;16(4):281–6.
6. Randelli F, Maglione D, Favilla S, et al. Os acetabuli and femoro-acetabular impingement: aetiology, incidence, treatment, and results. Int Orthop 2019; 43(1):35–8.
7. Chiamil SM, Abarca CA. Imaging of the hip: a systematic approach to the young adult hip. Muscles Ligaments Tendons J 2016;6(3):265.
8. Agten CA, Sutter R, Buck FM, et al. Hip imaging in athletes: sports imaging series1. Radiology 2016;280(2):351–69.
9. Sutter R, Zubler V, Hoffmann A, et al. Hip MRI: how useful is intraarticular contrast material for evaluating surgically proven lesions of the labrum and articular cartilage? Am J Roentgenol 2014;202(1):160–9.

10. Hegazi TM, Belair JA, McCarthy EJ, et al. Sports injuries about the hip: what the radiologist should know. Radiographics 2016;36(6):1717–45.

11. Tannast M, Kubiak-Langer M, Langlotz F, et al. Noninvasive three-dimensional assessment of femoroacetabular impingement. J Orthop Res 2007;25(1):122–31.

12. Christie-Large M, Tapp MJF, Theivendran K, et al. The role of multidetector CT arthrography in the investigation of suspected intra-articular hip pathology. Br J Radiol 2010;83(994):861–7.

13. Lerch TD, Todorski IAS, Steppacher SD, et al. Prevalence of femoral and acetabular version abnormalities in patients with symptomatic hip disease: a controlled study of 538 hips. Am J Sports Med 2018;46(1):122–34.

14. McKibbin B. Anatomical factors in the stability of the hip joint in the newborn. J Bone Joint Surg Br 1970;52(1):148–59.

15. Meyer NB, Jacobson JA, Kalia V, et al. Musculoskeletal ultrasound: athletic injuries of the lower extremity. Ultrasonography 2018;37(3):175–89.

16. Kong A, Vliet A, Zadow S. MRI and US of gluteal tendinopathy in greater trochanteric pain syndrome. Eur Radiol 2007;17(7):1772–83.

17. Dawes ARL, Seidenberg PH. Sonography of sports injuries of the hip. Sports Health 2014;6(6):531–8.

18. Deslandes M, Guillin R, Cardinal É, et al. The snapping iliopsoas tendon: new mechanisms using dynamic sonography. Am J Roentgenol 2008;190(3):576–81.

19. Blankenbaker DG, de Smet AA, Keene JS. Sonography of the iliopsoas tendon and injection of the iliopsoas Bursa for diagnosis and management of the painful snapping hip. Skeletal Radiol 2006;35(8):565–71.

20. Hoeber S, Aly AR, Ashworth N, et al. Ultrasound-guided hip joint injections are more accurate than landmark-guided injections: a systematic review and meta-analysis. Br J Sports Med 2016;50(7):392–6.

21. Pfirrmann CWA, Chung CB, Theumann NH, et al. Greater trochanter of the hip: attachment of the abductor mechanism and a complex of three bursae - MR imaging and MR bursography in cadavers and MR imaging in asymptomatic volunteers. Radiology 2001;221(2):469–77.

22. Lungu E, Michaud J, Bureau NJ. US assessment of sports-related hip injuries. Radiographics 2018;38(3):867–89.

Femoroacetabular Impingement and Management of Labral Tears in the Athlete

David A. Hankins, MD[a], Lucas Korcek, MD[b],
Dustin L. Richter, MD[c],*

KEYWORDS

- Hip impingement • Femoroacetabular impingement • FAI • Labral repair
- Labral reconstruction • Outcomes

KEY POINTS

- Femoroacetabular impingement can include altered bony morphology of the femoral head-neck junction (cam lesion), acetabular rim (pincer lesion), or both (mixed lesions). Restoring the labral seal is critical in restoring function and stability to the hip joint.
- A nonoperative treatment algorithm consisting of rest, nonsteroidal anti-inflammatory drugs, physical therapy, and consideration of a one-time image-guided intra-articular injection can successfully manage symptoms in many patients.
- It is critical to correct abnormal bony morphology in addition to treatment of labral pathology. We favor labral repair when enough competent tissue is available to restore the labral seal. Typically, reconstruction with allograft is preferred in a revision setting, for an ossified labrum, or if the labrum is irreparable.
- Correction of bony impingement and labral preservation techniques allow a high rate of RTP in recreational and elite athletes alike.

INTRODUCTION

The ball-in-socket articulation of the femoral head in the acetabulum is highly constrained, conferring stability from bony and soft tissue structures. Optimal function depends on sphericity of the femoral head, adequate (but not over) containment by the acetabulum, soft tissue stabilization, spinopelvic parameters, and neuromuscular integrity. Any conditions affecting these components can lead to hip impingement or instability, chondrolabral injury, and early joint degeneration.

[a] Lexington Orthopaedics, 146 East Hospital Drive, Suite 140, West Columbia, SC 29169, USA;
[b] Slocum Center for Orthopaedics and Sports Medicine, 55 Coburg Road, Eugene, OR 97401, USA; [c] Department of Orthopaedic Surgery, University of New Mexico, 1 University of New Mexico, MSC10 5600, Albuquerque, NM 87131, USA
* Corresponding author.
E-mail address: dustin.richter1818@gmail.com

Clin Sports Med 40 (2021) 259–270
https://doi.org/10.1016/j.csm.2020.11.003
0278-5919/21/© 2020 Elsevier Inc. All rights reserved.

The radius of curvature of the femoral head should hold constant until it increases at the transition to the femoral neck. The alpha angle, best measured on modified lateral hip radiographs (Dunn views) or advanced imaging, quantifies this point of transition (**Fig. 1**A, B). A premature increase in the radius of curvature causes a nonspherical femoral head and thus the term cam lesion morphology. A cam lesion is the most common abnormality leading to femoroacetabular impingement (FAI) and subsequent acetabular labral tears. Cam lesion morphology is largely idiopathic; however, some recent evidence supports the development of these lesions during adolescence in response to repetitive stress on the open proximal femoral physis. Palmer and colleagues[1] determined that sporting activity during adolescence is strongly associated with the development of cam morphology secondary to epiphyseal hypertrophy and extension with a dose-response relationship. Furthermore, males participating in competitive sport are at particularly elevated risk of developing cam morphology and secondary hip pathology.[1] Childhood disease, such as epiphyseal dysplasias,

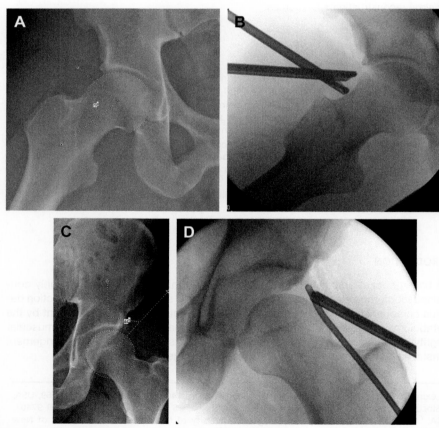

Fig. 1. (*A*) Dunn lateral radiograph of the right hip showing a moderate cam lesion morphology with an alpha angle of 79°. (*B*) Subsequent intraoperative fluoroscopic image demonstrating postfemoroplasty correction. (*C*) Anteroposterior radiograph of the left hip in a different patient showing an increased lateral center edge angle of 44° indicative of pincer lesion morphology secondary to prior healed anterior inferior iliac spine avulsion injury. (*D*) Intraoperative fluoroscopic image demonstrating resection of pincer lesion.

slipped capital femoral epiphysis, Legg-Calvé-Perthes disease, inflammatory conditions, and post-traumatic malformation can also create secondary cam morphology. Other sources of femoral-sided (cam-type) impingement include coxa vara, femoral retroversion, and osteophyte formation.[2–4]

On the acetabular side, the femoral head must be appropriately contained. Hip dysplasia describes undercontainment of the femoral head by the acetabulum and can lead to labral tearing from serial microinstability events. In contrast, pincer morphology describes a state of overcontainment of the femoral head by the acetabulum (**Fig. 1**C, D). This is from lateral and/or anterior overcoverage in the form of coxa profunda/protrusio, acetabular retroversion, prominence of the anterior inferior iliac spine, labral calcification, and osteophyte formation.[5–8]

Static soft tissue stability is conferred to the hip joint by the acetabular labrum and joint capsule. The hip labrum is a horseshoe-shaped structure contiguous with the transverse acetabular ligament. In normal hip joint biomechanics, the labrum is crucial in retaining a layer of pressurized intra-articular fluid for joint lubrication and load support/distribution. Its seal around the femoral head is further regarded as contributing to hip stability through its suction effect. The labrum also has fibers aiding in hip proprioception. Although traumatic labral injury can occur in the absence of FAI secondary to hip dislocation or subluxation events, labral tears are most commonly a result of repetitive bony impingement causing stress and tearing. Iatrogenic causes of instability caused by capsulectomy, labral resection, or overresection of a cam or pincer lesion have also been described.

Spinopelvic parameters and muscular coordination impact the development of FAI and are often the target of physical therapy for this condition. Lumbar hyperlordosis, low pelvic tilt, and high sacral slope can create functional pincer impingement by rotating the acetabulum forward in relation to the femoral head, creating abutment during hip flexion. Similarly, muscular imbalance, joint contracture, and deconditioning exacerbate FAI by altering hip kinesthetics. Physical therapy for FAI and labral injury involves posture and gait training and core and kinetic chain strengthening and coordination, as described in other articles in this issue.[9]

Given the comprehensive nature of the articles in this issue, the evaluation of the athlete with hip pain including patient presentation and physical examination have been thoroughly discussed. In addition, the interpretation of hip imaging and role for diagnostic and therapeutic injections has been covered. The diagnosis of the source of hip pain in the absence of arthritis is challenging, but a reproducible algorithm can make diagnosis and treatment more effective with improved patient outcomes. This article focuses on the management of FAI in the athlete with a suspected or documented labral tear including labral repair and reconstruction options, and discusses outcomes in this patient population.

CONSERVATIVE MANAGEMENT

Conservative treatment of FAI consisting of nonsteroidal anti-inflammatory drugs and conditioning to improve posture and gait mechanics is often successful for definitive management. Physical deconditioning, if present, should always be addressed before considering surgical intervention. Focused physical therapy for a minimum of 4 to 6 weeks is frequently efficacious, has limited downside, and can serve as effective prehabilitation before an arthroscopic procedure if pain and functional limitations persist. A single image-guided intra-articular injection (local anesthetic ± corticosteroid) is considered as a diagnostic and potentially therapeutic treatment option. At this time there continues to be limited evidence to support use of platelet-rich plasma, hyaluronic acid, or stem cell treatments for management of FAI or labral tears. Those patients that fail these conservative treatment measures and are deemed appropriate surgical candidates should be considered for hip arthroscopy.[10,11]

BONY TREATMENT

Osteoplasty of the femur and/or acetabulum to address cam and pincer morphology is critical in the setting of FAI and labral tears. This improves the kinematic conflict causing FAI and protects the labrum from reinjury.[12] Care must be taken to balance the risk of revision surgery (with underresection) with fracture risk or loss of labral seal (overresection of cam), or iatrogenic instability and early hip degeneration (over-resection of pincer). Use of intraoperative fluoroscopy or advanced imaging modalities is critical to avoid complications related to underresection or overresection of pincer and cam lesions.

LABRAL TREATMENT
Operative Management: Debridement, Repair, or Reconstruction

Open versus arthroscopic treatment
Although Burman was the first to perform and describe hip arthroscopy in 1931, it would take more than 75 years for hip arthroscopy to blossom. As such, arthroscopic management of patients with FAI and labral tears that have failed conservative treatment measures continues to increase in popularity worldwide. Favorable results have been demonstrated using open and arthroscopic approaches to treat FAI and labral tears.[13] Improved hip outcome score (HOS) sports subscale and higher nonarthritic hip scores at 2-year follow-up were observed in the arthroscopic cohort. Similarly, superior health-related quality of life score and trends toward faster recovery and return to sport have been shown with arthroscopic treatment of FAI and labral tears in studies when compared with open hip dislocation. Nonetheless, both procedures were found to have excellent patient-reported outcome measures and equivalent hip survival rates.[14,15]

Labral debridement
Historically, arthroscopic treatment primarily consisted of labral debridement only. Byrd and Jones[16] reported in 2009 on a cohort of 29 patients with osteoarthritis who underwent selective arthroscopic labral debridement and showed an increased Harris Hip Score (HHS) of 29 points (mean, 81 at 10-year follow-up). Of these patients, 88% with preoperative osteoarthritis progressed to a total hip arthroplasty (THA) at a mean of 63 months. However, there was limited correction of cam and/or pincer deformity in this cohort. Although labral debridement still remains a viable option for a select subset of patients, labral repair or labral reconstruction (LR) with correction of bony impingement is preferred for most symptomatic individuals.[17] Preserving and/or restoring as much native, functional labrum as possible is paramount to maintaining proper mechanics to approximate a "normal" hip.[18]

The first prospective study comparing labral debridement with repair in female patients was performed in 2013.[19] The postoperative HOS activity of daily living (HOS-ADL) was shown to be significantly higher in those undergoing labral repair with minimum 1-year follow-up. In another study, midterm (3.5 year) follow-up showed similar benefits comparing labral repair with debridement with the repair cohort having significantly greater improvements in HHS and SF-12 at final follow-up.[20] Limited long-term results comparing the procedures are available. Menge and colleagues[21] reported at 10-year follow-up no demonstrated differences in modified HHS (mHHS; 90 vs 85), HOS-ADL (96 vs 96), or HOS-Sport (89 vs 87) when comparing labral repair with debridement. They did note a higher rate of conversion to THA in older patients, those with acetabular microfracture, and hips with preoperative joint space less than 2 mm. The risk of poor outcomes and high rate of conversion to THA in patients with osteoarthritis undergoing hip arthroscopic procedures has been well documented previously.[22,23] However, the degree to which degenerative changes of the hip should preclude a patient from arthroscopic surgery has not been completely elucidated because those with Tonnis grade 1 arthritic changes have been found to have similar favorable short-term outcomes compared with those with no arthritis (Tonnis grade 0) in a matched-controlled study.[24]

With careful analysis of available literature, the authors favor primary acetabular labral repair over debridement whenever possible. Labral debridement could be considered in patients who are older, lower demand, with low radiographic or clinical risk of instability, or if the labrum is damaged beyond repair. Ideally the labral tear would be peripheral in nature without instability at its base and would have adequate functional size following debridement. However, this is a small subset of patients and if a labrum is irreparable, reconstruction should be strongly considered. Furthermore, the authors' preference is to typically avoid hip arthroscopic management in patients who have greater than Tonnis grade 1 arthritic changes given the less favorable results and increased conversion to THA.

Labral repair

Over the past decade the treatment paradigm for management of acetabular labral tears with or without FAI has shifted in favor of labral preservation. Most symptomatic patients in the primary setting typically undergo arthroscopic labral repair (**Fig. 2**). These patients are typically younger, active patients with an unstable labral base and adequate tissue quality to restore the labral suction seal following repair. Labral preservation is consistently associated with superior outcomes when compared with labral excision. An intact labrum not only restores the fluid suction seal but also increases articular surface contact area. This results in decreased articular friction, improved stability, and decreased contact pressure.

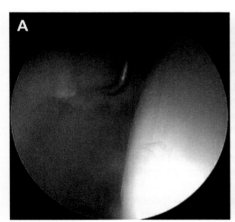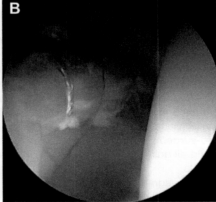

Fig. 2. (*A*) Arthroscopic images of a right hip demonstrating an anterior-superior labral tear with a small cartilage wave sign. (*B*) Arthroscopic repair of a torn native labrum with circumferential suture technique.

Although there are certainly many variations in terms of technique for fixation of labral tears, most revolve around similar premises. When performing fixation of labral tears, multiple anchor options exist allowing the surgeon to decide which design and suture type fit their need to perform the indicated surgical procedure. Anchors are generally placed 7 to 10 mm apart to allow for stable repair and limit risk of convergence of implants. The anchors should be placed as close to the acetabular rim as possible to recreate the labral seal and avoid eversion of the labrum during repair. The type of repair stitch (mattress vs circumferential or looped) and knotted versus knotless fixation to repair labral base tears has also been debated. Ultimately, it is up to treating surgeons to decide their preferred technique, although some recent studies have shown that a mattress stitch may better restore normal joint pressures and distractibility of the native hip.[25–27] Proposed advantages of knotless fixation are that it allows for easier and more reproducible labral repairs, decreased surgical time, and enhanced control of the desired tension with better labral positioning to avoid eversion. This was shown to be true for labral base fixation and circumferential repair.[28] These results suggest that the tensioning of the labral repair may actually be more important than the repair technique itself.

Labral reconstruction and augmentation

In hip LR, patient selection, graft type, and surgical technique are all important considerations. Good to excellent clinical outcomes have been described for reconstruction and augmentation of segmental and circumferential/complete labral defects.[29–33] However, when compared with reconstruction, primary labral repair was shown to better restore hip fluid suction seal in a cadaveric hip model.[34] Initial descriptions of LR were detailed by Philippon and colleagues[29] in 2010 using iliotibial band autograft. In their study, 9% of the reconstruction cohort progressed to THA at minimum 1-year follow-up. Those with less than 2 mm of joint space radiographically had worse outcomes and were more likely to require arthroplasty. However, improvement in mHHS averaged 23 points and mean patient satisfaction was 8 out of 10. Since that time, the implementation of augmentation and reconstruction techniques have become valuable resources in the toolbox of the more experienced hip arthroscopist.

Multiple different graft options for these procedures have been described over the previous decade using autograft and allograft tissue.[33,35,36] In a meta-analysis of 537 hips undergoing LR, Rahl and colleagues[37] showed a 76% to 100% survivorship of autografts and 86.3% to 90% survivorship of allografts at mean 29 months. Similar rates of conversion to THA (0%–13.2% and 0%–12.9%, respectively) and need for revision hip arthroscopy (0%–11.0% and 0%–10.0%, respectively) for autograft and allograft were reported. A mean improvement in mHHS of 29 was shown for LR in these studies. The authors concluded that LR resulted in clinically significant improvements in patient-reported outcome measures but that no graft type showed superiority.[37] These results were confirmed by Maldonado and colleagues who showed no difference in mHHS, NAHS (non-arthritic hip score), HOS sports-specific subscale, or VAS (visual analog scale) between autograft and allograft reconstruction.[38] Therefore, surgeon experience, patient preference, morbidity, operative time, and cost should all guide physicians in selecting the appropriate graft type for their individual patients.

Labral augmentation (LA) versus LR has also been a more recent topic of debate.[17] Philippon and colleagues[39] compared outcomes of LA with LR in patients with joint space greater than 2 mm and LCEA (lateral center edge angle) greater than 20° at 2-year follow-up. They showed significantly higher HOS-ADL, HOS-Sport, mHHS, and WOMAC scores in the LA group. Additionally, the percentage of patients who reached minimally clinically important difference regarding HOS-ADL and HOS-Sport was significantly higher for the LA group. Both LA and LR were found to have similar rates of revision (18% vs 14%) and conversion to THA (3% vs 4.25%).[39]

Although these techniques are generally reserved for the revision setting, it has been suggested that primary complete (or circumferential) acetabular LR may achieve results similar to primary repair in specific patients.[31] Nakashima and coworkers[40] reported that age greater than 45 years, body mass index greater than 23.1 kg/m^2, and vertical center anterior angle greater than 36° are risk factors for an unsalvageable labral tear at initial hip arthroscopy.[40] Additionally, Maldonado and coworkers[38] showed Tonnis grade 1 changes had a 2.5 times higher odds of necessitating primary reconstruction than grade 0.[38] In these patients with more severe pathology, primary LR has been shown to be a viable treatment option with promising short-term outcomes.[31] A survey of 12 high-volume hip arthroscopists outlined indications for LR in primary and revision settings.[41] Eleven of the 12 respondents would reconstruct in certain primary settings including poor-quality labral tissue, calcified labrum, and hypoplastic labrum. None of the surgeons favored reconstruction over repair when repair was a viable option in primary cases. Seven of the respondents favored reconstruction over debridement in primary cases with an irreparable labrum. In revision cases, 100% favored reconstruction over debridement. Eleven of the respondents preferred allograft versus autograft reconstruction and complete excision of the remnant labral tissue before reconstruction (ie, not augmentation). Most respondents performed segmental reconstruction as opposed to circumferential/complete reconstruction.

The authors prefer LR in younger patients without advanced arthritis who present with ossified, deficient, or incompetent labral tissue not amenable to repair. This may be in either a primary or revision setting, and we recommend discussion of allograft reconstruction preoperatively with all patients. We prefer the "kite technique" previously described by Bhatia and coworkers[42] with a tibialis anterior allograft (**Fig. 3**). We typically perform a segmental reconstruction, with repair of the graft to the native labrum when possible anteriorly and posteriorly. Of note, the term circumferential reconstruction is misleading because the labrum is horseshoe-shaped and we favor the term complete reconstruction.

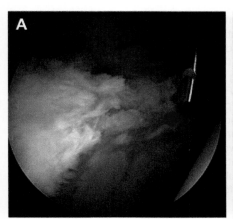 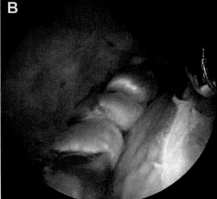

Fig. 3. (*A*) Arthroscopic image of a revision right hip arthroscopy demonstrating an irreparable labrum. (*B*) Arthroscopic image demonstrating LR using the kite technique with tibialis anterior allograft tissue. Notice restoration of the labral seal when traction is removed.

Capsular management

Capsular management has been an area of increased focus in recent years. This topic is discussed in depth elsewhere within this issue. Briefly, iatrogenic instability from capsular deficiency is an uncommon but real potential complication following hip arthroscopy. Dysplasia and hyperlaxity are well-known risk factors and caution should be exercised when considering surgery in this population. It is our belief that capsular closure should be performed whenever possible and in certain cases of hyperlaxity or microinstability capsular plication should be considered.

OUTCOMES

In general, results of arthroscopic labral repair in patients who have failed conservative management are favorable at 8 months postoperatively compared with a continued nonoperative course with regard to improved functional status and preservation of the native joint.[43] Poor outcomes are associated with increasing age, preexisting arthritic changes, and obesity. A recent cohort study demonstrated that surgical intervention early after the onset of symptoms (within 3–6 months) was associated with superior postoperative outcomes when compared with patients who underwent surgical intervention following a longer duration of symptoms.[44] Furthermore, economic modeling assessing cost-impact of arthroscopic surgery on society has shown cost-savings when compared with nonoperative treatment.[45]

As the number of hip arthroscopy procedures increases, especially in a younger and more active populations, more attention has been focused on return-to-play (RTP) for these individuals. Studies have been performed examining outcomes across a diverse group of athletes from yoga to military personnel to National Football League athletes.[14,46,47] Christian and colleagues[48] reported on RTP among 131 professional athletes (151 hips) from the four major North American sports leagues (National Football League, National Basketball Association, Major League Baseball, National Hockey League). They found a high rate of RTP at 88.7%; however, the median number of seasons played postoperatively was low (2.7, 2.3, 1.1, and 0.9 for National Football League, National Basketball Association, Major League Baseball, and National Hockey League, respectively). National Hockey League players in particular were found to have the worst prognosis with sustained decreases in games played and performance in the first 3 seasons postoperatively. Additionally, a recent systematic review and meta-analysis found that there is significant variability in RTP protocols because of a lack of standardization between institutions. Many protocols are not evidence-based relying heavily on expert opinion and no validated functional test currently exists to assess RTP. Despite this ambiguity, the overall rate of RTP and improvement in PROs (patient reported outcome) following surgery remains high.[49]

Guidelines and outcomes relating to RTP in patients following LR are also limited; however, short-term follow-up on these patients is promising. Philippon and co-workers[29] reported on 21 elite athletes undergoing LR with iliotibial band autograft, showing an RTP rate of 85.7% (81% returned to similar level) with average follow-up of 41.4 months. The authors also showed increases in mHHS (67–84) and HOS-Sport (56–77) in this cohort.[29] More recently, Maldonado and coworkers[50] reported on 1-year follow-up for athletes (high school, college, recreational, or amateur) undergoing primary LR with a 78% RTP at final follow-up.

SUMMARY

Conservative management of patients with FAI and labral tears is successful and should be attempted as a first-line treatment. In those who continue to be symptomatic, arthroscopic management has been demonstrated to have favorable outcomes for properly selected patients. Most patients benefit from early arthroscopic labral repair and appropriate correction of bony impingement. LR (segmental or complete/circumferential) or augmentation with autograft or allograft should typically be reserved for revision cases or in select primary settings. Correction of bony impingement and labral preservation techniques allow a high rate of RTP in recreational and elite athletes alike. Because hip arthroscopy is a rapidly evolving field, there is still much to be learned regarding appropriate patient selection, treatment algorithms, expected return to activities/sport, and long-term outcomes in these patients.

CLINICS CARE POINTS

- FAI is frequently associated with labral tears. It is important to treat the abnormal bony morphology and restore the labral seal through either repair or reconstruction for optimal outcomes.
- Labral repair is favored over labral debridement. Multiple options exist regarding type of suture anchor and repair technique without clear evidence showing superiority for any given technique.
- Labral repair and reconstruction demonstrate significant improvements in patient outcomes. Reconstruction is typically reserved for the revision setting, presence of ossified labrum, or when there is deficient or incompetent labral tissue not amenable to repair.
- Capsular closure should be performed when possible, particularly in cases with concomitant hip dysplasia or hyperlaxity.
- Hip arthroscopic correction of bony impingement and labral preservation techniques allow a high rate of RTP in recreational and elite athletes alike.

DISCLOSURE

No outside research support or funding is pertinent to this review. The authors have no conflicts of interest to disclose.

REFERENCES

1. Palmer A, Fernquest S, Gimpel M, et al. Physical activity during adolescence and the development of cam morphology: a cross-sectional cohort study of 210 individuals. Br J Sports Med 2018;52(9):601–10.
2. Clohisy JC, Baca G, Beaulé PE, et al. Descriptive epidemiology of FAI. Am J Sports Med 2013;41(6):1348–56.
3. Siebenrock KA, Ferner F, Noble PC, et al. The cam-type deformity arises in childhood in response to vigorous sporting activity. Clin Orthop Relat Res 2011; 469(11):3229–40.
4. Ejnisman L, Philippon MJ. Femoral acetabular impingement: the femoral side. Clin Sports Med 2011;30(2):317–29.
5. Hadeed MM, Cancienne JM, Gwathmey FW. Pincer impingement. Clin Sports Med 2016;35(3):405–18.
6. Ferguson SJ, Bryant JT, Ganz R, et al. An in vitro investigation of the labral seal in hip joint mechanics. J Biomech 2003;36(2):171–8.

7. Hlavácek M. The influence of the labrum seal and synovial fluid thixotropy on squeeze-film lubrication of a spherical synovial joint. J Biomech 2002;35(10): 1325–35.

8. Seldes RM, Tan V, Hunt J, et al. Anatomy, histologic features, and vascularity of the adult acetabular labrum. Clin Orthop Relat Res 2001;(382):232–40.

9. Nepple JJ, Goljan P, Briggs KK, et al. Hip strength deficits in patients with symptomatic FAI and labral tears. Arthroscopy 2015;32(11):2106–11.

10. Mardones RM, Gonzalez C, Chen Q, et al. Surgical treatment of femoroacetabular impingement: evaluation of the effect of the size of the resection. Surgical technique. J Bone Joint Surg Am 2006;88(Suppl 1 PT 1):84–91.

11. Al Mana L, Coughlin RP, Desai V, et al. The hip labrum reconstruction: indications and outcomes-an updated systematic review. Curr Rev Musculoskelet Med 2019; 12(2):156–65.

12. Bedi A, Dolan M, Hetsroni I, et al. Surgical treatment of femoroacetabular impingement improves hip kinematics: a computer-assisted model. Am J Sports Med 2011;39(Suppl):43S–439S.

13. Domb BG, Stake CE, Botser I, et al. Surgical dislocation of the hip versus arthroscopic treatment of femoroacetabular impingement: a prospective matched-pair study with average 2-year follow-up. Arthroscopy 2013;29(9):1506–13.

14. Nwanchukwu BU, Bedi A, Premkumar A, et al. Characteristics and outcomes of arthroscopic femoroacetabular impingement surgery in the National Football League. Am J Sports Med 2018;46(1):144–8.

15. Botser IB, Jackson TJ, Smith TW, et al. Open surgical dislocation versus arthroscopic treatment of femoroacetabular impingement. Am J Orthop 2014;43(5): 209–14.

16. Byrd JWT, Jones KS. Hip arthroscopy for labral pathology: prospective analysis with 10-year follow-up. Arthroscopy 2009;25(4):365–8.

17. Woyski D, Mather RC III. Surgical treatment of labral tears: debridement, repair, reconstruction. Curr Rev Musculoskelet Med 2019;12(3):291–9.

18. Wolff AB, Grossman J. Management of the acetabular labrum. Clin Sports Med 2016;35(3):345–60.

19. Krych AJ, Thompson M, Knutson Z, et al. Arthroscopic labral repair versus selective labral debridement in female patients with femoroacetabular impingement: a prospective randomized study. Arthroscopy 2013;29(1):46–53.

20. Larson CM, Giveans MR, Stone RM. Arthroscopic debridement versus refixation of the acetabular labrum associated with femoroacetabular impingement: mean 3.5 year follow-up. Am J Sports Med 2012;40(5):1015–21.

21. Menge TJ, Briggs KK, Dornan GJ, et al. Survivorship and outcomes 10 years following hip arthroscopy for femoroacetabular impingement: labral debridement compared with labral repair. J Bone Joint Surg Am 2017;99(12):997–1004.

22. Schairer WW, Nwachukwu BU, McCormick F, et al. Use of hip arthroscopy and risk of conversion to total hip arthroplasty: a population-based analysis. Arthroscopy 2016;32(4):587–93.

23. McCormick F, Nwanchukwu BU, Alpaugh K, et al. Predictors of hip arthroscopy outcomes for labral tears at minimum 2-year follow-up: the influence of age and arthritis. Arthroscopy 2012;28(10):1359–64.

24. Chandrasekaran S, Darwish N, Lodhia P, et al. Outcomes of hip arthroscopic surgery in patients with Tonnis grade 1 osteoarthritis with a minimum 2-year follow-up: evaluation using a matched-pair analysis with a control group with Tonnis grade 0. Am J Sports Med 2016;44(7):1781–8.

25. Philippon MJ, Nepple JJ, Campbell KJ, et al. The hip fluid seal-part 1: the effect of an acetabular labral tear, repair, resection, and reconstruction on hip fluid pressurization. Knee Surg Sports Traumatol Arthrosc 2014;22:722–9.
26. Nepple JJ, Philippon MJ, Campbell KJ, et al. The hip fluid seal-part 2: the effect of an acetabular labral tear, repair, resection, and reconstruction hip stability to distraction. Knee Surg Sports Traumatol Arthrosc 2014;22:730–6.
27. Sawyer GA, Briggs KK, Dornan GJ, et al. Clinical outcomes after arthroscopic hip labral repair using looped versus pierced suture techniques. Am J Sports Med 2015;43(7):1683–8.
28. Jackson TJ, Hammarstedt JE, Vemula SP, et al. Acetabular labral base repair versus circumferential suture repair: a matched-paired comparison of clinical outcomes. Arthroscopy 2015;31(9):1716–21.
29. Philippon MJ, Briggs KK, Hay CJ, et al. Arthroscopic labral reconstruction in the hip using iliotibial band autograft: technique and early outcomes. Arthroscopy 2010;26(6):750–6.
30. Chandrasekaran S, Darwish N, Close MR, et al. Arthroscopic reconstruction of segmental defects of the hip labrum: results in 22 patients with mean 2-year follow up. Arthroscopy 2017;33(9):1685–93.
31. Scanaliato JP, Christensen DL, Salfiti C, et al. Primary circumferential acetabular labral reconstruction: achieving outcomes similar to primary labral repair despite more challenging patient characteristics. Am J Sports Med 2018;46(9):2079–88.
32. White BJ, Patterson J, Herzog MM. Revision arthroscopic acetabular labral treatment: repair or reconstruct? Arthroscopy 2016;32(12):2513–20.
33. Matsuda DK, Burchette RJ. Arthroscopic hip labral reconstruction with a Gracilis autograft versus labral refixation: 2-year minimum outcomes. Am J Sports Med 2013;41(5):980–7.
34. Cadet ER, Chan AK, Vorys GC, et al. Investigation of the preservation of the fluid seal effect in the repaired, partially resected and reconstructed acetabular labrum in a cadaveric hip model. Am J Sports Med 2012;40(10):2218–23.
35. Rathi R, Mazek J. Arthroscopic acetabular labral reconstruction with rectus femoris tendon autograft: our experiences and early results. J Orthop 2018;15(3):783–6.
36. Redmond JM, Cregar WM, Martin TJ, et al. Arthroscopic labral reconstruction of the hip using semitendinosus allograft. Arthrosc Tech 2015;4(4):e323–9.
37. Rahl MD, LaPorte C, Steinl GK, et al. Outcomes after arthroscopic hip labral reconstruction: a systematic review and meta-analysis. Am J Sports Med 2019. https://doi.org/10.1177/0363546519878147. 363546519878147.
38. Maldonado DR, Lall AC, Laseter JR, et al. Primary hip arthroscopic surgery with labral reconstruction: is there a difference between an autograft and allograft? Orthop J Sports Med 2019;7(3). 2325967119833715.
39. Philippon MJ, Bolia IK, Locks R, et al. Labral preservation: outcomes following labrum augmentation versus labrum reconstruction. Arthroscopy 2018;34(9):2604–11.
40. Nakashima H, Tsukamoto M, Ohnishi Y, et al. Clinical and radiographic predictors for unsalvageable labral tear at the time of initial hip arthroscopic management for femoroacetabular impingement. Am J Sports Med 2019;47(9):2029–37.
41. Maldonado DR, Lall AC, Walker-Santiago R, et al. Hip labral reconstruction: consensus study on indications, graft type and technique among high-volume surgeons. J Hip Preserv Surg 2019;6(1):41–9.
42. Bhatia S, Chahla J, Dean CS, et al. Hip labral reconstruction: the "kite technique" for improved efficiency and graft control. Arthrosc Tech 2016;5(2):e337–42.

43. Palmer AJR, Ayyar Gupta V, Fernquest S, et al. Arthroscopic hip surgery compared with physiotherapy and activity modification for the treatment of symptomatic femoroacetabular impingement: multicentre randomised controlled trial. BMJ 2019;364:l185.

44. Kunze KN, Beck EC, Nwachukwu BU, et al. Early hip arthroscopy for femoroacetabular impingement syndrome provides superior outcomes when compared with delaying surgical treatment beyond 6 months. Am J Sports Med 2019;47(9): 2038–44.

45. Mather RC 3rd, Nho SJ, Federer A, et al. Effects of arthroscopy for femoroacetabular impingement syndrome on quality of life and economic outcomes. Am J Sports Med 2018;46(5):1205–13.

46. Frank RM, Ukwuani G, Allison B, et al. High rate of return to yoga for athletes after hip arthroscopy for femoroacetabular impingement syndrome. Sports Health 2019;10(5):434–40.

47. Thomas DD, Bernhardson AS, Bernstein E, et al. Hip arthroscopy for femoroacetabular impingement in a military population. Am J Sports Med 2017;45(14): 3298–304.

48. Christian RA, Lubbe RJ, Chun DS, et al. Prognosis following hip arthroscopy varies in professional athletes based on sport. Arthroscopy 2019;35(3):837–42.

49. O'Connor M, Minkara AA, Westermann RW, et al. Return to play after hip arthroscopy: a systematic review and meta-analysis. Am J Sports Med 2018;46(11): 2780–8.

50. Maldonado DR, Chen SL, Yelton MJ, et al. Return to sport and athletic function in an active population after primary arthroscopic labral reconstruction of the Hip. Orthop J Sports Med 2020;8(2). 2325967119900767.

Hip Dysplasia

Joshua D. Harris, MD[a,b,c,d],*, Brian D. Lewis, MD[e], Kwan J. Park, MD[a]

KEYWORDS

- Dysplasia • Hip • Instability • Version • Acetabulum • Borderline • Arthroscopy
- Periacetabular osteotomy

KEY POINTS

- Acetabular dysplasia is a 3-dimensional osseous structural insufficiency of acetabular coverage of the femoral head.
- Acetabular dysplasia is characterized with a variety of 2- and 3-dimensional imaging modalities, including plain radiographs, MRI, and computed tomography scans.
- Acetabular dysplasia management includes a variety of different nonsurgical and surgical treatment options.
- Surgical treatment of acetabular dysplasia includes periacetabular osteotomy, with or without concurrent hip arthroscopy.
- The long-term natural history of untreated acetabular dysplasia is early hip osteoarthritis.

INTRODUCTION

Acetabular dysplasia represents a multiplanar structural pathomorphology associated with hip pain, instability, and osteoarthritis. The wide spectrum of dysplasia anatomically refers to a shallow acetabulum and is further classified based on the magnitude and location of undercoverage. Analogous to the Warwick agreement for femoroacetabular impingement (FAI) syndrome,[1] the diagnosis of hip dysplasia requires the assessment and interpretation of patient symptoms, physical examination signs, and imaging. The definition of dysplasia has been and continues to be controversial, especially regarding its mild version, frequently termed "borderline" dysplasia or "transitional acetabular coverage."[2] Although many trials, articles, books, presentations, and guidelines often define dysplasia dichotomously via a lateral center edge angle (LCEA) of less than 20°, this is a shallow interpretation of a highly complex 3-

[a] The Houston Methodist Hip Preservation Program, Houston Methodist Orthopedics and Sports Medicine, 6445 Main Street, Suite 2500, Houston, TX 77030, USA; [b] Houston Methodist Academic Institute; Houston Methodist Orthopedics & Sports Medicine, Houston, TX, USA; [c] Weill Cornell Medical College, New York, NY, USA; [d] Texas A&M University, College Station, TX, USA; [e] Department of Orthopedics, Duke University Medical Center, Box 3389, Durham, NC 27710, USA
* Corresponding author. The Houston Methodist Hip Preservation Program, Houston Methodist Orthopedics and Sports Medicine, 6445 Main Street, Suite 2500, Houston, TX 77030.
E-mail address: joshuaharrismd@gmail.com

Clin Sports Med 40 (2021) 271–288
https://doi.org/10.1016/j.csm.2020.11.004
0278-5919/21/© 2020 Elsevier Inc. All rights reserved.

dimensional volumetric- and surface area-based insufficiency in coverage. The natural history of dysplasia leads to chondral injury secondary to the shallow cup and upsloping sourcil, with a resultant increased risk of early hip arthritis.[3] Thus, in symptomatic individuals with dysplasia, the cornerstone of treatment addresses coverage with increased structural stability via periacetabular osteotomy (PAO). The goals of PAO are multifaceted, with improvements in pain, function, and the natural history via arthritis risk reduction. With an increased recognition of structural hip abnormalities, especially cam morphology, concomitant simultaneous or staged hip arthroscopy has significant advantages to address intra-articular pathology, including the labrum, articular cartilage, head–neck offset, subspine impingement, and iliofemoral ligament. In nonarthritic individuals, there is evidence that PAO alters the natural history of dysplasia and reduces the risk of hip arthritis and subsequent total hip arthroplasty.[4]

PATIENT PRESENTATION
History

The presentation of patients with acetabular dysplasia typically includes atraumatic, insidious (97%) onset groin (72%) or lateral hip (66%) pain.[5] The pain location is usually deep in the hip, with a "C" sign or "between the fingers" sign frequently exhibited.[6] As with most intra-articular problems, like FAI syndrome or arthritis, position- and motion-dependent pain with prolonged seated or deep flexion and rotational maneuvers is common.[1] Activity-related (88%), weight-bearing lateral hip pain with ambulating may manifest with increasing load, often termed "abductor fatigue."[5] Objective abnormalities in gait include a limp (48%),[5] apprehension with terminal hip extension at the end of stance phase,[7] and Trendelenburg gait. These symptoms are largely due to structural instability owing to deficient acetabular coverage with resultant femoral head edge loading the acetabular rim, and subsequent increased long-term secondary osteoarthritis. Twisting and pivoting exacerbate pain, mainly with extension and external rotation. Hip flexor symptoms, including painful internal snapping (audible, palpable), occur owing to the anterior head instability seen with anterior undercoverage. Painful external snapping (visible, palpable), owing to the iliotibial band, also frequently occurs. Anterior undercoverage typically manifests as anterior hip and groin pain, whereas posterior dysplasia manifests as anterior and/or posterior hip pain (often concomitant diagnoses include sacroiliac dysfunction, piriformis syndrome, deep gluteal syndrome, sciatica, low back pain); and lateral dysplasia manifests as deep lateral pain.[8]

Skeletally mature individuals with symptomatic dysplasia are typically young and active. In a group of 982 consecutive hips that underwent PAO, patients were primarily female (83%), with a mean age of 25.3 years (range, 9–54 years), mean body mass index of 24.6 kg/m[2], 87% Caucasian, family history of hip disease (27%), and significant preoperative low scores on validated hip-specific (the Hip injury and Osteoarthritis Outcome Score, modified Harris Hip Score), activity (University of California at Los Angeles), and general health (Short Form-12) patient-reported outcome scores.[9] Interestingly, 71% of patients in the latter study had symptoms for at least 1 year, 30% for at least 3 years, and 17% for at least 5 years. In addition, 35% had undergone previous hip surgery (15% ipsilateral, 20% contralateral), with 50% of ipsilateral cases being hip arthroscopy. In a similar investigation of 65 symptomatic skeletally mature hips diagnosed with dysplasia, the mean time from symptom onset to diagnosis was 61.5 months (range, 5 months to 29 years), the mean number of health care providers seen before diagnosis was 3.3 (range, 0–11), and most patients had tried multiple treatments before diagnosis (rest [75%], oral nonsteroidal medications [57%], physical therapy [43%], activity modification [42%], surgery [18%], and opioids [8%]).[5] These numbers are similar to that of FAI syndrome: patients saw 4.0 health care providers, had 3.4 imaging tests, had 3.1 previous treatments, spent $2456.97, and waited 32 months before diagnosis.[10]

Physical Examination

A proper systematic physical examination in a patient with dysplasia should include observation (including gait), inspection, palpation, motion (supine, lateral, prone, and seated), strength, and special testing. Gait assessment should evaluate for a Trendelenburg gait (common with abductor fatigue), antalgic gait (concern for effusion, stress fracture), in-toeing or out-toeing (significant version abnormalities), and the use of gait aides (eg, crutches, cane, wheelchair). Inspection is frequently normal, without cutaneous abnormalities, such as atrophy or deformities. Palpation evaluates all osseous and soft tissue structures around the hip, thigh, pelvis, and lumbosacral spine. An obvious tenet to this evaluation mandates absolute consideration for modesty and genitourinary and gastrointestinal systems. A pre-examination discussion with the patient and their family (eg, parents, if applicable) about the latter ensures professionalism and decreases the risk of misperceived examination techniques, especially palpation. The hip joint is a deep structure impossible to palpate. Specific areas to be palpated and documented for tenderness include the greater trochanteric facets, abductor tendons, iliac crest (from anterior superior to posterior superior iliac spines), inguinal canal (including inguinal hernia evaluation), pubic symphysis, pubic bone, rectus abdominis, sacroiliac joint, spinous processes (including asymmetry in coronal and sagittal plane alignment [scoliosis, kyphosis, and lordosis], and rib humps with forward bend), deep gluteal space, ischiofemoral space (lateral to ischium), sciatic nerve (plus Tinel evaluation), proximal hamstring, ischial tuberosity, adductor longus, quadriceps muscle, and iliotibial band (from the hip to tibia Gerdy's tubercle).

Hip (flexion, extension, abduction, adduction, and internal and external rotation) and knee (flexion, extension) motion should be measured and compared with the contralateral side. Importantly, hip flexion should be measured with the contralateral hip at 0° flexion (anterior pelvic tilt) and maximal hip flexion (posterior pelvic tilt).[11] Hip rotation should also be measured in both the supine and prone (obviates cam morphology engagement) positions.[12] Hip internal rotation is affected more by femoral version, whereas hip flexion is affected more by cam morphology.[13] Frequently in dysplasia, hip internal rotation is significantly increased and external rotation is decreased with increased version.[9] Strength (Medical Research Council classification, x/5) of the paraspinal muscles and all lower extremity muscles is measured. Special testing should include log roll, axial load (while supine), axial distraction, external rotation recoil, dial test, impingement testing (anterior via flexion, adduction, internal rotation; subspine via straight sagittal plane maximal flexion; lateral via straight coronal plane maximal abduction; and posterior via external rotation [pain for impingement; apprehension for instability]; and flexion, abduction, external rotation distance to table asymmetry [>4 cm for FAI syndrome] vs sacroiliac joint pain), iliopsoas evaluation (Ludloff, Stinchfield, iliopsoas test, and iliopsoas snap [audible pop]), iliotibial band snap (visible pop), Ober test, long- and short-lever adductor squeeze, resisted sit-up/crunch, and Valsalva examination (hernia, sports hernia, or core muscle injury). Most, but not all, patients with dysplasia demonstrate either a positive anterior (76%) or posterior impingement (27%) sign.[9] A positive impingement test implies an intra-articular location of the pain, but is not the sine qua non for FAI syndrome.[9] Thus, the impingement test is often positive in dysplasia as well. In patients with dysplasia, an assessment of hypermobility should always be performed; the Beighton score is the most common tool (x/9; >4/9 indicates hypermobility).

Imaging

Plain radiographs

Imaging evaluation for individuals with dysplasia should include a combination of high-quality 2- and 3-dimensional modalities. Initial evaluation includes plain radiographs of the hip and pelvis. A weight-bearing anteroposterior (AP) pelvis and a variety of lateral views are typically performed. The AP pelvis and false profile views are the 2 primary views to characterize acetabular morphology. The LCEA is the most common measurement used to characterize dysplasia on the AP view, but should not be used to diagnose in isolation. The normal range of LCEA is 25° to 40°.[14] Using a computed tomography (CT) scan as the reference standard in 474 asymptomatic hips, mean lateral coverage represents a mean LCEA of 31° ± 1°.[15] The LCEA described by Wiberg[16] is measured to the lateral edge of the sourcil. However, the LCEA may also be measured to the lateral edge of acetabular bone, which may be significantly different from the sourcil lateral edge (**Fig. 1**). Using a 3-dimensional CT scan, the lateral edge of the sourcil (anterosuperior) is more anterior than the lateral edge of acetabular bone (superolateral) (1:30 ± 0:42 vs 12:06 ± 0:30, respectively).[17] The bone LCEA has been reported to be as much as greater than 13° more than the sourcil LCEA (mean, 4°–5°; range, −4° to 13°).[17,18] In a study by Hanson and colleagues,[18] out of the 14 patients with a sourcil LCEA of less than 20°, only 4 (29%) also had a bone LCEA of less than 20°; similarly, out of the 54 patients with a sourcil LCEA of less than 25° (dysplasia or borderline dysplasia), 32 (59%) had a bone LCEA of greater than 25° (normal coverage); further, 6 patients had a sourcil LCEA of less than 20°, but a bone LCEA of greater than 25°. This significant variation in the LCEA measurements alone can dramatically alter diagnostic and treatment decisions. Lateral coverage may also be assessed by the femoral head extrusion index, with values of greater than 20% to 25% indicating dysplasia.[3]

The Tonnis angle, also known as the sourcil angle or acetabular index, is a measure that represents the slope of the weight-bearing surface of the acetabular dome from the medial to lateral sourcil (**Fig. 2**A). The normal range of Tonnis angle is typically 0° to 10°, with borderline from 10° to 15°.[14] However, studies have shown a significantly increased risk of arthritis progression in patients with a Tonnis angle of more than even 7° to 8°,[3] and a significantly increased risk of reoperation after

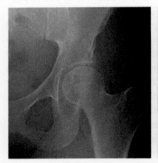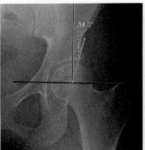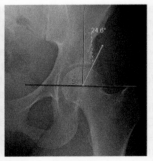

Fig. 1. Weight-bearing AP pelvis plain radiograph with focus on left hip in 17-year-old girl (*left*) showing an LCEA of 14.3° measured to the lateral sourcil (*middle*) and 24.6° measured to the lateral acetabular bone (*right*).

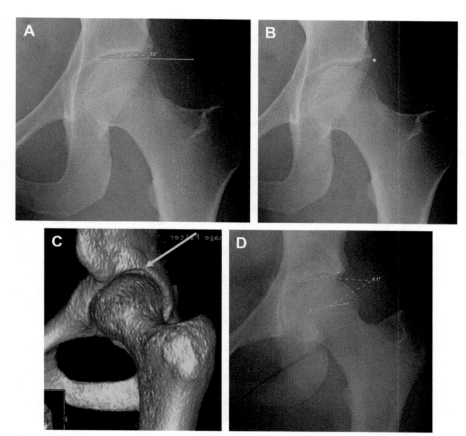

Fig. 2. (*A*) Weight-bearing AP pelvis plain radiograph with focus on left hip in 19-year-old woman showing a Tonnis angle of 10°. (*B*) An upsloping lateral sourcil (*asterisk*). (*C*) Upsloping lateral sourcil in the same patient visualized on 3-dimensional computed tomography scan; and (*D*) a FEAR Index of 4.1°.

arthroscopy (mean, 6.7° [range, 5.3°–8.1°] in the reoperation group vs 4.8° [range, 4.4°–5.3°] in the nonreoperation group).[19] For every increased degree in Tonnis angle, the odds ratio was 1.12 for reoperation.[19] In patients with a Tonnis angle of greater than 10°, the risk of reoperation was 84%.[19] The upsloping sourcil places excessive shearing force on the acetabular articular cartilage with weight-bearing, hence the increased arthritis risk. In addition to the Tonnis angle measurement itself, an upsloping lateral sourcil (**Fig. 2**B, C) is significantly associated with generalized joint hypermobility (59% prevalence).[20] Thus, an upsloping lateral sourcil may represent more than just osseous structural instability. A relatively recent measure of stability is the femoroepiphyseal acetabular roof (FEAR) index (**Fig. 2**D).[21] The FEAR index has value in the evaluation of hip instability (femoral head migration on conventional plain radiographs or head recentering on an AP abduction view) in patients with transitional acetabular coverage. In patients with the latter (also known as borderline dysplasia), a FEAR index of less than 5° is likely to be stable (sensitivity, 78%; specificity, 80%; the stable borderline group's mean FEAR index was −2.1°

± 8.4° vs the unstable group, 13.3° ± 15.2°). A greater degree of instability may be associated with head lateralization and incongruity, which can radiographically be observed with a broken Shenton's line.

Although the LCEA represents lateral (or global) acetabular coverage, it largely ignores anterior and posterior coverage.[8,22] A variety of measures can be visualized on plain radiographs to characterize the magnitude of anterior coverage. On the false profile view, the anterior center edge angle (ACEA) is analogous to the LCEA in that there is commonly a discrepancy between its measurement at the anterior sourcil versus anterior bone (**Fig. 3**).[18] However, the magnitude of discrepancy in the ACEA measurement is much greater than in the LCEA. The bone ACEA has been reported to be as much as 22° more than sourcil ACEA (mean, 10°; range, −2° to 22°). An ACEA discrepancy of greater than 5° was observed in 78% of patients (107/137). All the patients with a sourcil ACEA less than 20° (7/7) had a bone ACEA of greater than 20°. The false profile view has the advantage of the ability to concurrently assess the anterior and inferomedial joint space and the anterior inferior iliac spine morphology. A disadvantage of the false profile is the significant challenge in patient positioning during the radiograph.[23] The latter leads to large variation and low reliability in ACEA measurement, even with small changes in pelvic rotation during image acquisition.[24] Thus, a low-dose pelvis CT scan (effective dose as low as 0.97–1.46 mSv) may obviate the false-profile view (1.0 mSv) altogether, with the addition of all the advantages of 3-dimensional analysis of coverage.[25,26] The low-dose CT protocol can result in a 90% decrease in the total effective dose radiation exposure versus a traditional CT scan.[26]

Additional measures of anterior coverage include the anterior wall index (AWI) and percent anterior coverage. The AWI radiographically quantifies anterior acetabular coverage (**Fig. 4**).[27] The mean normal AWI is 0.41 (range, 0.30–0.51). In dysplasia, the mean AWI is 0.28 (range, −0.06 to 0.52). Anterior coverage is the percentage of the femoral head covered by the acetabulum in the AP direction[28] and can be measured via CT scan or a variety of computerized collision detection software programs.[15] Normal anterior coverage is 18.6% (range, 6.7%–28.9%). In dysplasia, the mean anterior coverage is 9.8% (range, 0%–22.2%). Using surface area regional coverage of the femoral head, anterior coverage of 40% ± 2% for a large asymptomatic group (474 hips; 61% ± 3% for superior coverage, 48% ± 3% for posterior coverage).[15]

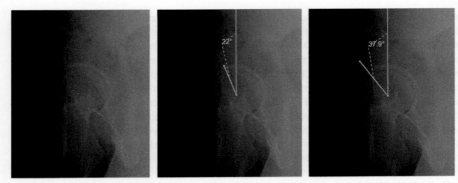

Fig. 3. False profile plain radiograph of right hip in 21-year-old woman (*left*) showing an ACEA of 22° measured to the anterior sourcil (*middle image*) and 37.9° measured to the anterior acetabular bone (*right*).

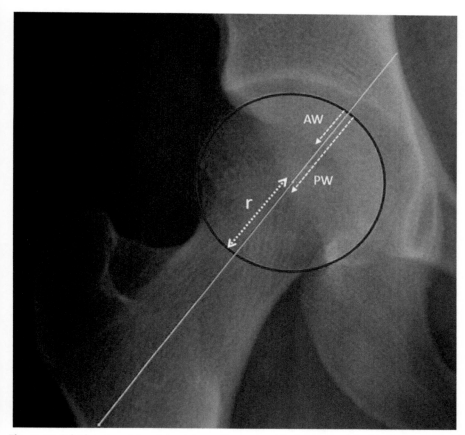

Fig. 4. Weight-bearing AP pelvis plain radiograph with focus on right hip in 24-year-old man showing the measurements needed to calculate the AWI and the PWI. A best-fitting perfect circle is drawn around the femoral head. A line is drawn connecting the femoral neck center intersecting with the head center. AWI = AW/r; PWI = PW/r.

Analogous to the AWI, the posterior wall index (PWI) radiographically quantifies posterior acetabular coverage (see **Fig. 3**).[27] The mean normal PWI is 0.91 (range, 0.81–1.14). In dysplasia, the mean PWI is 0.81 (range, 0.35–1.04). Posterior coverage is the percentage of femoral head covered by the acetabulum in the posteroanterior direction.[28] Normal posterior coverage 42.9% (range, 31.6%–59.1%). In dysplasia, the mean posterior coverage is 36.6% (range, 15.3%–53.0%). A further analysis of posterior coverage includes an evaluation of the posterior wall and ischial spine signs, which indicate global acetabular retroversion, with or without dysplasia (**Fig. 5**).[29] Although the crossover sign has been used to characterize focal acetabular retroversion, its accuracy is poor given the frequent (50%) false-positive rate owing to a prominent anterior inferior iliac spine.[30] In a study of 474 normal hips evaluated with a CT scan, only 15% of hips with true cranial retroversion displayed a crossover sign.[15]

In addition to traditional static measures of coverage, pelvic incidence is an unmodifiable plain radiographic (lateral sacral, EOS) or CT (lateral scout view) measure used to characterize pelvic tilt and the sacral slope that plays a significant dynamic role in

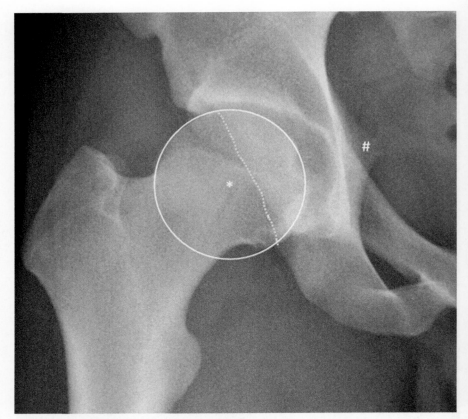

Fig. 5. Weight-bearing AP pelvis plain radiograph with focus on right hip in 31-year-old man demonstrating a positive posterior wall sign (*) and positive ischial spine sign (#).

dysplasia. In patients with an elevated pelvic incidence, there is increased lumbar lordosis, which forces posterior pelvic tilt to maintain sagittal balance, which anteverts and uncovers the anterior acetabulum, exacerbating dysplasia.[31,32] In patients with a low pelvic incidence, there is less lumbar lordosis and, to maintain sagittal balance, anterior pelvic tilt occurs, which covers the anterior acetabulum, improving the structural instability associated with anterior undercoverage. However, this factor may also exacerbate anterior impingement and posterior instability.[33]

Computed tomography scans
A CT scan is an excellent imaging modality to evaluate dysplasia. The optimal way to assess acetabular coverage and version is via CT scanning. In the largest study to date of asymptomatic trauma pelvis CT scans, the mean acetabular version for male and female hips (n = 878) was 15.5° and 18.3° at 1 o'clock; 21.5° and 24.0° at 2 o'clock; and 20.2° and 24.3° at 3 o'clock, respectively (**Fig. 6**).[34] The coverage spectrum analysis (from dysplasia to pincer) of a patient's hip may be compared with these normative reference values. In addition to acetabular version, femoral version must be assessed. Unfortunately, there is wide discrepancy and variation in the technique and reported normative reference femoral version values. There are at least 5 common

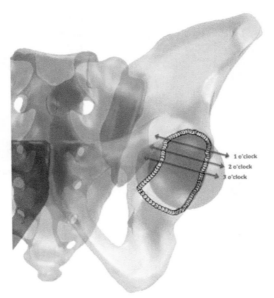

Fig. 6. Clock-face positions of version measurements. This 3-dimensional model depicts the 3 different locations we used to measure focal acetabular version (1, 2, and 3 o'clock). (*From* Tannenbaum EP, Zhang P, Maratt JD, et al. A Computed Tomography Study of Gender Differences in Acetabular Version and Morphology: Implications for Femoroacetabular Impingement. Arthroscopy 2015;31:1247–54; with permission.)

methods used for measurement (**Fig. 7**).[35] In patients with symptomatic dysplasia, abnormalities and a wide variation in femoral version are more of the rule, rather than the exception. In a study of 90 symptomatic hips using the method described by Murphy and colleagues[36] (the most accurate of the femoral version measurement methods, although it does overestimate femoral version by 3.5° to 6.3°), Lerch and colleagues[37] reported femoral version at 25° ± 15° (range, −9° to 84°), with greater version in females (27° ± 16°) than males (19° ± 12°). Further, 63% of hips' femoral version was either greater than 25° or less than 10°; and 26% was either greater than 35° or less than 0°. Excessive femoral anteversion (greater than 25°) was more common (47%) than retroversion (17%). Although a CT scan is the most accurate and reproducible method for measuring femoral version, an axial MRI may be an excellent alternative because it results in less than a 2° difference from true version, but obviates ionizing radiation concerns.[38] The issue of ionizing radiation is an especially important one for young patients, because the number needed to harm (lifetime attributable risk of cancer) for the preoperative and postoperative average dose CT is 952 (male) and 564 (female) patients, with a relative risk of 17.5 (male) and 16.1 (female).[39]

Combining the acetabular and femoral versions may be done in a variety of ways. Traditionally, the McKibbin index is the most commonly used.[40] Unfortunately, as other investigators have suggested,[41] the study that developed the Instability Index of McKibbin[40] was based on a study of newborn cadaveric specimens and adult dried osteological specimens from an anatomy department (some held together with wire) using a simple protractor. Because most assessments of the femoral and acetabular versions in modern hip preservation surgery uses a CT scan, a more updated term, the COmbined femoral Torsion and Acetabular Version (COTAV) Index is growing in use.[12] The COTAV index, analogous to the McKibbin index, is simply the sum of acetabular

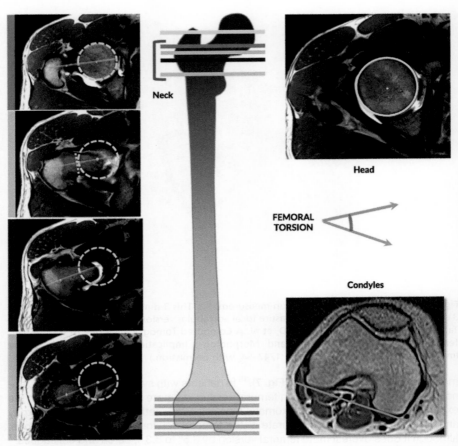

Fig. 7. Assessment of femoral torsion on cross-sectional imaging. On consecutive strict axial images over the proximal femur, determine the femoral head center (FHC) (*yellow circle* and *yellow line*). Defining the femoral neck axis (*green line*) can be done by several methods. Lee method *(red bar):* A line is drawn on the first image on which the FHC can be connected with the most cephalic junction of the greater trochanter and the femoral neck; Reikeras method (*light blue bar*): A line connecting the FHC with the femoral neck center is drawn on an image where the anterior and posterior cortices run parallel to each other; Jarret method (not shown): A line is drawn on a single image that runs from the FHC trough the center of the femoral neck; Tomczak method (*dark blue bar*): The FHC is connected with the center of the greater trochanter at the base of the femoral neck; and Murphy method (*orange bar*): The FHC is connected with the center of the base of the femoral neck directly superior to the lesser trochanter. Then, over the distal femur, draw a tangent to the posterior aspect of the femoral condyles (*blue line;* choosing the slice where the condyles are more prominent). The angle between both lines represents the femoral torsion. Although some of these reference points are located on different adjacent slices, modern workstations should allow drawing and modifying a line across multiple images in 1 series or, alternatively, different slices can be superimposed on a single image with the help of postprocessing software. (*From* Mascarenhas VV, Ayeni OR, Egund N, et al. Imaging Methodology for Hip Preservation: Techniques, Parameters, and Thresholds. Semin Musculoskelet Radiol 2019;23:197-226; with permission.)

(equatorial/central; at approximately the 3 o'clock position) and femoral version measurements. A normal COTAV index is between 20° and 45°, with excessive at greater than 45° and decreased if less than 20°.[12] In addition to these summative indices of femoral and acetabular version, the omega surface[42] and the omega zone[43] have been described to account for both femoral and acetabular versions, alpha angle, LCEA, and neck shaft angle. These CT scan-based measures are more applicable to patients with FAI syndrome, rather than dysplasia. A simple and useful classification, called the Morphologic Matrix, can help surgeons to dichotomize a borderline dysplastic patient's symptoms and mechanical diagnosis into either impingement or instability.[44,45] The Morphologic Matrix has 3 imaging-based criteria: the LCEA, alpha angle, and femoral version. The LCEA is subdivided into 4 groups: 1 (<18°), 2 (18°–25°), 3 (26°–40°), and 4 (>40°). The alpha angle is subdivided into 4 groups: 1 (<50°), 2 (50°–65°), 3 (66°–80°), and 4 (>80°). Femoral version is subdivided into 3 groups: 1 (>25°), 2 (5°–25°), and 3 (<5°). Lower numbers (eg, 111) indicate dysplasia and instability, whereas higher numbers (eg, 333) indicate impingement.

MRI

In patients with dysplasia, MRI has immense value in the evaluation of multiple soft tissue causes of hip pain. MRI typically reveals a hypertrophic labrum.[46] In addition, periarticular muscles also reveal hypertrophy, including the iliocapsularis and abductors.[47] Capsular thickness should be assessed as well, especially the anterior capsule (iliofemoral ligament), posterior recess, and zona orbicularis. A thin or patulous capsule may frequently be present in individuals with instability.[48] Although the femoroacetabular articular cartilage thickness has also been shown to be thicker in patients with dysplasia,[49] this finding is nonspecific. A more specific finding of an inside-out acetabular articular cartilage defects has been shown with greater frequency in dysplasia (88% arthroscopic incidence in patients with an LCEA of <20°) as opposed to the outside-in defects observed with cam FAI (90% arthroscopic incidence in patients with an LCEA of >20°).[50] Ligamentum teres integrity also plays a significant role. However, its role in either the cause of symptoms in the presence of dysplasia or the effect of the dysplasia is unclear.[51] Advanced imaging techniques, such as delayed gadolinium-enhanced MRI of cartilage, may have excellent value in the prediction of early stages of arthritis and hip preservation surgery outcome prediction. Unfortunately, delayed gadolinium-enhanced MRI of cartilage is primarily a research tool currently, and less clinically relevant, even in most tertiary hip preservation referral centers and programs.

TREATMENT

The management of patients with acetabular dysplasia is multifactorial. Patient-specific variables that mandate consideration in treatment selection include age, occupation, body mass index, smoking status, symptom type (instability vs impingement), symptom duration, symptom severity, expectations, concomitant periarticular symptoms (eg, low back, knee, pelvic floor), current and desired activity levels, previous treatments (including oral medications, including opioids), and unilaterality or bilaterality. Structural hip-specific variables include imaging-based hip, lumbopelvic, and lower extremity shape, grade of arthritis, chondrolabral junction status, and the coexistence of cam, pincer, or subspine morphology.

Nonsurgical Treatment

The initial management of individuals with acetabular dysplasia is primarily nonsurgical. However, in symptomatic dysplasia, the natural history predicts arthritis treatment with total hip arthroplasty at an earlier age than in FAI syndrome or normal hips.[3,52] Thus, most surgeons recommend structural correction with PAO in patients with more than mild symptoms or without symptoms. Nonsurgical measures include rest, activity modification, oral nonopioid over-the-counter or prescription medications (eg, nonsteroidal anti-inflammatory drugs), and physical therapy. Although the role of injections is limited, they can help diagnostically in cases with multiple pain sources or therapeutically in mild cases. Given the structural instability present with dysplasia, periarticular muscle dysfunction can be managed with high-quality physical therapy, focusing on strength of the hip, low back, lower extremity, pelvic floor, and core. Because the abductors are frequently weak, focus on gait normalization (eg, walking or endurance loading or running) and Trendelenburg elimination is critically important. Because the iliopsoas is often involved in anterior head stability (analogous to the long head biceps tendon in anterior shoulder instability), addressing hip flexion strength is also of immense value. A key concept of any nonsurgical program should be education—understanding the pathology and symptomatology for patients requires a care team that provides patient education to encourage pain improving modalities and avoids pain-provoking activities and interventions. Analogous to the FAI syndrome, a motion- and position-dependent entity like dysplasia should contraindicate forced stretching or supraphysiological motion goals. Short-term (1-year) improvements in pain and function can be achieved in patients with symptomatic dysplasia.[53]

Surgical Treatment

In patients with persistent unsatisfactory symptoms after a trial of nonsurgical treatment, surgery is indicated. In patients with dysplasia, per the American Academy of Orthopedic Surgeons Appropriate Use Criteria for the Management of Osteoarthritis of the Hip (adopted by the American Academy of Orthopedic Surgeons Board of Directors in December 2017),[54] hip preservation surgery is appropriately indicated in young patients (<40 years of age) with function-limiting pain, minimal to no osteoarthritis, with or without range of motion limitations, with or without modifiable risk factors, and without contraindications to surgery. In middle-aged patients (41–64 years of age) with function-limiting pain, minimal to no arthritis, with or without range of motion limitations, with or without modifiable risk factors, and without contraindications to surgery, hip preservation surgery may be appropriate or rarely appropriate. Hip preservation surgery can be either arthroscopic in isolation, open (eg, PAO, proximal femoral osteotomy) in isolation, or both.

Arthroscopy

Arthroscopic hip preservation surgery in patients with dysplasia plays a controversial role. Key concepts of arthroscopic treatments include the following: do not use arthroscopy in isolation to treat an instability problem associated with structural acetabular deficiency, the labrum must be preserved (ie, repair, reconstruction, augmentation) and not debrided, the iliopsoas must not be cut, the acetabular rim should not be further resected (ie, iatrogenic dysplasia), the capsule (iliofemoral ligament, zona orbicularis) should be preserved (eg, repair, plication, augmentation, reconstruction) and not left open, abnormalities in femoral version should be corrected (either staged or simultaneous), and the ligamentum teres should be preserved.[55]

A universal agreed-upon clear definition of borderline dysplasia does not exist. Although it does imply a well-known spectrum of pathology associated with dysplasia and structural instability, it leaves surgeons in a gray zone of decision making. More recently, the phrase transitional acetabular coverage has been introduced[2] to better describe the in-between pathomorphologic nature of this group of individuals who have too mild of deformity for PAO but too unpredictable for arthroscopy.[45] Although arthroscopy may seems to be more appealing owing to its minimally invasive approach, it should never be tried first if dysplasia is the underlying mechanical diagnosis, because the ultimate PAO outcome as a revision procedure after arthroscopy is inferior to that of the PAO outcome as a primary procedure.[56] A potential indication for isolated arthroscopy in the setting of transitional acetabular coverage may be when the clinical examination is more impingement (ie, position- or motion-dependent [deep flexion and rotation] pain, seated pain more than when ambulating, associated with stiffness) than instability (ie, abductor fatigue, mechanical overload with walking, snapping [both internal and external], weakness, apprehension, giving out, hip flexor symptoms). In the latter situation, secondary signs of instability should be sought on imaging (eg, hypertrophic labrum, hypertrophic iliocapsularis, thin or patulous capsule) and clinical examination (eg, Beighton score, Brighton, Hakim-Grahamme). Another potential indication for isolated arthroscopy is when the cam morphology (eg, elevated alpha angle on multiple views, including AP for posterolateral cam; elevated omega angle) is the clear mechanical problem, when the femoral head simply does not fit in the acetabulum.

The optimal timing of arthroscopy and PAO is debatable, with limited to no data to recommend which one first and when. In simultaneous surgery, arthroscopy first is advantageous because the distraction will be pulling on an intact pelvis, but this will cloud open surgery tissue planes, complicating the PAO technique. PAO first is advantageous because the technique will be clean as if performed in isolation, but then distraction necessary for arthroscopy may disrupt the PAO fragment fixation. A planned staged surgery can be as short as the same hospitalization (2–3 days) or as long as more than 12 months. If perform arthroscopy first, followed by staged PAO, then overcorrection to pincer FAI may occur and would necessarily require another operation to correct. The latter is an important consideration, knowing that appropriate acetabular orientation (more specifically, the absence of retroversion and normalization of the ACEA) enhances the longevity of the hip after PAO.[57,58] If performing PAO first and overcorrection occurs, then subsequent arthroscopy can accurately address this complication.

The outcomes of isolated arthroscopy in the setting of dysplasia have been historically poor, with high rates of failure (up to nearly 1 in 3).[59] In the setting of borderline dysplasia, different clusters of patients can be typically observed: in females, ACEA (55%), FEAR index (42%), and AWI (34%) were the common abnormal imaging findings, whereas in males, PWI (48%) was the most common.[60] Multiple recent systematic reviews have yielded a variety of findings regarding the diagnosis, treatment, and outcomes at short- and mid-term follow-up in patients with borderline dysplasia. Kraeutler and colleagues[61] reported that the LCEA is an unreliable isolated marker for dysplasia, there is a wide spectrum of instability in patients with borderline dysplasia, and properly chosen patients can achieve good outcomes with careful selection based on history, physical examination, and imaging. Kuroda and colleagues[62] defined borderline dysplasia simply via LCEA 20° to 25°, showed an 80% to 87% rate of achieving a minimal clinically important difference with the modified Harris Hip Score, and demonstrated an increased risk of femoral head articular cartilage defects, with poor outcomes observed in those more than 40 years of age and with more than 20° of femoral version. Ding and colleagues[63] reported significant short-term improvements in validated subjective outcomes, with a reoperation rate of 8.5%, including a PAO conversion rate of 4.0%, with the most important outcome predictors being bipolar articular cartilage defects, arthritis (Tonnis 2, 3), and ligamentum teres tears.

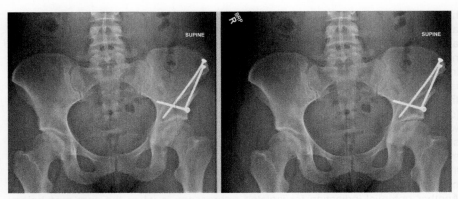

Fig. 8. Postoperative AP pelvis plain radiograph following PAO of left hip in 20-year-old woman with an LCEA of 34° (*left*) and a Tonnis angle of 3° (*right*).

Periacetabular osteotomy

There are several different techniques for pelvic osteotomy to treat dysplasia. Most current PAO techniques and their modifications are all based on the one that Ganz originally described nearly 40 years ago, the Bernese PAO (**Fig. 8**).[64] Long-term follow-up investigations after PAO have revealed excellent survivorship. Lerch and colleagues[65] showed that 29% of patients did not progress in arthritis grade or convert to total hip arthroplasty at 30 years after PAO (performed 1984–1987). In the latter, postoperative anterior acetabular overcoverage or acetabular retroversion were associated with inferior survival. PAO does truly alter the natural history of dysplasia. Patients with more advanced arthritis (Tonnis 2) at the time of surgery are at an increased risk of early total hip arthroplasty conversion (within 10 years).[4] In nonarthritic individuals, survivorship approaches 90% and 60% at 10 and 20 years, respectively.[66] Further, there is a 10-year survivorship of 93%, 90%, 82%, and 63% at ages 20, 30, 40, and 50 years, respectively. Although the treatment of an intra-articular pathology is intuitively indicated with PAO, the evidence to support its routine use is limited to low levels of evidence and short-term follow-up. The efficacy of the addition of arthroscopy to PAO is the subject of a current randomized trial, with clinically important outcomes and costs both being investigated.[67]

CLINICS CARE POINTS

- Acetabular dysplasia is a complex multiplanar structural pathomorphology associated with hip pain, instability, and osteoarthritis.

- The natural history of dysplasia leads to chondral injury secondary to the highly complex 3-dimensional volumetric- and surface area-based insufficiency in coverage.

- Dysplasia can be characterized by its location: anterior, posterior, or lateral (or global).

- Evaluation of dysplasia requires plain radiographs and either MRI or CT scan (or both) to properly measure coverage and version.

- Isolated arthroscopy should not be used to treat structural instability observed in moderate or severe dysplasia.

- In properly selected patients with transitional acetabular coverage, or borderline dysplasia, good outcomes can be achieved at short- and mid-term follow-up.

- PAO and hip arthroscopy can be used together, either simultaneous or staged, to accurately correct both dysplasia and FAI syndrome.
- In nonarthritic individuals, PAO alters the natural history of dysplasia and reduces the risk of hip arthritis and subsequent THA.

DISCLOSURE

J.D. Harris: AAOS: Board or committee member; American Orthopaedic Society for Sports Medicine: Board or committee member; Arthroscopy: Editorial or governing board; Arthroscopy Association of North America: Board or committee member; International Society of Arthroscopy and Knee Orthopedic Surgery (ISAKOS): Board or committee member; PatientPop: Stock or stock options; Arthrex/Medinc of Texas: Research support; DePuy, A Johnson & Johnson Company: Research support; Frontiers In Surgery: Editorial or governing board; NIA Magellan: Paid consultant; SLACK Incorporated: Publishing royalties, financial or material support; Smith and Nephew: Paid presenter or speaker, Paid consultant, Research support; Ossur: Paid speaker. B.D. Lewis: Stryker, Paid consultant; Zimmer, Paid consultant. K.J. Park: Journal of Bone and Joint Surgery, British: Editorial/governing board.

REFERENCES

1. Griffin DR, Dickenson EJ, O'Donnell J, et al. The Warwick Agreement on femoroacetabular impingement syndrome (FAI syndrome): an international consensus statement. Br J Sports Med 2016;50:1169–76.
2. Nepple JJ. Editorial commentary: at the intersection of borderline dysplasia and femoroacetabular impingement-which way should we turn? Arthroscopy 2020;36:1185–8.
3. Wyles CC, Heidenreich MJ, Jeng J, et al. The John Charnley award: redefining the natural history of osteoarthritis in patients with hip dysplasia and impingement. Clin Orthop Relat Res 2017;475:336–50.
4. Wyles CC, Vargas JS, Heidenreich MJ, et al. Natural history of the dysplastic hip following modern periacetabular osteotomy. J Bone Joint Surg Am 2019;101:932–8.
5. Nunley RM, Prather H, Hunt D, et al. Clinical presentation of symptomatic acetabular dysplasia in skeletally mature patients. J Bone Joint Surg Am 2011;93(Suppl 2):17–21.
6. Harris J. Hypermobile hip syndrome. Oper Tech Sports Med 2019;27(3):108–18.
7. Kraeutler MJ, Garabekyan T, Pascual-Garrido C, et al. Hip instability: a review of hip dysplasia and other contributing factors. Muscles Ligaments Tendons J 2016;6:343–53.
8. Bali K, Smit K, Ibrahim M, et al. Ottawa classification for symptomatic acetabular dysplasia assessment of interobserver and intraobserver reliability. Bone Joint Res 2020;9:242–9.
9. Sankar WN, Duncan ST, Baca GR, et al. Descriptive epidemiology of acetabular dysplasia: the academic network of conservational hip outcomes research (ANCHOR) periacetabular osteotomy. J Am Acad Orthop Surg 2017;25:150–9.
10. Kahlenberg CA, Han B, Patel RM, et al. Time and cost of diagnosis for symptomatic femoroacetabular impingement. Orthop J Sports Med 2014;2. 2325967114523916.
11. Harris JD, Mather RC, Nho SJ, et al. Reliability of hip range of motion measurement among experienced arthroscopic hip preservation surgeons. J Hip Preserv Surg 2020;7:77–84.

12. Chadayammuri V, Garabekyan T, Bedi A, et al. Passive Hip Range of Motion Predicts Femoral Torsion and Acetabular Version. J Bone Joint Surg Am 2016;98: 127–34.

13. Kraeutler MJ, Chadayammuri V, Garabekyan T, et al. Femoral version abnormalities significantly outweigh effect of cam impingement on hip internal rotation. J Bone Joint Surg Am 2018;100:205–10.

14. Vaudreuil NJ, McClincy MP. Evaluation and treatment of borderline dysplasia: moving beyond the lateral center edge angle. Curr Rev Musculoskelet Med 2020;13:28–37.

15. Larson CM, Moreau-Gaudry A, Kelly BT, et al. Are normal hips being labeled as pathologic? A CT-based method for defining normal acetabular coverage. Clin Orthop Relat Res 2015;473:1247–54.

16. Wiberg G. The anatomy and roentgenographic appearance of a normal hip joint. Acta Chir Scand 1939;83:7–38.

17. Wylie JD, Kapron AL, Peters CL, et al. Relationship between the lateral center-edge angle and 3-dimensional acetabular coverage. Orthop J Sports Med 2017;5. 2325967117700589.

18. Hanson JA, Kapron AL, Swenson KM, et al. Discrepancies in measuring acetabular coverage: revisiting the anterior and lateral center edge angles. J Hip Preserv Surg 2015;2:280–6.

19. McQuivey KS, Secretov E, Domb BG, et al. A multicenter study of radiographic measures predicting failure of arthroscopy in borderline hip dysplasia: beware of the Tönnis angle. Am J Sports Med 2020;48:1608–15.

20. Wong TY, Jesse MK, Jensen A, et al. Upsloping lateral sourcil: a radiographic finding of hip instability. J Hip Preserv Surg 2018;5:435–42.

21. Wyatt M, Weidner J, Pfluger D, et al. The Femoro-Epiphyseal Acetabular Roof (FEAR) index: a new measurement associated with instability in borderline hip dysplasia? Clin Orthop Relat Res 2017;475:861–9.

22. Nepple JJ, Wells J, Ross JR, et al. Three patterns of acetabular deficiency are common in young adult patients with acetabular dysplasia. Clin Orthop Relat Res 2017;475:1037–44.

23. Li RT, Neral M, Gould H, et al. Assessing precision and accuracy of false-profile hip radiographs. Hip Int 2019. https://doi.org/10.1177/1120700019877848. 1120700019877848.

24. Li RT, Hu E, Gould H, et al. Does pelvic rotation alter radiologic measurement of anterior and lateral acetabular coverage? Arthroscopy 2019;35:1111–6.e1.

25. Haddad FS, Garbuz DS, Duncan CP, et al. CT evaluation of periacetabular osteotomies. J Bone Joint Surg Br 2000;82:526–31.

26. Su AW, Hillen TJ, Eutsler EP, et al. Low-dose computed tomography reduces radiation exposure by 90% compared with traditional computed tomography among patients undergoing hip-preservation surgery. Arthroscopy 2019;35: 1385–92.

27. Siebenrock KA, Kistler L, Schwab JM, et al. The acetabular wall index for assessing anteroposterior femoral head coverage in symptomatic patients. Clin Orthop Relat Res 2012;470:3355–60.

28. Tannast M, Mistry S, Steppacher SD, et al. Radiographic analysis of femoroacetabular impingement with Hip2Norm-reliable and validated. J Orthop Res 2008; 26:1199–205.

29. Werner CM, Copeland CE, Ruckstuhl T, et al. Radiographic markers of acetabular retroversion: correlation of the cross-over sign, ischial spine sign and posterior wall sign. Acta Orthop Belg 2010;76:166–73.

30. Zaltz I, Kelly BT, Hetsroni I, et al. The crossover sign overestimates acetabular retroversion. Clin Orthop Relat Res 2013;471:2463–70.
31. Imai N, Miyasaka D, Tsuchiya K, et al. Evaluation of pelvic morphology in female patients with developmental dysplasia of the hip using three-dimensional computed tomography: a cross-sectional study. J Orthop Sci 2018;23:788–92.
32. Okuzu Y, Goto K, Okutani Y, et al. Hip-spine syndrome: acetabular anteversion angle is associated with anterior pelvic tilt and lumbar hyperlordosis in patients with acetabular dysplasia: a retrospective study. JB JS Open Access 2019;4: e0025.
33. Gebhart JJ, Streit JJ, Bedi A, et al. Correlation of pelvic incidence with cam and pincer lesions. Am J Sports Med 2014;42:2649–53.
34. Tannenbaum EP, Zhang P, Maratt JD, et al. A computed tomography study of gender differences in acetabular version and morphology: implications for femoroacetabular impingement. Arthroscopy 2015;31:1247–54.
35. Mascarenhas VV, Ayeni OR, Egund N, et al. Imaging methodology for hip preservation: techniques, parameters, and thresholds. Semin Musculoskelet Radiol 2019;23:197–226.
36. Murphy SB, Simon SR, Kijewski PK, et al. Femoral anteversion. J Bone Joint Surg Am 1987;69:1169–76.
37. Lerch TD, Todorski IAS, Steppacher SD, et al. Prevalence of femoral and acetabular version abnormalities in patients with symptomatic hip disease: a controlled study of 538 hips. Am J Sports Med 2018;46:122–34.
38. Beebe MJ, Wylie JD, Bodine BG, et al. Accuracy and reliability of computed tomography and magnetic resonance imaging compared with true anatomic femoral version. J Pediatr Orthop 2017;37:e265–70.
39. Wylie JD, Jenkins PA, Beckmann JT, et al. Computed tomography scans in patients with young adult hip pain carry a lifetime risk of malignancy. Arthroscopy 2018;34:155–63.e3.
40. McKibbin B. Anatomical factors in the stability of the hip joint in the newborn. J Bone Joint Surg Br 1970;52:148–59.
41. Garabekyan T, Mei-Dan O. Editorial commentary: treating hip impingement without a computed tomography scan? you might as well operate with a blindfold. Arthroscopy 2020;36:1872–4.
42. Bouma H, Hogervorst T, Audenaert E, et al. Combining femoral and acetabular parameters in femoroacetabular impingement: the omega surface. Med Biol Eng Comput 2015;53:1239–46.
43. Bouma HW, Hogervorst T, Audenaert E, et al. Can combining femoral and acetabular morphology parameters improve the characterization of femoroacetabular impingement? Clin Orthop Relat Res 2015;473:1396–403.
44. Kelly B. Borderline dysplasia. San Diego (CA): AOSSM Annual Meeting; 2018.
45. Kelly B. The Morphologic Matrix: mechanical factors associated with early hip disease. Bern Hip Symposium. Bern, Switzerland, February 4, 2016.
46. Henak CR, Abraham CL, Anderson AE, et al. Patient-specific analysis of cartilage and labrum mechanics in human hips with acetabular dysplasia. Osteoarthritis Cartilage 2014;22:210–7.
47. Babst D, Steppacher SD, Ganz R, et al. The iliocapsularis muscle: an important stabilizer in the dysplastic hip. Clin Orthop Relat Res 2011;469:1728–34.
48. Harris JD. Capsular management in hip arthroscopy. Clin Sports Med 2016;35: 373–89.
49. Ashwell ZR, Flug J, Chadayammuri V, et al. Lateral acetabular coverage as a predictor of femoroacetabular cartilage thickness. J Hip Preserv Surg 2016;3:262–9.

50. Kraeutler MJ, Goodrich JA, Fioravanti MJ, et al. The "outside-in" lesion of hip impingement and the "inside-out" lesion of hip dysplasia: two distinct patterns of acetabular chondral injury. Am J Sports Med 2019;47:2978–84.

51. Bardakos NV, Villar RN. The ligamentum teres of the adult hip. J Bone Joint Surg Br 2009;91:8–15.

52. Ganz R, Leunig M, Leunig-Ganz K, et al. The etiology of osteoarthritis of the hip: an integrated mechanical concept. Clin Orthop Relat Res 2008;466:264–72.

53. Hunt D, Prather H, Harris Hayes M, et al. Clinical outcomes analysis of conservative and surgical treatment of patients with clinical indications of prearthritic, intra-articular hip disorders. PM R 2012;4:479–87.

54. Clinical practice guideline on the management of osteoarthritis of the hip. Rosemont (IL): AAOS; 2017. Available at: https://aaos.org/quality/quality-programs/lower-extremity-programs/osteoarthritis-of-the-hip/. Accessed August 29, 2020.

55. Duplantier NL, McCulloch PC, Nho SJ, et al. Hip dislocation or subluxation after hip arthroscopy: a systematic review. Arthroscopy 2016;32(7):1428–34.

56. Ricciardi BF, Fields KG, Wentzel C, et al. Early functional outcomes of periacetabular osteotomy after failed hip arthroscopic surgery for symptomatic acetabular dysplasia. Am J Sports Med 2017;45:2460–7.

57. Wyles CC, Vargas JS, Heidenreich MJ, et al. Hitting the target: natural history of the hip based on achieving an acetabular safe zone following periacetabular osteotomy. J Bone Joint Surg Am 2020;102(19):1734–40.

58. Tannast M, Pfander G, Steppacher SD, et al. Total acetabular retroversion following pelvic osteotomy: presentation, management, and outcome. Hip Int 2013;23(Suppl 9):S14–26.

59. Larson CM, Ross JR, Stone RM, et al. Arthroscopic management of dysplastic hip deformities: predictors of success and failures with comparison to an arthroscopic FAI cohort. Am J Sports Med 2016;44:447–53.

60. McClincy MP, Wylie JD, Yen YM, et al. Mild or borderline hip dysplasia: are we characterizing hips with a lateral center-edge angle between 18° and 25° appropriately? Am J Sports Med 2019;47:112–22.

61. Kraeutler MJ, Safran MR, Scillia AJ, et al. A contemporary look at the evaluation and treatment of adult borderline and frank hip dysplasia. Am J Sports Med 2020; 48:2314–23.

62. Kuroda Y, Saito M, Sunil Kumar KH, et al. Arthroscopy and borderline developmental dysplasia of the hip: a systematic review. Arthroscopy 2020;36(9): 2550–67.e1.

63. Ding Z, Sun Y, Liu S, et al. Hip arthroscopic surgery in borderline developmental dysplastic hips: a systematic review. Am J Sports Med 2019;47:2494–500.

64. Ganz R, Klaue K, Vinh TS, et al. A new periacetabular osteotomy for the treatment of hip dysplasias. Technique and preliminary results. Clin Orthop Relat Res 1988;26–36.

65. Lerch TD, Steppacher SD, Liechti EF, et al. One-third of Hips After Periacetabular Osteotomy Survive 30 Years With Good Clinical Results, No Progression of Arthritis, or Conversion to THA. Clin Orthop Relat Res 2017;475:1154–68.

66. Ziran N, Varcadipane J, Kadri O, et al. Ten- and 20-year survivorship of the hip after periacetabular osteotomy for acetabular dysplasia. J Am Acad Orthop Surg 2019;27:247–55.

67. Wilkin GP, Poitras S, Clohisy J, et al. Periacetabular osteotomy with or without arthroscopic management in patients with hip dysplasia: study protocol for a multicenter randomized controlled trial. Trials 2020;21:725.

Hip Instability in the Athlete

Anatomy, Etiology, and Management

Kevin C. Parvaresh, MD, Jonathan Rasio, BS*, Eric Azua, BS,
Shane J. Nho, MD, MS

KEYWORDS

- Hip • Instability • Microinstability • Femoroacetabular impingement • Traumatic
- Laxity

KEY POINTS

- Hip instability may be a source of significant hip dysfunction and pain.
- The etiology of hip instability may be traumatic or atraumatic, including microinstability, iatrogenic instability, and femoroacetabular impingement-induced instability.
- Surgical options for the management of instability include open and arthroscopic approaches and are targeted toward correction of the individual pathology.
- Early results suggest significant improvement in patient reported outcomes after surgical management of hip instability.

INTRODUCTION

Hip instability is becoming increasingly recognized as a source of significant pain and functional impairment. Historically, instability was thought to occur secondary to direct trauma, although more recently atraumatic causes have been described.[1] Atraumatic instability may be further defined as macroinstability, microinstability, iatrogenic instability, or femoroacetabular impingement (FAI)-induced instability.[2] Treatment encompasses both operative and nonoperative treatment modalities directed toward the underlying etiology. In this review, we outline the anatomic factors that contribute to hip stability and summarize the clinical presentation of hip instability in athletes. We particularly evaluate the recent literature regarding traumatic and atraumatic instability, focusing on surgical treatment options and outcomes.

ANATOMIC CONSIDERATIONS FOR HIP STABILITY

The normal native hip joint is an intrinsically stable structure owing to contributions from both static and dynamic stabilizers. Static stabilizers include osseous, chondrolabral, and ligamentous structures, whereas dynamic stabilization is provided by the

Department of Orthopedic Surgery, Rush University Medical Center, 1611 West Harrison Street, Suite 300, Chicago, IL 60612, USA
* Corresponding author.
E-mail address: Nho.research@rushortho.com

Clin Sports Med 40 (2021) 289–300
https://doi.org/10.1016/j.csm.2020.11.005
0278-5919/21/© 2020 Elsevier Inc. All rights reserved.

surrounding musculature (**Fig. 1**). The osseous morphology includes a highly congruent acetabulum and femoral head. The acetabulum provides an average of 170° of head coverage and is oriented with 48° of coronal abduction and 21° of anteversion, whereas the femur has an average of 10° of anteversion and a neck-shaft angle of 130°.[1] Variations in the osseous development of the acetabulum or femur, including undercoverage, overcoverage, or changes in orientation, may significantly affect hip stability. Depending on the degree of acetabular coverage, the orientation of the acetabulum and/or proximal femur and the articular geometry may affect the osseous contribution to the static stabilizing structures.

The chondrolabral junction has recently been highlighted as a significant contributor to hip stability through the suction seal. Ferguson and colleagues[3] initially described the importance of the labrum in maintaining a pressurized fluid environment in the hip joint. Cadet and colleagues[4] further described the negative pressure effect of the fluid seal, showing that the suction seal was lost in conditions of labral tear and resection. Suppauksorn and colleagues[5] recently showed restoration of the suction seal after labral repair. Subsequent biomechanical studies have validated the contributions of the fluid seal to hip stability, demonstrating increased femoral head rotation and translation with loss of the chondrolabral suction seal.[6–8]

Other major contributors to hip stability include the capsuloligamentous structures surrounding the hip joint. The iliofemoral ligament is the largest and strongest ligament, resisting anterior hip translation as well as rotation.[9,10] The ischiofemoral and pubofemoral ligaments also provide significant resistance to internal and external rotation, respectively.[11] Other smaller ligamentous structures, including the zona orbicularis and ligamentum teres, additionally provide a component of stability to the hip joint.[12,13] Together, these static structures work with the dynamic musculature to control hip stability throughout motion.

CLINICAL EVALUATION

An evaluation of hip instability encompasses the typical sequence of history, physical examination, and imaging workup. Particular questioning should be performed to elucidate the nature of pain and mechanical symptoms, as well as the avoidance of particular motions. Patients may describe mechanical symptoms or apprehension in certain positions.[14] A thorough assessment of any prior hip surgery with operative data should be performed. The medical history, particularly any familial collagen disorders, should be obtained. The physical examination should include an assessment of the Beighton criteria, posterior impingement with extension, the hip dial test, and the axial distraction test.[15] Imaging usually involves a standard hip series of

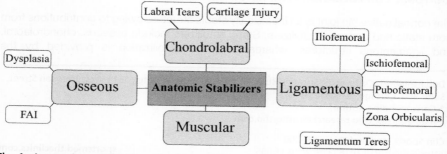

Fig. 1. Anatomic considerations for hip stability.

radiographs (anteroposterior pelvis, false profile view, and Dunn lateral). Specific radiographic findings, including the vacuum sign on splits radiographs[16] and the femoral head cliff sign,[17] have been described as diagnostic tools for instability. MRI with or without MR arthrography may additionally be used to better assess soft tissue pathology, particularly of the labrum and capsuloligamentous structures. A 3-dimensional computed tomography scan may also be obtained to identify any relevant bony morphology.

DISCUSSION
Hip Macroinstability

Hip macroinstability or traumatic hip instability is the result of a relatively high-energy impact to the hip joint resulting in gross hip instability. The spectrum of injury may include hip subluxation to dislocation along with damage to the surrounding capsulo-ligamentous structures, labrum, and cartilage (**Fig. 2**).[18,19] Simultaneous fractures may also occur in the acetabulum, femur, or both.[20] The mechanism of injury in athletes is typically a direct posterior force to a flexed and adducted hip, most commonly occurring in sports such as football, rugby, soccer, and gymnastics.[2] Although posterior dislocations occur most commonly, anterior dislocations have also been described.[21]

In cases of acute dislocation, management involves urgent reduction with a subsequent computed tomography scan to confirm a concentric reduction and rule out any concomitant fractures or intra-articular loose bodies.[22] Isolated dislocations with confirmed concentric reduction, although rare, may be treated nonoperatively. Dislocations with acetabular fractures of the posterior wall are typically examined for instability under anesthesia, with fixation recommended in cases of posterior instability.[23] Large acetabular fractures, femoral fractures involving the weight-bearing region of the head or neck, or intra-articular loose bodies require surgical intervention for fixation. There should be a high suspicion for loose bodies after hip dislocation; 1 study involving patients who underwent arthroscopy found loose bodies in 92% of patients, with 78% of those having negative imaging preoperatively.[24] Postinjury and postoperative weight-bearing restrictions and rehabilitation vary depending on pathology, although they usually include initial hip precautions to prevent recurrent dislocation. Additionally, MRI should be considered 6 weeks after injury to rule out the development of avascular necrosis.[25]

Although recurrence rates are low after an initial traumatic dislocation, there is a high rate of long-term sequelae associated with injury. Dreinhofer and colleagues[26] reported on 50 hip dislocations all reduced within 3 hours of injury and still found

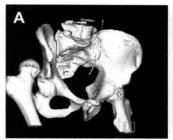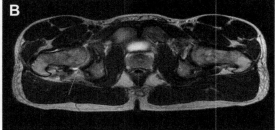

Fig. 2. A traumatic posterior hip dislocation. (*A*) A 3-dimensional computed tomography reconstruction of a posterior hip dislocation. (*B*) A traumatic posterior capsular tear. The arrow points to a traumatic posterior capsular tear.

complication rates of 4% for osteonecrosis, 18% for post-traumatic arthritis, and 8% for heterotopic ossification, with 38% of patients reporting fair or poor results. In a similar study, Sahin and colleagues[27] found a 16.1% rate of post-traumatic arthritis and a 9.6% rate of osteonecrosis with 71% of patients reporting very good to medium satisfaction. Bhandari and colleagues[28] reported on 109 hip dislocations with acetabular fractures managed operatively and found anatomic reduction was essential to limit post-traumatic arthritis, but still found a rate of post-traumatic arthritis of 25.5%, even with anatomic reduction. Reported factors that may influence prognosis include the direction of the dislocation, the extent of the injury, and the time to reduction.[21] A recognition of the relatively high rates of these sequelae are important for discussing overall outcomes and return to sport goals in the athletic population.

Recurrent dislocation, subluxation, or continued symptomatic instability after trauma, although rare, requires a further workup for an assessment of any soft tissue pathology. A traumatic injury to the ligamentous capsule, labrum, or cartilage has been described previously.[18,19] Although the initial treatment involves formal therapy for dynamic stabilization, refractory instability may necessitate a surgical intervention. Surgical management may be approached via an open or arthroscopic route to address labral repair, capsular repair, plication, or reconstruction, or cartilage restoration.[24,29–31] The literature regarding the outcomes of surgical intervention in recurrent traumatic instability is limited to a few case reports[31] and thus further research is needed to delineate specific results.

Hip Microinstability

The concept of hip microinstability emerged more recently as a clinical entity characterized by extraphysiologic motion resulting in hip pain or dysfunction with or without gross symptomatic instability.[32,33] A diagnosis of instability may be challenging, because there are no objective criteria that are universally accepted for microinstability.[15] In contrast with traumatic instability, patients with microinstability typically do not define a discrete mechanism of injury. Provocative examination maneuvers, however, may be similarly present in both traumatic instability and microinstability.

The pathology is thought to be due to repetitive microtrauma in the presence of underlying osseous and soft tissue abnormalities.[15] Numerous etiologies have been described causing microinstability, typically classified based on the following 6 groups: osseous abnormalities, connective tissue disorders, traumatic injuries, repetitive microtrauma, iatrogenic injury, and idiopathic (**Fig. 3**).[34] Common bony abnormalities occur with developmental dysplasia of the hip, including a flattened aspherical femoral head, a shortened femoral beck, a shallow acetabulum, loss of anterolateral coverage, and excessive anteversion of the acetabulum and femur.[35,36] Connective tissue disorders such as Ehlers–Danlos syndrome, Marfan syndrome, and Down syndrome, as well as joint hypermobility syndrome, can also contribute to microinstability.[33,37,38] Both traumatic and microtraumatic injuries may occur in athletes from a direct event or repetitive impact, respectively. Iatrogenic sources are further discussed elsewhere in this article. The identification of the underlying pathology, when present, is crucial for appropriate management.

The management of microinstability includes both operative and nonoperative treatments. As a newer diagnosis, there are no primary publications regarding the nonoperative management of microinstability. Nonetheless, most experts agree that traditional nonoperative modalities, such as activity modification, physical therapy, anti-inflammatory medications, and injections, may be used as a first-line treatment or before surgery for in-season athletes.[15,33] Targeted neuromuscular rehabilitation with sport-specific strengthening may address any functional deficits or allow

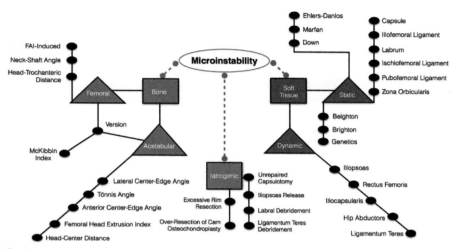

Fig. 3. Anatomic and etiologic considerations for microinstability. (*From* Harris JD, Gerrie BJ, Lintner DM, Varner KE, McCulloch PC. Microinstability of the Hip and the Splits Radiograph. *Orthopedics.* 2016;39(1):e169-e175; with permission.)

satisfactory compensation.[39] In refractory cases or those with severe pathology, open or arthroscopic surgery may be indicated.

The surgical treatment options are directed toward correcting the underlying pathologic etiology. In cases of severe dysplasia, correction with an osteotomy may be necessary. However, in athletes with borderline hip dysplasia, capsular plication has been shown to be sufficient for stabilization and improved clinical outcomes.[40,41] Capsular plication may also be used for patients with connective tissue disease,[37,42] with capsular reconstruction reserved for extreme ligamentous insufficiency.[43] Thermal capsulorraphy has also been proposed as a means of reducing capsular volume, although concerns related to intra-articular thermal injury have limited its widespread acceptance.[44] A labral pathology is typically treated similar to FAI, with repair, reconstruction, and augmentation as options depending on the labral integrity.[45,46] The management of ligamentum teres pathology remains controversial in the literature, although options for reconstruction have been described.[47]

The literature on surgical outcomes for treatment of microinstability are limited, but early studies have supported improved patient-reported outcomes. A recent study by Cancienne and colleagues[48] evaluating arthroscopic management of borderline hip dysplasia showed significant improvements in the modified Harris Hip Score (mHHS), Hip Outcome Score–Sport-Specific Subscale, and Hip Outcome Score–Activity of Daily Living without significant differences between patients with borderline hip dysplasia and those without borderline hip dysplasia. A subgroup analysis also showed that patients with borderline hip dysplasia were as likely to reach the minimal clinically important difference for patient-reported outcomes as patients without borderline hip dysplasia.[48] Domb and colleagues[41] also found significant improvements in the mHHS, Hip Outcome Score–Activity of Daily Living, Hip Outcome Score–Sport-Specific Subscale, Non-Arthritic Hip Score, and visual analog scale for pain in patients with hip instability and underlying borderline hip dysplasia at a mean of 2 years postoperatively. Similarly, Kalisvaart and Safran[40] found significant improvements in the mHHS and the International Hip Outcome Tool score at a minimum of 12 months postoperatively. They also showed that 9 of the 11 collegiate or professional athletes were able to return to sport. Notably, poor surgical prognostic factors for patients with dysplastic microinstability include a broken Shenton's line, a femoral neck-shaft angle of greater than 140°, a lateral center-edge angle of less than 19°, and a body mass index of greater than 23 kg/m^2.[49] In patients with Ehler-Danlos syndrome and hip instability, Larson and colleagues[37] reported significant improvements for the mHHS, 12-Item Short Form Health Survey, and visual analog scale pain score at a mean of 45 months. Unfortunately, long-term outcomes and larger studies on sports performance remain to be determined for athletes with microinstability.

Iatrogenic Hip Instability

Iatrogenic hip instability is a newly recognized cause of hip pain and dysfunction in patients that may involve gross instability or microinstability. Multiple case reports of anterior, posterior, and superolateral instability have been documented after hip arthroscopy.[16,50,51] Iatrogenic injury can occur in any of the stabilizing structures of the hip or may involve multiple structures resulting in significant symptomatic instability. Common sources include excessive cam or pincer resection, iliopsoas release, excessive labral debridement, and capsular injury.[16]

Because prior studies have identified the hip capsule as a major stabilizing structure, the surgical management of the capsule is recognized as an integral component of operative treatment. Additionally, biomechanical studies have demonstrated that capsulotomy size inversely affects the force required for hip distraction[52] and directly affects hip stability.[53,54] Evidence of capsular defects has been reported after capsulotomy during hip arthroscopy.[55] In fact, capsular insufficiently has been shown to be one of the most common indications for revision hip arthroscopy.[56] Accordingly, the literature on iatrogenic instability has focused on the identification of the capsular status and the treatment of capsular defects to restore stability and hip function (**Fig. 4**).

Capsular repair and plication have been shown to be effective procedures for restoring native hip stability in cases of capsular defects with sufficient tissue integrity.[52,57] The traditional techniques involved open approaches,[14] although with recent advances in technology the majority of cases can now be managed arthroscopically. The decision to repair or plicate depends on a number of factors, although plication is typically preferred in cases of instability.[58] In cases of insufficient capsule, a capsular reconstruction may be performed with an allograft or autograft tissue.[43] Although the

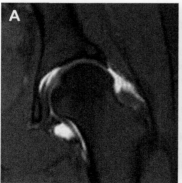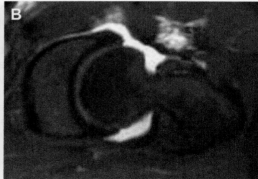

Fig. 4. (*A*) Coronal and (*B*) axial MRI of a left hip after a hip arthroscopy with a large interportal capsulotomy without repair.

long-term evidence is limited, early results show significant improvements in patient-reported outcomes after the correction of capsular defects in patients with iatrogenic instability.[40,59,60]

Similar to the capsule, the surgical management of other sources is tailored to the individual pathology. In cases of excessive cam resection, augmentation with a soft tissue autograft or allograft may be used to restore the chondrolabral junction and suction seal.[61] Iatrogenic instability with acetabular undercoverage corrected with periacetabular osteotomy has also been reported.[62] Segmental labral defects may be treated with reconstruction or augmentation to restore the suction seal effect for hip stability.[46] As an emerging concept, the outcomes literature regarding these individual pathologic entities is limited.

Femoroacetabular Impingement–Induced Hip Instability

Initial case series evaluating athletes with low energy hip dislocations found a high rate of radiographic FAI.[18,63–65] A systematic review of these case series found that rates of cam lesions (73%) and relative acetabular retroversion (72%) were notably higher in these athletic dislocations than the general population (**Fig. 5**).[66] More recently, studies have subsequently validated these correlations with a direct cohort

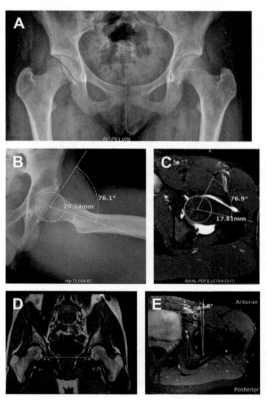

Fig. 5. (A) An anteroposterior pelvis radiograph with right hip crossover sign. (B) A Dunn lateral radiograph with an alpha angle of 76.1°. (C) An axial proton density fat suppressed (PDFS) sequence straight section hip MRI with an alpha angle of 76.9°. (D) A T1 coronal sectioned and (E) a T2 axial sectioned hip MRI demonstrates 3.8° of acetabular version based on previously described MRI measurement techniques.[72]

analysis.[30,67] Based on these findings, it is theorized that bony impingement occurring at extremes of motion in athletes with underlying FAI syndrome predisposes the hip to instability. In effect, the anterior cam impingement creates a fulcrum resulting in posterolateral instability of the femoral head, similar to prosthetic hip impingement.[68]

Imaging studies have further evaluated the concept of FAI-induced instability. Using 3-dimensional models based on MRIs in ballet dancers, Charbonnier and colleagues[69] showed that significant subluxation of the femoral head was present at the extremes of motion and always directly correlated with impingement. A high rate of posterior subluxation (70%) was also found by Wassilew and colleagues[70] in positions of impingement on dynamic computed tomography scans. Cvetanovich and colleagues[71] recently demonstrated significant posteroinferior translation in patients with FAI in the flexion–abduction–external rotation position compared with neutral positioning that was directly related to the size of the cam lesion. Together, these motion-based investigations further support FAI syndrome as a predisposing factor for hip instability.

The outcomes evidence for operative and nonoperative management for FAI-induced hip instability is limited to a case series by Krych and colleagues.[64] Their study included 22 athletes with imaging evidence of a posterior rim fracture from a low-energy sports mechanism. Management included nonoperative treatment with posterior hip precautions and protected weight bearing for 6 weeks in 11 patients, and standard hip arthroscopy for FAI management in the other 11 patients. All nonoperative patients reported return to sport at their prior level, although only 9 of the 11 operative patients were able to do so. Unfortunately, surgical indications were not standardized and thus may have biased treatment groups. Nonetheless, it still provides a basis for treatment of athletes with FAI-induced hip instability.

SUMMARY

Hip instability in the athlete may be caused by macrotrauma such as high-energy trauma or low-energy mechanisms in hips with predisposing factors for instability. Microinstability of the hip is a newly recognized diagnosis caused by osseous abnormalities, connective tissue disease, iatrogenic injury, or repetitive microtrauma that can result in hip pain and dysfunction. Both operative and nonoperative treatment options may provide significant improvements, with modalities targeted toward the underlying etiology. Capsular defects are a major source of iatrogenic instability and may be managed with plication or reconstruction. Further research is needed to better delineate treatment principles and long-term outcomes particular to athletic hip instability.

CLINICS CARE POINTS

- A thorough understanding of the anatomic components of hip stability is integral to the appropriate recognition and treatment of clinical hip instability.

- The etiology of microinstability includes osseous abnormalities, connective tissue disorders, traumatic injury, repetitive microtrauma, iatrogenic injury, and idiopathic disease.

- Capsular defects are a major source of iatrogenic instability and may be managed with plication or reconstruction.

- FAI morphology, particularly cam lesions and a retroverted acetabulum, may predispose athletes to posterior hip instability.

- Early results support the improvement of pain and the restoration of hip function with arthroscopic management of hip instability in athletes.

DISCLOSURES

K.C. Parvaresh (none), J. Rasio (none), E. Azua (none), S.J. Nho (Received $53,225.00 for Consulting Fees, $2949.86 for Food and Beverage, and $2780.15 for Travel and Lodging from Stryker Corporation in 2018; $2191.00 for Education from Elite Orthopedics, L.L.C., in 2017; $43,425.00 for Consulting Fees, $2093.15 for Food and Beverage, and $1168.69 for Travel and Lodging from Stryker Corporation in 2017; $33,475.00 in Consulting Fees, $5045.44 for Food and Beverage, and $2998.43 for Travel and Lodging from Stryker Corporation in 2016; and $34,400.00 for Consulting Fees, $5053.88 for Food and Beverage, and $4433.88 for Travel and Lodging from Stryker Corporation in 2015.)

REFERENCES

1. Boykin RE, Anz AW, Bushnell BD, et al. Hip instability. J Am Acad Orthop Surg 2011;19(6):340–9.
2. Smith MV, Sekiya JK. Hip instability. Sports Med Arthrosc Rev 2010;18(2):108–12.
3. Ferguson SJ, Bryant JT, Ganz R, et al. An in vitro investigation of the acetabular labral seal in hip joint mechanics. J Biomech 2003;36(2):171–8.
4. Cadet ER, Chan AK, Vorys GC, et al. Investigation of the preservation of the fluid seal effect in the repaired, partially resected, and reconstructed acetabular labrum in a cadaveric hip model. Am J Sports Med 2012;40(10):2218–23.
5. Suppauksorn S, Beck EC, Chahla J, et al. Comparison of suction seal and contact pressures between 270 degree labral reconstruction, labral repair, and the intact labrum. Arthroscopy 2020;36(9):2433–42.
6. Philippon MJ, Nepple JJ, Campbell KJ, et al. The hip fluid seal—part I: the effect of an acetabular labral tear, repair, resection, and reconstruction on hip fluid pressurization. Knee Surg Sports Traumatol Arthrosc 2014;22(4):722–9.
7. Nepple JJ, Philippon MJ, Campbell KJ, et al. The hip fluid seal—part II: the effect of an acetabular labral tear, repair, resection, and reconstruction on hip stability to distraction. Knee Surg Sports Traumatol Arthrosc 2014;22(4):730–6.
8. Johannsen AM, Ejnisman L, Behn AW, et al. Contributions of the capsule and labrum to hip mechanics in the context of hip microinstability. Orthop J Sports Med 2019;7(12). 232596711989084.
9. Hewitt JD, Glisson RR, Guilak F, et al. The mechanical properties of the human hip capsule ligaments. J Arthroplasty 2002;17(1):82–9.
10. Myers CA, Register BC, Lertwanich P, et al. Role of the acetabular labrum and the iliofemoral ligament in hip stability: an in vitro biplane fluoroscopy study. Am J Sports Med 2011;39(Suppl):85S–91S.
11. Martin HD, Savage A, Braly BA, et al. The function of the hip capsular ligaments: a quantitative report. Arthroscopy 2008;24(2):188–95.
12. Ito H, Song Y, Lindsey DP, et al. The proximal hip joint capsule and the zona orbicularis contribute to hip joint stability in distraction. J Orthop Res 2009;27(8):989–95.
13. Jo S, Hooke AW, An K-N, et al. Contribution of the ligamentum teres to hip stability in the presence of an intact capsule: a cadaveric study. Arthroscopy 2018;34(5):1480–7.

14. Bellabarba C, Sheinkop MB, Kuo KN. Idiopathic hip instability: an unrecognized cause of coxa saltans in the adult. Clin Orthop 1998;355:261–71.
15. Kalisvaart MM, Safran MR. Microinstability of the hip–it does exist: etiology, diagnosis and treatment. J Hip Preserv Surg 2015;2(2):123–35.
16. Harris JD, Gerrie BJ, Lintner DM, et al. Microinstability of the hip and the splits radiograph. Orthopedics 2016;39(1):e169–75.
17. Packer JD, Cowan JB, Rebolledo BJ, et al. The cliff sign: a new radiographic sign of hip instability. Orthop J Sports Med 2018;6(11). 2325967118807176.
18. Philippon MJ, Kuppersmith DA, Wolff AB, et al. Arthroscopic findings following traumatic hip dislocation in 14 professional athletes. Arthroscopy 2009;25(2): 169–74.
19. Mandell JC, Marshall RA, Banffy MB, et al. Arthroscopy after traumatic hip dislocation: a systematic review of intra-articular findings, correlation with magnetic resonance imaging and computed tomography, treatments, and outcomes. Arthroscopy 2018;34(3):917–27.
20. Moorman CT, Warren RF, Hershman EB, et al. Traumatic posterior hip subluxation in American football. J Bone Joint Surg Am 2003;85(7):1190–6.
21. Clegg TE, Roberts CS, Greene JW, et al. Hip dislocations—epidemiology, treatment, and outcomes. Injury 2010;41(4):329–34.
22. Shindle MK, Ranawat AS, Kelly BT. Diagnosis and management of traumatic and atraumatic hip instability in the athletic patient. Clin Sports Med 2006;25(2): 309–26.
23. Moed BR, Ajibade DA, Israel H. Computed tomography as a predictor of hip stability status in posterior wall fractures of the acetabulum. J Orthop Trauma 2009; 23(1):7–15.
24. Mullis BH, Dahners LE. Hip arthroscopy to remove loose bodies after traumatic dislocation. J Orthop Trauma 2006;20(1):22–6.
25. Poggi JJ, Callaghan JJ, Spritzer CE, et al. Changes on magnetic resonance images after traumatic hip dislocation. Clin Orthop 1995;(319):249–59. NA.
26. Dreinhofer K, Schwarzkopf, Haas N, et al. Isolated traumatic dislocation of the hip. Long-term results in 50 patients. J Bone Joint Surg Br 1994;76-B(1):6–12.
27. Sahin V, Karakas ES, Aksu S, et al. Traumatic dislocation and fracture-dislocation of the hip: a long-term follow-up study. J Trauma 2003;54(3):520–9.
28. Bhandari M, Matta J, Ferguson T, et al. Predictors of clinical and radiological outcome in patients with fractures of the acetabulum and concomitant posterior dislocation of the hip. J Bone Joint Surg Br 2006;88-B(12):1618–24.
29. Podeszwa DA, Rocha ADL, Larson AN, et al. Surgical hip dislocation is safe and effective following acute traumatic hip instability in the adolescent. J Pediatr Orthop 2015;35(5):435–42.
30. Novais EN, Heare TC, Hill MK, et al. Surgical hip dislocation for the treatment of intra-articular injuries and hip instability following traumatic posterior dislocation in children and adolescents. J Pediatr Orthop 2016;36(7):673–9.
31. Weber M, Ganz R. Recurrent traumatic dislocation of the hip: report of a case and review of the literature. J Orthop Trauma 1997;11(5):382–5.
32. Bolia I, Chahla J, Locks R, et al. Microinstability of the hip: a previously unrecognized pathology. Muscles Ligaments Tendons J 2016;6(3):354–60.
33. Safran MR. Microinstability of the hip—gaining acceptance. J Am Acad Orthop Surg 2019;27(1):12–22.
34. Shu B, Safran MR. Hip instability: anatomic and clinical considerations of traumatic and atraumatic instability. Clin Sports Med 2011;30(2):349–67.

35. Greenhill BJ, Hugosson C, Jacobsson B, et al. Magnetic resonance imaging study of acetabular morphology in developmental dysplasia of the hip. J Pediatr Orthop 1993;13(3):314–7.
36. Sugano N, Noble PC, Kamaric E, et al. The morphology of the femur in developmental dysplasia of the hip. J Bone Joint Surg Br 1998;80(4):9.
37. Larson CM, Stone RM, Grossi EF, et al. Ehlers-Danlos syndrome: arthroscopic management for extreme soft-tissue hip instability. Arthroscopy 2015;31(12): 2287–94.
38. Bennet G, Rang M, Roye D, et al. Dislocation of the hip in trisomy 21. J Bone Joint Surg Br 1982;64-B(3):289–94.
39. Torry MR, Schenker ML, Martin HD, et al. Neuromuscular hip biomechanics and pathology in the athlete. Clin Sports Med 2006;25(2):179–97, vii.
40. Kalisvaart MM, Safran MR. Hip instability treated with arthroscopic capsular plication. Knee Surg Sports Traumatol Arthrosc 2017;25(1):24–30.
41. Domb BG, Stake CE, Lindner D, et al. Arthroscopic capsular plication and labral preservation in borderline hip dysplasia: two-year clinical outcomes of a surgical approach to a challenging problem. Am J Sports Med 2013;41(11):2591–8.
42. Chandrasekaran S, Vemula SP, Martin TJ, et al. Arthroscopic technique of capsular plication for the treatment of hip instability. Arthrosc Tech 2015;4(2): e163–7.
43. Mei-Dan O, Garabekyan T, McConkey M, et al. Arthroscopic anterior capsular reconstruction of the hip for recurrent instability. Arthrosc Tech 2015;4(6):e711–5.
44. Philippon MJ. The role of arthroscopic thermal capsulorrhaphy in the hip. Clin Sports Med 2001;20(4):817–29.
45. Woyski D, Chad Mather R. Surgical treatment of labral tears: debridement, repair, reconstruction. Curr Rev Musculoskelet Med 2019;12(3):291–9.
46. Philippon MJ, Bolia IK, Locks R, et al. Labral preservation: outcomes following labrum augmentation versus labrum reconstruction. Arthroscopy 2018;34(9): 2604–11.
47. Bajwa AS, Villar RN. Editorial commentary: arthroscopic hip ligamentum teres reconstruction-reality or mythology? Arthroscopy 2018;34(1):152–4.
48. Cancienne JM, Beck EC, Kunze KN, et al. Functional and clinical outcomes of patients undergoing revision hip arthroscopy with borderline hip dysplasia at 2-year follow-up. Arthroscopy 2019;35(12):3240–7.
49. Uchida S, Utsunomiya H, Mori T, et al. Clinical and radiographic predictors for worsened clinical outcomes after hip arthroscopic labral preservation and capsular closure in developmental dysplasia of the hip. Am J Sports Med 2016;44(1):28–38.
50. Matsuda DK. Acute iatrogenic dislocation following hip impingement arthroscopic surgery. Arthroscopy 2009;25(4):400–4.
51. Ranawat AS, McClincy M, Sekiya JK. Anterior dislocation of the hip after arthroscopy in a patient with capsular laxity of the hip: a case report. J Bone Joint Surg Am 2009;91(1):192–7.
52. Khair MM, Grzybowski JS, Kuhns BD, et al. The effect of capsulotomy and capsular repair on hip distraction: a cadaveric investigation. Arthroscopy 2017; 33(3):559–65.
53. Wuerz TH, Song SH, Grzybowski JS, et al. Capsulotomy size affects hip joint kinematic stability. Arthroscopy 2016;32(8):1571–80.
54. Bayne CO, Stanley R, Simon P, et al. Effect of capsulotomy on hip stability— a consideration during hip arthroscopy. Am J Orthop(Belle Mead NJ) 2014;43: 160–5.

55. McCormick F, Slikker W, Harris JD, et al. Evidence of capsular defect following hip arthroscopy. Knee Surg Sports Traumatol Arthrosc 2014;22(4):902–5.
56. Cvetanovich GL, Harris JD, Erickson BJ, et al. Revision hip arthroscopy: a systematic review of diagnoses, operative findings, and outcomes. Arthroscopy 2015;31(7):1382–90.
57. Chahla J, Mikula JD, Schon JM, et al. Hip capsular closure: a biomechanical analysis of failure torque. Am J Sports Med 2017;45(2):434–9.
58. Domb BG, Philippon MJ, Giordano BD. Arthroscopic capsulotomy, capsular repair, and capsular plication of the hip: relation to atraumatic instability. Arthroscopy 2013;29(1):162–73.
59. Wylie JD, Beckmann JT, Maak TG, et al. Arthroscopic capsular repair for symptomatic hip instability after previous hip arthroscopic surgery. Am J Sports Med 2016;44(1):39–45.
60. Fagotti L, Soares E, Bolia IK, et al. Early outcomes after arthroscopic hip capsular reconstruction using iliotibial band allograft versus dermal allograft. Arthroscopy 2019;35(3):778–86.
61. Frank JM, Chahla J, Mitchell JJ, et al. Remplissage of the femoral head-neck junction in revision hip arthroscopy: a technique to correct excessive cam resection. Arthrosc Tech 2016;5(6):e1209–13.
62. Sheean AJ, Barrow AE, Burns TC, et al. Iatrogenic hip instability treated with periacetabular osteotomy. J Am Acad Orthop Surg 2017;25(8):594–9.
63. Berkes MB, Cross MB, Shindle MK, et al. Traumatic posterior hip instability and femoroacetabular impingement in athletes. Am J Orthop 2012;41:166–71.
64. Krych AJ, Thompson M, Larson CM, et al. Is posterior hip instability associated with cam and pincer deformity? Clin Orthop Relat Res 2012;470(12):3390–7.
65. Steppacher SD, Albers CE, Siebenrock KA, et al. Femoroacetabular impingement predisposes to traumatic posterior hip dislocation. Clin Orthop 2013; 471(6):1937–43.
66. Canham CD, Yen Y-M, Giordano BD. Does femoroacetabular impingement cause hip instability? a systematic review. Arthroscopy 2016;32(1):203–8.
67. Mayer SW, Abdo JCM, Hill MK, et al. Femoroacetabular impingement is associated with sports-related posterior hip instability in adolescents: a matched-cohort study. Am J Sports Med 2016;44(9):2299–303.
68. Malik A, Maheshwari AV, Dorr LD. Impingement with total hip replacement. J Bone Joint Surg Am 2007. https://doi.org/10.2106/JBJS.F.01313.
69. Charbonnier C, Kolo FC, Duthon VB, et al. Assessment of congruence and impingement of the hip joint in professional ballet dancers: a motion capture study. Am J Sports Med 2011;39(3):557–66.
70. Wassilew GI, Janz V, Heller MO, et al. Real time visualization of femoroacetabular impingement and subluxation using 320-slice computed tomography. J Orthop Res 2013;31(2):275–81.
71. Cvetanovich GL, Beck EC, Chalmers PN, et al. Assessment of hip translation in vivo in patients with femoroacetabular impingement syndrome using 3-dimensional computed tomography. Arthrosc Sports Med Rehabil 2020;2(2):e113–20.
72. Muhamad AR, Freitas JM, Bomar JD, et al. Acetabular version on magnetic resonance imaging: analysis of two different measuring techniques. HIP Int 2012; 22(6):672–6.

Hip Flexor Injuries in the Athlete

Zachary K. Christopher, MD*, Jeffrey D. Hassebrock, MD, Matthew B. Anastasi, MD,
Kostas J. Economopoulos, MD

KEYWORDS

• Athlete • Hip flexor • Injuries • Epidemiology • Treatment • Diagnosis

KEY POINTS

- Hip flexor anatomy is intricate and relies on combination of history, physical examination, and advanced imaging for early and accurate diagnosis.
- Most hip flexor injuries can be treated conservatively; however, operative indications exist for those who fail conservative therapy alone.
- Most hip flexor injuries result in minimal time loss from sport, despite a relatively high incidence in athletic populations.

INTRODUCTION

Athletic injuries to the hip flexors and iliopsoas have been described in populations across all levels of competitive sports.[1–5] Overall estimates of hip flexor pathology in the literature have ranged from 5% of injuries all the way to 28% of injuries among high-risk sport-specific groups.[3–5] Although most of these injuries are successfully treated with conservative management, and high rates of return to play are observed, significant rehabilitation time can be involved.[3,6] As understanding of hip pathology with imaging modalities such as MRI has advanced, greater importance has been placed on accurately diagnosing hip flexor injuries and initiating rehabilitation protocols early to minimize time loss from sport and maximize long-term function.[3]

ANATOMY OF THE HIP FLEXORS

In order to accurately diagnose and treat hip flexor injuries in athletes, it is critical to understand their anatomy and function. The hip flexors consist of 6 key muscles that contribute to hip flexion: iliacus, psoas major, psoas minor, pectineus, rectus femoris, and sartorius. The iliacus is a triangular muscle arising from the wing of the ilium and inserting on the lateral psoas tendon and lesser trochanter of the femur.[7,8] The

Mayo Clinic Arizona, Orthopedics, Sports Medicine Department, 5777 East Mayo Boulevard, Phoenix, AZ 85054, USA
* Corresponding author.
E-mail address: Christopher.zachary@mayo.edu

Clin Sports Med 40 (2021) 301–310
https://doi.org/10.1016/j.csm.2020.11.006
0278-5919/21/© 2020 Elsevier Inc. All rights reserved.

psoas major originates from the transverse processes and vertebral margins of T12-L5 and merges at the L5-S2 level with the iliacus to travel beneath the inguinal ligament and form the iliopsoas.[8] The psoas minor is a normal anatomic variant present in approximately 60% of people.[9,10] It originates from the T12 to L1 vertebral bodies, lies anterior to the psoas major, and inserts into the iliopectineal eminence.[7] The iliacus and psoas muscles are often grouped together as the iliopsoas musculotendinous unit secondary to overlapping function and anatomic proximity.[11] The action of this group is to flex the femur at the hip joint and provide secondary lateral flexion to the lower vertebrae. In addition, these muscles contribute to postural stability while standing erect and elevating the torso from a supine position. The iliopsoas has an associated bursa that is the largest bursa in the body and lies between the iliopsoas and the hip capsule/pubis.[12] The psoas major and iliacus are innervated by the L2-L3 nerve roots of the femoral nerve, while the psoas minor is supplied by L1 alone.[7]

The rectus femoris acts as a hip flexor with 2 distinct anatomic origins—the direct and indirect heads of the rectus. The direct head originates at the anterior inferior iliac spine, and the indirect head originates on the anterior/superior acetabular rim and hip capsule.[13] Distally, it becomes a part of the quadriceps tendon and ultimately inserts on the proximal pole of the patella, providing the primary force for knee extension. The sartorius, the longest muscle in the body, crosses the hip and the knee joints. It originates at the anterior superior iliac spine and inserts superficially on the pes anserinus as a broad fascial insertion. It functions to flex the hip, and secondarily to adduct the thigh and externally rotate the leg.[14] Finally, the pectineus acts as a hip flexor and secondary adductor from its origin on the superior pubic ramus and insertion on the pectineal line of the femur.[15] All 3 of these hip flexors are innervated by branches of the femoral nerve and are supplied by distinct arterial branches off the femoral artery.

EPIDEMIOLOGY OF HIP FLEXOR INJURIES

The epidemiology of hip flexor injuries can be challenging to delineate. However, some studies have described incidences at differing levels of athletic competition. Because of the high degree of functional overlap and compact anatomic space, they are often described together as hip flexor injuries and not separated by specific hip flexor muscle pathology. Iliopsoas or rectus femoris injuries may occasionally be specified uniquely, especially with advanced imaging. Another limitation in characterizing these injuries is that they are often grouped with groin injuries to the adductor muscles.

Overall, injuries to the hip have been shown to represent 9.3% of all injuries in high school athletes and 17.3% of all injuries in college athletes.[5] A 2018 study demonstrated that hip and groin injuries occurred at a rate of 53.06 injuries per 100,000 athlete-exposures (AEs) in college athletes.[3] Men's soccer players have been shown to have the highest rates of hip flexor strains (3.77 injuries per 10,000 AEs).[16] At the professional level, muscle strains are the most common hip injury in National Football League players (59%), and strains of the hip flexors account for 63% of these injuries.[2] Strains of the hip flexors are the second most common college football hip injury (28.55%).[4]

HIP FLEXOR INJURIES IN THE ATHLETE

The diagnosis of these injuries can be particularly difficult because of the numerous pain generators surrounding the hip. Pain in this location can be referred from many different structures including the lumbar spine, intra-abdominal organs, genitourinary tract, hip joint, surrounding capsule, ligaments, and crossing muscles and tendons. As mentioned previously, most athletic injuries to the hip flexors are muscle strains in nature.[2] Muscle strains often occur in larger muscles, especially ones that cross multiple joints during an eccentric contraction. Muscle strains and tears most frequently occur at the myotendinous junction, but may also occur in the muscle belly.[17] In the pediatric population, avulsion injuries can occur at the apophysis, especially of the anterior superior and inferior iliac spines, as there is a mismatch in apophyseal strength versus musculotendinous strength. The large iliopsoas bursa can also contribute to bursitis pain in this anatomic region. This article will focus on several of the most common hip flexor injuries in athletes individually.

Iliopsoas Pathologies: Strains, Tears, Tendinosis, and Bursitis

Strains, tears, tendinosis, and bursitis of the iliopsoas muscle can all present similarly. Strains or tears are often the result of overuse or eccentric hip flexion against resistance. Bursitis or tendinosis is caused by overuse of the iliopsoas tendon resulting in friction as the tendon glides over the iliopectineal eminence.[18] The most common symptom of an iliopsoas strain or tear is typically groin or proximal medial thigh pain. These symptoms are exacerbated by actively flexing the hip against resistance. There is also pain with passive extension of the hip by placing the iliopsoas tendon on stretch regardless of knee position. Tenderness over the femoral triangle and swelling may also be appreciated. Rarely a palpable muscle defect maybe noted. Qualitative strength assessment is important but often limited secondary to pain. In addition, the surrounding uninjured muscles may compensate for weakness in the injured muscle. This makes these injuries difficult for the patient to localize and for the physician to assess. It takes an average of 31 to 42 months from the onset of symptoms for a diagnosis to be made in most of these cases.[19] A specific test for iliopsoas injury can be performed by having the patient lie supine and raise his or her heels 15° up from the table. In this position, the only hip flexor active is the iliopsoas.[19]

When an iliopsoas injury is suspected, imaging studies are helpful in making the diagnosis. Plain radiographs are often normal, but can reveal avulsion injuries in the skeletally immature patient.[19] MRI is often the imaging study of choice. Axial images typically give the best view for detailed evaluation; however, the muscle and tendon can be appreciated on sagittal and coronal images as well.[20] Magnetic resonance is sensitive enough to detect other less common pathologies within the iliopsoas, including myositis ossificans or an acute hematoma. Tendinosis presents on MRI as attenuation of the tendon along its course or even at the insertion site on the lesser trochanter, and it is best appreciated on an axial image. High-intensity signal on T2 weighted images ischaracteristic.[20,21] MRI has been shown to be an accurate method of detecting iliopsoas bursitis also.[22] The bursa can be appreciated as an elongated fluid collection medial and posterior to the iliopsoas muscle. It will appear hypointense on T1 and hyperintense on T2 weighted images. If enlarged, it may displace the muscle laterally and can sometimes extend into the pelvis.[20] Distinct tears of the muscle can be visualized on axial, coronal, or sagittal images and are associated with edema around the muscle and a defect with attenuation.

Treatment of iliopsoas injuries is typically conservative in nature, initially with rest, stretching, strengthening, physical therapy, oral anti-inflammatory drugs, and possibly ultrasound-guided injection therapy. There is sparse literature evaluating specific therapy regimens for iliopsoas bursitis and tendinosis. Some centers have attempted to develop specific treatment protocols, but data are limited and mostly anecdotal.[19] There have not been any randomized studies evaluating conservative management of iliopsoas bursitis, tendinopathy, or strains/tears.

Corticosteroid injections may have a role in treatment of these pathologies. Studies are limited to case reports and small series.[23–25] Vaccaro demonstrated good results in 7 of 8 patients who underwent bursal injections with up to 2 years of symptomatic relief. However, 4 of these patients ultimately underwent surgery. Further studies comparing injection versus physical therapy alone are warranted prior to definitive recommendations.

Surgical management of iliopsoas strains/tears or tendinosis is not usually indicated unless patients have persistent disabling symptoms despite an adequate trial of conservative therapy. Patients who have persistent symptoms of iliopsoas pain greater than 6 months who have failed conservative measures may be surgical candidates. Most often, surgery involves the release of the iliopsoas tendon from its insertion on the lesser trochanter and can be performed open or endoscopically (**Fig. 1**). Symptom alleviation and return to play data for high-level athletes are limited after this surgical procedure; however, recreational athletes seem to have high rates of return to play.[26–28]

Coxa Sultans Interna (Internal Snapping Hip)

Internal snapping hip is a cause of groin pain in athletes that presents often with pain and a snapping sensation that can be perceived or audible. The snapping is often appreciated with activity, especially with hip flexion while running. Snapping hip syndrome can be broken down into external, internal, or intra-articular. An external snapping hip is caused by the iliotibial band snapping over the greater trochanter. An intra-articular snapping hip is caused by loose bodies, labral tears, synovial chondromatosis, synovial folds, or fracture fragments.[11] An internal snapping hip, also

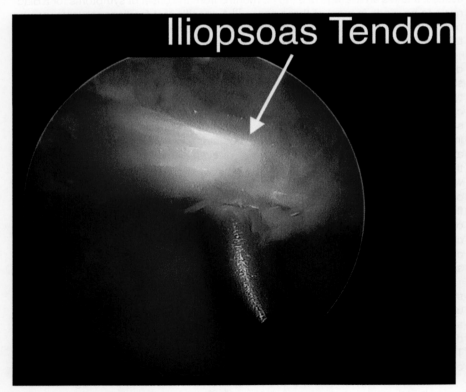

Fig. 1. Endoscopic view of iliopsoas tendon.

known as coxa sultans interna, is caused by the iliopsoas snapping over the iliopectineal eminence or the femoral head. Specifically, it occurs when the hip extends and the tendon travels from an anterolateral to a posteromedial position. An internal snapping hip is often associated with chronic iliopsoas bursitis,[8] likely caused by the motion of the tendon irritating the underlying bursa. The ideal imaging modality to appreciate the snapping hip is a dynamic ultrasound.[29] It allows the physician to visualize the pathology and correlate this with the patient's symptoms. The iliopsoas tendon is visualized under ultrasound with the patient supine and the hip moved from external rotation and slight flexion/abduction to extension and adduction. In addition, diagnostic injections can be utilized at the time of imaging. Bursography can also be performed, which allows visualization of the movement of the tendon, although this is less common.[30]

Treatment begins with conservative management. This consists of activity modification and physical therapy for stretching, especially if the patient has decreased hip extension. Previous studies have demonstrated success with conservative management with specific stretching routines.[31] Injection therapy with corticosteroids may also have a role, but evidence is limited to case reports and small series.[8,23,32] Wahl and colleagues[33] reported a 4-week return to play in 2 high-level athletes who underwent corticosteroid ultrasound-guided injection for an internal snapping hip, with long-term resolution at 26 months.

Surgical management may be considered if the patient fails 3 months of conservative management. There are 2 methods of surgical management, surgical release of the iliopsoas tendon[32,34] or lengthening of the tendon.[30,31,35,36] Endoscopic surgical release has been described in several studies with good results; however, some of the studies are confounded by simultaneous intra-articular arthroscopy for concomitant pathology or transcapsular release (Fig. 2). Ilizaliturri reported on 6 patients who underwent this procedure and had complete symptom resolution but loss of hip flexion.[37] Contreras and colleagues[38] reported similar results with no residual hip snapping in 7 patients. Other literature has demonstrated good results with complete return of strength at 3 months.[39] Byrd[40] evaluated 9 patients who underwent endoscopic release from the lesser trochanter and reported 100% success; however, more than half of the patients had concomitant intra-articular hip pathology. In a second study, Ilizaturri compared 2locations of release, at the level of the capsule versus at the lesser trochanter, and found no difference.[41]

Lengthening of the iliopsoas tendon has been shown to be another effective surgical strategy. This is commonly performed arthroscopically at the level of the iliopectineal groove, and only the tendinous portion of the iliopsoas is released, leaving the muscular portion intact.[42,43] Multiple studies have demonstrated its efficacy in relieving symptoms of internal snapping hip. Gruen and colleagues[36] demonstrated symptom relief in 11 of 11 patients with fractional lengthening; however, 45% of patients had subjective weakness with hip flexion postoperatively. In contrast, Dobbs and colleagues[44] demonstrated similar clinical results but with only 1 of 11 patients reporting weakness. More recently, Perets and colleagues[43] compared patients who underwent iliopsoas fractional lengthening with a control group, and determined that there were statistically significant improvement is Harris Hip Scores, VAS scores, Non-Arthritic Athletic Hip Scores, and Hip Outcome Score- Sports Specific Subscale (HOS-SSS) compared with the control group at a minimum of 2 years postoperatively. Painful snapping was relieved in 91.7% of athletes, and the authors demonstrated that 65% of players returned to sport with no subjective weakness among any patients. Overall, both endoscopic release of the iliopsoas and fractional lengthening are good surgical options that can alleviate symptoms in athletes with internal snapping

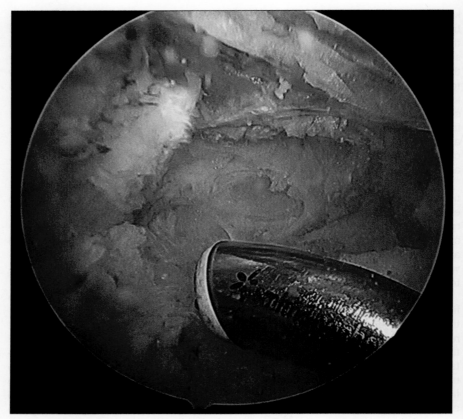

Fig. 2. Endoscopic release of the iliopsoas tendon.

hip who failed conservative management. However, there is limited evidence to suggest 1 surgical method over another, and further studies are warranted to answer this question.

Rectus Femoris Strains and Tears

Muscular injuries to the rectus femoris may also lead to groin pain in athletes. Patients can present with similar symptoms to other hip flexor strains or tears with groin pain, including focal tenderness about 8 to 10 cm below the ASIS, possible swelling, or less commonly a palpable defect.[6] Rectus strains typically occur from an eccentric strain during hip flexion or during an explosive hip flexion moment. Often times this is during kicking or sprinting in soccer players or runners. Like other muscle strains, these most commonly occur at the myotendinous junction. Workup initially involves a focused physical examination regarding hip strength and range of motion. Assessment for femoral nerve palsies should be performed. Imaging may consist of plain radiographs of the hip and pelvis to rule out an avulsion fracture. MRI can be utilized to assess for tears versus strains, especially in patients with prolonged symptoms that fail to improve with conservative management. MRI features may include a bulls-eye sign, muscular retraction, longitudinal scar, or hematoma (**Fig. 3**).[13] Management for rectus femoris strains or tears is conservative and consists of rest, icing, stretching, progressive

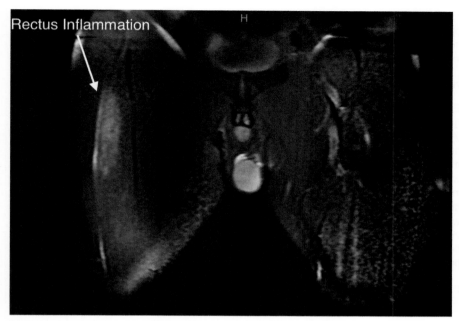

Fig. 3. Rectus strain as visualized on T2 sequencing MRI coronal view.

range-of-motion activities and strengthening. Management for most muscle injuries has not changed significantly over time despite medical advancement, and there remains limited evidence demonstrating an ideal rehabilitation method for these muscle strains.[45]

Avulsion Fractures

Avulsion fractures can lead to significant hip and groin pain in athletes, and occur primarily in skeletally immature patients. They can occur at any major muscle attachment and are typically caused by a forceful eccentric muscle contraction. Regarding primary hip flexors, the most common sites are avulsions of anterior inferior iliac spine (AIIS), and less commonly, the lesser trochanter or anterior superior iliac spine. AIIS avulsions are caused by forceful contraction of the direct head of the rectus femoris, and lesser trochanter avulsions can be caused by contraction of the iliopsoas muscle. On physical examination, patients will assume a position that reduces tension on the avulsed fragment and affected muscle. For avulsion fractures of hip flexors, this is most commonly hip flexion, and pain is elicited with passive hip extension. The diagnosis can be confirmed with plain radiographs. However, in skeletally immature patients, these ossification centers may not be visible, so one must have a high index of suspicion. In children and adolescents, the periosteum often limits significant displacement.[6] Management is almost always nonoperative,[46] and conservative management is recommended initially for most patients. Many nonoperative protocols exist, but most consist of a brief period of rest followed by protected weight bearing, progressive stretching, and strengthening with gradual return to sports and activities.[46–48] Schuett and colleagues[48] retrospectively reviewed 228 pelvic apophyseal avulsion fractures and found 97% were treated with nonoperative management. They determined displacement greater than 20 mm was an independent risk factor for nonunion. In their series, 1 patient of the 112 with AIIS avulsion fractures underwent open reduction and internal fixation, and only 2% of all patients required steroid injections for chronic pain at the fracture site. Furthermore, the authors reported an excellent union rate of 98% in patients treated nonoperatively.[48]

FUTURE DIRECTIONS

Examination of the literature demonstrates an increasing trend in arthroscopic hip surgeries being performed specifically among the American Board of Orthopedic Surgery (ABOS) candidates.[49,50] This relative increase is likely secondary to an increasing number of fellowship programs including hip arthroscopy among their training regimens.[50] This increased focus on intra-articular and pericapsular hip anatomy along with increased imaging resolution has led to a renewed focus on diagnosing and treating hip flexor pathology. With an increasing number of athletic participants annually and a steady incidence of hip flexor pathology, early and correct diagnoses along with appropriate rehabilitation protocol will remain crucial for the athletic care provider.[3,5] Future studies examining specific rehabilitation protocols for the varied hip flexor injuries are warranted, as are additional studies comparing surgical treatment hip flexor pathology with conservative management controls.

CLINICS CARE POINTS

- Hip flexor anatomy is intricate and relies on combination of history, physical examination and advanced imaging for early and accurate diagnosis.
- Most hip flexor injuries can be treated conservatively; however, operative indications exist for those who fail conservative therapy alone
- Most hip flexor injuries result in minimal time loss from sport, despite a relatively high incidence in athletic populations.

DISCLOSURE

The authors have nothing to disclose.

REFERENCES

1. DeLee JC, Farney WC. Incidence of injury in Texas high school football. Am J Sports Med 1992;20(5):575–80.
2. Feeley BT, Powell JW, Muller MS, et al. Hip injuries and labral tears in the National Football League. Am J Sports Med 2008;36(11):2187–95.
3. Kerbel YE, Smith CM, Prodromo JP, et al. Epidemiology of hip and groin injuries in collegiate athletes in the United States. Orthop J Sports Med 2018;6(5). Available at: https://doi.org/10.1177/2325967118771676.
4. Makovicka JL, Chhabra A, Patel KA, et al. A decade of hip injuries in national collegiate athletic association football players: an epidemiologic study using National Collegiate Athletic Association surveillance data. J Athl Train 2019;54(5): 483–8.
5. Shankar PR, Fields SK, Collins CL, et al. Epidemiology of high school and collegiate football injuries in the United States, 2005-2006. Am J Sports Med 2007; 35(8):1295–303.

6. Anderson K, Strickland SM, Warren R. Hip and Groin Injuries in Athletes. Am J Sports Med 2001;29(4):521–33.
7. Drake RL, Gray H, editors. Gray's atlas of anatomy: study smart with student consult. 2nd edition. Edinburgh (United Kingdoms): Elsevier, Churchill Livingstone; 2015.
8. Tatu L, Parratte B, Vuillier F, et al. Descriptive anatomy of the femoral portion of the iliopsoas muscle. Anatomical basis of anterior snapping of the hip. Surg Radiol Anat 2002;23(6):371–4.
9. Guerra DR, Reis FP, Bastos A de A, et al. Anatomical study on the Psoas minor muscle in human fetuses. Int J Morphol 2012;30(1):136–9.
10. Van Dyke JA, Holley HC, Anderson SD. Review of iliopsoas anatomy and pathology. Radiographics 1987;7(1):53–84.
11. Blankenbaker DG, Tuite MJ. Iliopsoas musculotendinous unit. Semin Musculoskelet Radiol 2008;12(1):13–27.
12. Meaney JF, Cassar-Pullicino VN, Etherington R, et al. Ilio-psoas bursa enlargement. Clin Radiol 1992;45(3):161–8.
13. Gyftopoulos S, Rosenberg ZS, Schweitzer ME, et al. Normal anatomy and strains of the deep musculotendinous junction of the proximal rectus femoris: MRI features. Am J Roentgenol 2008;190(3):W182–6.
14. Dziedzic D, Bogacka U, Ciszek B. Anatomy of sartorius muscle. Folia Morphol 2014;73(3):359–62.
15. Lytle WJ. Inguinal anatomy. J Anat 1979;128(Pt 3):581–94.
16. Eckard TG, Padua DA, Dompier TP, et al. Epidemiology of hip flexor and hip adductor strains in National Collegiate Athletic Association Athletes, 2009/2010-2014/2015. Am J Sports Med 2017;45(12):2713–22.
17. Garrett WE. Muscle strain injuries. Am J Sports Med 1996;24(6 Suppl):S2–8.
18. Morelli V, Smith V. Groin injuries in athletes. Am Fam Physician 2001;64(8):1405–14.
19. Johnston CAM, Wiley JP, Lindsay DM, et al. Iliopsoas bursitis and tendinitis. Sports Med 1998;25(4):271–83.
20. Shabshin N, Rosenberg ZS, Cavalcanti CFA. MR Imaging of Iliopsoas Musculotendinous Injuries. Magn Reson Imaging Clin N Am 2005;13(4):705–16.
21. Tsukada S, Niga S, Nihei T, et al. Iliopsoas disorder in athletes with groin pain. JB JS Open Access 2018;3(1). Available at: https://doi.org/10.2106/JBJS.OA.17.00049.
22. Wunderbaldinger P, Bremer C, Schellenberger E, et al. Imaging features of iliopsoas bursitis. Eur Radiol 2002;12(2):409–15.
23. Silver SF, Connell DG, Duncan CP. Case report 550: Snapping right iliopsoas tendon. Skeletal Radiol 1989;18(4):327–8.
24. Staple TW, Jung D, Mork A. Snapping tendon syndrome: hip tenography with fluoroscopic monitoring. Radiology 1988;166(3):873–4.
25. Vaccaro JP, Sauser DD, Beals RK. Iliopsoas bursa imaging: efficacy in depicting abnormal iliopsoas tendon motion in patients with internal snapping hip syndrome. Radiology 1995;197(3):853–6.
26. Anderson SA, Keene JS. Results of arthroscopic iliopsoas tendon release in competitive and recreational athletes. Am J Sports Med 2008;36(12):2363–71.
27. Barlow B. Editorial commentary: iliopsoas fractional lengthening: treating a disease or a symptom? Arthroscopy 2019;35(5):1441–4.
28. Fabricant PD, Bedi A, De La Torre K, et al. Clinical outcomes after arthroscopic psoas lengthening: the effect of femoral version. Arthroscopy 2012;28(7):965–71.
29. Deslandes M, Guillin R, Cardinal É, et al. The snapping iliopsoas tendon: new mechanisms using dynamic sonography. Am J Roentgenol 2008;190(3):576–81.

30. Yen Y-M, Lewis CL, Kim Y-J. Understanding and treating the snapping hip. Sports Med Arthrosc 2015;23(4):194–9.
31. Jacobson T, Allen WC. Surgical correction of the snapping iliopsoas tendon. Am J Sports Med 1990;18(5):470–4.
32. Taylor GR, Clarke NM. Surgical release of the "snapping iliopsoas tendon. J Bone Joint Surg Br 1995;77(6):881–3.
33. Wahl CJ, Warren RF, Adler RS, et al. Internal coxa saltans (snapping hip) as a result of overtraining: a report of 3 cases in professional athletes with a review of causes and the role of ultrasound in early diagnosis and management. Am J Sports Med 2004;32(5):1302–9.
34. Harper MC, Schaberg JE, Allen WC. Primary iliopsoas bursography in the diagnosis of disorders of the hip. Clin Orthop Relat Res 1987;221:238–41.
35. Flanum ME, Keene JS, Blankenbaker DG, et al. Arthroscopic treatment of the painful "internal" snapping hip. Am J Sports Med 2007;35(5):770–9.
36. Gruen GS, Scioscia TN, Lowenstein JE. The surgical treatment of internal snapping hip. Am J Sports Med 2002;30(4):607–13.
37. Ilizaliturri VM, Villalobos FE, Chaidez PA, et al. Internal snapping hip syndrome: treatment by endoscopic release of the iliopsoas tendon. Arthroscopy 2005; 21(11):1375–80.
38. Contreras MEK, Dani WS, Endges WK, et al. Arthroscopic treatment of the snapping iliopsoas tendon through the central compartment of the hip: a pilot study. J Bone Joint Surg Br 2010;92(6):777–80.
39. Wettstein M, Jung J, Dienst M. Arthroscopic psoas tenotomy. Arthroscopy 2006; 22(8):907.e1-4.
40. Byrd JWT. Evaluation and management of the snapping iliopsoas tendon. Tech Orthop 2005;20(1):45–51.
41. Ilizaliturri VM, Buganza-Tepole M, Olivos-Meza A, et al. Central compartment release versus lesser trochanter release of the iliopsoas tendon for the treatment of internal snapping hip: a comparative study. Arthroscopy 2014;30(7):790–5.
42. Chandrasekaran S, Close MR, Walsh JP, et al. Arthroscopic technique for iliopsoas fractional lengthening for symptomatic internal snapping of the hip, iliopsoas impingement lesion, or both. Arthrosc Tech 2018;7(9):e915–9.
43. Perets I, Hartigan DE, Chaharbakhshi EO, et al. Clinical outcomes and return to sport in competitive athletes undergoing arthroscopic iliopsoas fractional lengthening compared with a matched control group without iliopsoas fractional lengthening. Arthroscopy 2018;34(2):456–63.
44. Dobbs MB, Gordon JE, Luhmann SJ, et al. Surgical correction of the snapping iliopsoas tendon in adolescents. J Bone Joint Surg Am 2002;84(3):420–4.
45. Järvinen TAH, Järvinen TLN, Kääriäinen M, et al. Muscle injuries: biology and treatment. Am J Sports Med 2005;33(5):745–64.
46. McKinney BI, Nelson C, Carrion W. Apophyseal avulsion fractures of the hip and pelvis. Orthopedics 2009;32(1):42.
47. Howard FM, Piha RJ. Fractures of the apophyses in adolescent athletes. JAMA 1965;192(10):842–4.
48. Schuett DJ, Bomar JD, Pennock AT. Pelvic apophyseal avulsion fractures: a retrospective review of 228 cases. J Pediatr Orthop 2015;35(6):617–23.
49. Bozic KJ, Chan V, Valone FH, et al. Trends in hip arthroscopy utilization in the United States. J Arthroplasty 2013;28(8, Supplement):140–3.
50. Colvin AC, Harrast J, Harner C. Trends in hip arthroscopy. J Bone Joint Surg Am 2012;94(4):e23.

Hip Abductor and Peritrochanteric Space Conditions

Alexander E. Weber, MD*, Jennifer A. Bell, MD,
Ioanna K. Bolia, MD, MS, PhD

KEYWORDS

- Peritrochanteric space • Greater trochanteric pain syndrome • Endoscopy
- Gluteus medius • Outcomes

KEY POINTS

- Disorders of the peritrochanteric space are common in middle-aged individuals and are sometimes associated with intra-articular hip pathology, which warrants further diagnostic testing.
- Greater trochanteric pain syndromes (GTPS) refers to pain generated by one or multiple disorders of the peritrochanteric space, such as trochanteric bursitis, gluteus medius and minimus tendinopathy or tear, and disorders of the proximal iliotibial band.
- Conservative management of GTPS may include physical therapy; oral medication; and/or local injection with corticosteroids, anesthetic, or platelet-rich plasma.
- Endoscopic management of the greater trochanteric pain syndrome results in resolution of pain and significant improvement in function at midterm follow-up.

BACKGROUND

Basic Anatomy of the Peritrochanteric Space of the Hip

The most superficial layer of the peritrochanteric space consists of the fibromuscular sheath of the gluteus maximus, tensor fascia lata, and iliotibial band (ITB).[1] The greater trochanter is considered the deep boundary of this anatomic region, which contains the following structures: trochanteric bursa, tendinous insertions of the gluteal muscles, and the origin vastus lateralis.[2] **Table 1** summarizes the anatomy and function of the gluteal muscles. The trochanteric bursa is superficial to the hip abductor muscles and deep to the ITB.

Endoscopic Evaluation of the Peritrochanteric Space

With the rapid expansion of minimally invasive surgical techniques in orthopedics, most of the peritrochanteric space disorders can be addressed endoscopically.[2,3]

USC Epstein Family for Sports Medicine at Keck Medicine of USC, 1520 San Pablo Street, #2000, Los Angeles, CA 90033, USA
* Corresponding author.
E-mail address: weberae@usc.edu

Clin Sports Med 40 (2021) 311–322
https://doi.org/10.1016/j.csm.2021.01.001
0278-5919/21/© 2021 Elsevier Inc. All rights reserved.

Table 1
Anatomy and function of the gluteal muscles

Muscle	Origin	Insertion	Action	Innervation	Arterial Supply
Gluteus minimus	Dorsal ilium between inferior and anterior gluteal lines Edge of greater sciatic notch	Anterior surface of greater trochanter	Hip abduction and internal rotation	Superior gluteal nerve	Superior gluteal artery
Gluteus medius	Dorsal ilium inferior to iliac crest	Lateral and superior surfaces of greater trochanter	Hip abduction; hip internal rotation (anterior fibers); hip external rotation (posterior fibers)	Superior gluteal nerve	Superior gluteal artery
Gluteus maximus	Posterior aspect of dorsal ilium posterior to posterior gluteal line posterior superior iliac crest Posterior inferior aspect of sacrum and coccyx Sacrotuberous ligament	Fascia lata at the iliotibial band Gluteal tuberosity on posterior femoral surface	Hip extension; assists in hip external rotation and abduction	Inferior gluteal nerve	Inferior and superior gluteal arteries First perforating branch of the profunda femoris artery

Lall and colleagues[4] described a classification system that is useful in the diagnosis and management of greater trochanteric space pain syndrome (GTPS; type I-V) primarily based on endoscopic findings (**Table 2**), and by taking into account the physical examination and imaging diagnosis.

Trochanteric Bursitis

Inflammation of the trochanteric bursa is commonly diagnosed in middle aged or older individuals, and stems from the repetitive friction of the bursa between the greater trochanter and ITB during hip motion.[5] Patients with this condition present with lateral hip or buttock pain and peritrochanteric tenderness is characteristic on physical examination.[6] Although some patients present with isolated trochanteric bursitis, this condition might be associated with intra-articular hip joint pathology (femoroacetabular impingement, arthritis) or gluteal tendinopathy or tear.[7,8] Because of this, imaging testing of the hip joint with radiograph and possibly MRI must be considered to reveal the diagnosis.[6–9] The initial, nonoperative management of trochanteric bursitis may include rest, activity modification, physical therapy, oral medication (nonsteroidal anti-inflammatory), or local injection therapy (corticosteroids, local anesthetic, platelet-rich plasma).[8,10,11]

Surgical management consists of the excision of the inflamed trochanteric bursa, and it is the preferred treatment in cases of failure of conservative measures. Excellent clinical outcomes have been reported in patients undergoing trochanteric bursectomy (isolated or in combination with arthroscopic femoroacetabular impingement (FAI) surgery or gluteal tendon repair) using previously described open or endoscopic surgical techniques.[9,12,13] The endoscopic approach offers the advantages of smaller skin incision and reduced normal tissue violation, which might accelerate the postoperative recovery of the patient.[13–18]

Snapping Hip Syndrome

Patients with coxa saltans or snapping hip syndrome often describe a "click" that is heard or felt during movement of the hip joint, and is sometimes accompanied by hip pain.[19] This condition is common among dancers and is categorized into three types, based on the cause.[19,20] External snapping hip is caused by sliding of the ITB over the greater trochanter, whereas internal snapping hip is most commonly the result of iliopsoas tendon sliding over the femoral head, prominent iliopectineal ridge, lesser trochanter, or the iliopsoas bursa. Intra-articular snapping hip syndrome is associated with the presence of loose bodies in the hip joint or labral tears.[19,21]

Table 2
Classification of GTPS based on endoscopic examination

GTPS Type	
I	Isolated trochanteric bursitis
II	Trochanteric bursitis + fraying
III	IIIa: Abductor tendon partial-thickness tear <25%
	IIIB: Abductor tendon partial-thickness tear <25%
IV	Full-thickness abductor tendon tear
V	Full-thickness abductor tendon tear ± retraction

Adapted from Lall AC, Schwarzman GR, Battaglia MR, et al. Greater Trochanteric Pain Syndrome: An Intraoperative Endoscopic Classification System with Pearls to Surgical Techniques and Rehabilitation Protocols. Arthroscopy techniques. 2019;8(8):e889-e903; with permission.

In patients with external snapping syndrome, applying pressure over the greater trochanter with the patient's hip in flexion often stops snapping.[19,22] Reproduction of internal hip snapping during physical examination is achieved by passive movement of the hip from flexion and external rotation to extension and internal rotation.[23] Radiographic evaluation may include an anteroposterior hip radiograph (which is normal in most patients), but MRI is useful in cases where additional intra-articular hip or peritrochanteric pathology are suspected.[24]

Physical therapy with or without local injection therapy is the first-line therapy for snapping hip syndrome, regardless of type. Patients with external snapping hip syndrome who fail to improve with conservative measures may undergo surgical excision of the trochanteric bursa in combination with Z plasty of ITB. In cases of internal snapping hip syndrome that is resistant to nonoperative therapy, iliopsoas tendon release might be performed.[25] Psoas tenotomy can also be performed in patients with internal snapping hip following total hip replacement with satisfactory outcomes.[26] In patients with intra-articular snapping hip syndrome, treatment must focus on the correction of the existing the intra-articular hip pathology, which might result in the resolution of snapping without additional intervention.[27]

Gluteal Tendinopathy

Diagnosis

Careful history and physical examination must be completed when evaluating patients with lateral-sided hip pain and suspected gluteal tendinopathy or tear. Patients commonly report insidious onset of lateral hip pain associated with weight bearing, lying on affected hip, and/or difficulty with ascending or descending stairs.[2] Gluteal tendinopathy occurs four times more often in women than men and is most prevalent between the ages of 50 and 80.[21,28] Patients will have often attempted and failed nonoperative treatments of trochanteric bursitis.[29] Physical examination findings including tenderness to palpation of the greater trochanter, decreased abduction strength, and abductor atrophy may be notable.[30] Patients may also walk with an antalgic and/or Trendelenburg gait.[21,31]

The most commonly used imaging includes plain radiographs, ultrasonography, and MRI.[2,32] Patients with gluteal tendinopathy and abductor tears often have unremarkable plain films, although radiographs are important at ruling out other differentials including degenerative joint disease, femoroacetabular impingement, and dysplasia.[5,33] Walsh and colleagues[28] evaluated the plain radiographs of 72 patients with surgically treated abductor tendon tears. Patients with long-standing symptoms were more likely to have spurs in superior and inferior facet with a normal-appearing lateral margin of the trochanter, and new boney growth over anterior facet.[28]

MRI is the most sensitive and specific study to confirm a gluteal tendinopathy and rule out other intra-articular and extra-articular disorders (**Fig. 1**).[34] Similar to rotator cuff injuries of the shoulder, tears can range from partial thickness to full thickness. Increased signal intensity of the gluteal tendon on T2-weighted images is consistent with a partial tear.[35] Full-tendon tears show discontinuity of the tendon, with or without atrophy.[35] The Goutallier-Fuchs classification is frequently used to classify fatty infiltration of the gluteal muscles (0 = normal muscle; 1 = some fatty streaks; 2 = moderate fatty streaks, although more muscle than fat; 3 = severe fatty muscle with equal amounts muscle and fat; and 4 = muscle contains more fat than muscle).[36]

More recently in the literature, there has been increasing evidence that amount of fatty muscle atrophy is correlated with decreased postoperative outcomes.[36,37] Thaunat and colleagues[37] evaluated the short-term outcomes of patients with endoscopically repaired partial- and full-thickness tears of gluteus medius. Preoperative MRIs

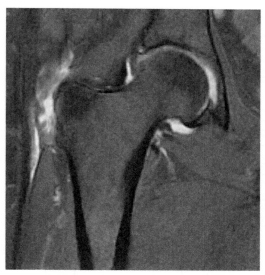

Fig. 1. MRI study of the right hip (coronal view) showing tear of the gluteus minimums and gluteus medius tendons with subgluteus bursal fluid collection.

were graded using the gluteus medius fatty degeneration index and found to be strongly negatively correlated with postoperative modified Harris hip score (mHHS), nonarthritic hip score, and visual analog scale for pain (VAS pain) and patient-rated overall satisfaction.[37]

Management of gluteal tendinopathy or tear

Initial treatment should start with a trial of nonoperative treatments including nonsteroidal anti-inflammatory drugs, physical therapy, activity modification, and corticosteroid injections.[5] Nonoperative management often fails and patients endorse persistent pain and abduction weakness on physical examination. Surgical indications have been suggested for patients who failed to improve with conservative treatment, exhibit 6 months of symptoms, MRI-confirming gluteal tendon tear, pain relief with injection, and/or the evolving fatty degeneration of the gluteus medius or minimus muscle.[37] Increased time to intervention could have negative effects on outcomes in patients with retracted tendons or fatty degeneration.

Surgical interventions include open versus endoscopic gluteal tendon repair (**Table 3**). Both have been reported to improve patient pain, limp, and abduction strength.[29] Advantages of the arthroscopic approach (**Fig. 2**) include assessing or treating concomitant periarticular pathology. Open procedures have easier visualization of the pathology. Such factors as size of the tear, retraction of the tendon, amount of fatty degeneration, atrophy of the muscle, and bone mineral density may affect the outcome of surgery. Maslaris and colleagues[38] found that patients with larger tears and fatty degeneration were more likely to be treated open. Ebert and colleagues[39] completed an extensive literature review of surgically treated gluteus tendon surgical repair method and patient outcomes and concluded that there is sufficient evidence to recommend gluteal tendon repairs treated either open or endoscopically.

Gluteal tendon repair can either be performed by using transosseus sutures or suture anchors and be performed open or endoscopically (see **Table 3**). **Fig. 3**

Table 3
Clinical outcomes following gluteal tendon repair using open or endoscopic technique

Author, Year	Surgery	Repair Method	Conclusion
Maslaris et al,[38] 2020	Endoscopic vs open	Suture anchors in 1 or 2 rows. Average of 1.8 vs 2.5 anchors used for endoscopic vs open.	All treatment groups mean different before and after treatment: VAS (−3.9), limp (−0.9), abduction (+0.4), analgesics (−1.2), and opioids (−0.3).
Perets et al,[21] 2017	Endoscopic	Partial thickness: side-to-side repair with 5.5-mm BioComposite Corkscrew anchor into the lateral facet. Full thickness: suture bridge with two 5.5-mm BioComposite Corkscrew anchors in the proximal row and distal row fixed with two 4.75-mm SwiveLock anchors.	Improvement in all patient-reported outcomes at 5-y follow-up: mHHS (52.4 vs 81.2), NAHS (48.0 vs 82.5), HOS-SS (30.1 vs 66.4), VAS score (6.2 vs 2.6).
Saltzman et al,[30] 2018	Endoscopic	5.5-mm BioComposite Corkscrew anchors. Tears <2 cm repaired in a single row with 1–2 anchors. Tears >2 cm repaired in double-row suture bridge fashion.	Repair w/o PRFM: VAS pain (6.4 vs 1.92), HOS-ADL (57.8 vs 82.79), HOS-SS (37.21 vs 72.31), and mHHS (55.96 vs 78.72). Repair w/PRFM: VAS pain (7.17 vs 2.51), HOS-ADL (53.74 vs 82.73), HOS-SS (30.44 vs 68.04), and mHHS (50.87 vs 77.01).
McCormick et al,[45] 2013	Endoscopic	Transosseous suture and suture anchors.	Average follow-up 22.6 mo with postoperative: HHS (84.7), HOS-ADL (89.1), patient satisfaction (90%).
Davies et al,[41] 2013	Open	Transosseous suture or suture anchors.	Preoperative to average follow-up of 70.8, HSS (53 vs 88). LEAS (6.7–8.8).
Bucher et al,[46] 2014	Open	Transosseous tunnel with suture anchors, augmented with LARS.	Significant improvement from preoperative to 12-mo follow-up in OHS (22.4 vs 4.1), VAS (7.1 vs 1.6), SF-36 PCS (29.7–44.4), and SF-36 MCS (45.8 vs 52.5).
Thaunat et al,[37] 2013	Endoscopic	Side-to-side repair using 1 or 2 U-shaped anchors and full-thickness tears, double-row repair with suture bridging was used.	Preoperative vs postoperative scores at 31.7 mo follow-up mHHS (33.7 vs 80.2), NAHS (47.7 vs 76.8), and VAS (7.2 vs 3.2).
Walsh et al,[28] 2011	Open	Transosseous tunnel with 5-Ethibond sutures.	MDP decreased significantly from preoperative (10.85), 6-mo (16.66), and 12-mo (16.65).

Abbreviations: ADL, activities of daily living; HOS, Hip Outcome Score; LARS, ligament augmentation and reconstruction system; LEAS, lower-extremity activity scale; MDP, Merle D'Aubigné Postel score; MCS, mental component score; MMSH, manual muscle strength assessment; NAHS, Nonarthritic Hip Score; OHS, oxford hip score; PCS, physical component score; PRFM, platelet rich fibrin matrix; SF, Short Form; SS, sport specific.

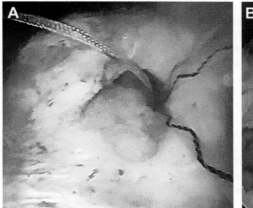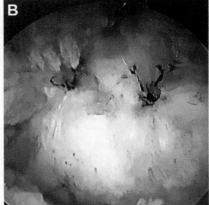

Fig. 2. (*A*) Arthroscopic depiction of gluteus medius tear (right hip). (*B*) Arthroscopic repair of gluteus medius tear (right hip).

demonstrates a gluteus medius tear (see **Fig. 3**A) and subsequent repair (see **Fig. 3**B) via an open surgical approach. Davies and colleagues[40,41] described their approach to open gluteal tendon repair. They evaluated 22 patients with 23 hips treated with open gluteal tendon over a 5-year follow-up.[41] For grade I and II tears, they frequently used sutures anchors, whereas for grade III and IV tears they used transosseus tunnels. HHS improved from 53 to 88 and lower-extremity activity scale improved from 6.7 to 8.9 at 5-year follow-up at preoperative and 5-year follow-up, respectively. A posterolateral approach was used, and an incision was made through the gluteus maximums fascia and then the ITB.[41] Next, a trochanter bursectomy was performed, the gluteus medius bluntly dissected, and the osseous bed on the greater trochanter

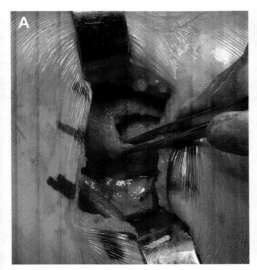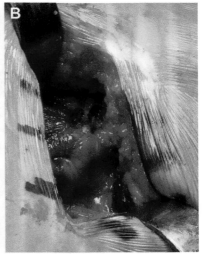

Fig. 3. (*A*) gluteus medius tear on a right hip. (*B*) Repair of a right-sided gluteus medius tear via open surgical approach.

was prepared with superficial burring.[41] Larger grade tears were repaired with a transosseus tunnel using a curvilinear drill. Small repairs were undertaken with 6.5-mm suture anchors with number-2 FiberWire (Arthrex, Naples, FL).[41]

For patients with chronic, retracted tears of the gluteus tendons or in complex revision cases where the gluteal tendons are irreparable, tendon repair with dermal allograft augmentation is an option (**Fig. 4**).

Multiple authors have described their endoscopic approach to gluteus medius repairs.[2,21,42] Similar to open approach, most authors describe bursectomy, debridement of the torn abductor tendon, and decortication of the insertion on the greater trochanter.[21,28,30,31,38,42–44] Saltzman and colleagues[30] described repairing small or medium tears (<2 cm) with single-row fashion with one or two anchors, and larger tears (>2 cm) with double-row suture anchors. However, tear pattern largely dictates the number, size, and orientation of the anchors.[2] Three lateral-based portals are commonly used for gluteal repairs that include a viewing portal just posterior to vastus lateralis, a working portal just distal to ridge, and proximal portal for anchor insertion. One benefit to endoscopic repair is to address intra-articular pathology. Other studies have reviewed gluteus medius repairs with simultaneous intra-articular correction.[21,29] Chandrasekaran and colleagues[29] reviewed 34 patients with intra-articular intervention at the time of surgical repair and found significant improvement in all patient-reported outcomes and decrease in pain score. The clinical outcomes following open and endoscopic gluteal repair procedures are presented in **Table 3**.

DISCUSSION

Multiple studies report that 65% to 70% of patients experience relief of symptoms following operative management of GTPS (see **Table 3**).[28,29,31,42] Recently in the literature, patient-reported outcomes have become an important tool in measuring postoperative improvements.[42] The minimally clinically important difference (MCID) and

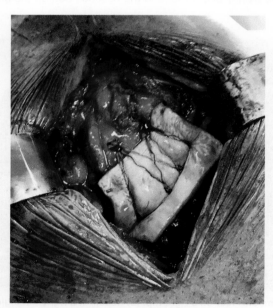

Fig. 4. Gluteus medius repair with dermal allograft augmentation on a right hip.

patient-acceptable symptomatic state are used to evaluate what are meaningful improvements postoperatively. Okoroha and colleagues[42] evaluated 60 patients with gluteus medius repairs with a minimum of 2-year follow-up. Activities of daily living (ADL) and sport-specific (SS) subscales of Hip Outcome Score (HOS) and mHHS were assessed preoperatively and at the final follow-up.[42] Preoperative scores and 2-year follow-up showed statistically significant improvement in HOS-ADL (48.4 vs 79.3), HOS-SS (24.5 vs 64.5), and mHHS (46.2 vs 75.6) preoperatively versus 2-year follow-up, respectively. A 70.7% reached MCID HOS-ADL, 75.5% reached MCID-HOS-SS, and 75.7% reached MCID mHHS; 56.4%, 50%, and 50% achieved pass, respectively. They concluded that 76.7% of patients were able to achieve meaningful outcomes. Perets and colleagues[21] retrospectively reviewed 16 patients with gluteus medius repair at 5-year follow-up. From preoperative to 5-year follow-up, all outcomes showed statistically significant improvement with mHHS (52.4 vs 81.2), Nonarthritic Hip Score (48.0 vs 82.5), HOS (30.1 vs 66.4), and VAS (6.2 vs 2.6). Mean satisfaction rating was 8.4 and there was 92.9% survivorship (one patient converted to total hip arthroplasty). HOS did not decrease between 2-year and 5-year follow-up.[21]

Use of Biologics in the Treatment of Greater Trochanteric Pain Syndrome

Platelet-rich plasma continues to be a topic of interest in tendinopathy and ligament injury. Saltzman and colleagues[30] retrospectively reviewed 18 patients who received preoperative platelet-rich fibrin matrix (PRFM), a fibrin matrix that acts as a scaffold for cell migration and slow release of growth factors, versus 29 treated without. Outcome scores for patients treated without PRFM improved as follows: VAS pain (6.4 vs 1.92), HOS-ADL (57.8 vs 82.79), HOS-SS (37.21 vs 72.31), and mHHS (55.96 vs 78.72). Outcome scores for patients treated with PRFM improved as follows: VAS pain (7.17 vs 2.51), HOS-ADL (53.74 vs 82.73), HOS-SS (30.44 vs 68.04), and mHHS (50.87 vs 77.01). One patient in the PRFM (5.6%) and three in the untreated group (10.3%) had clinical retears. Postoperative Short Form-12 and International Hip Outcome Tool-12 were 45.5 versus 28.09 and 64.61 versus 44.03 in patients treated with versus without PRFM. They concluded that platelet-rich plasma had no difference in pain or the rate of retear, although it may improve subjective outcomes.[30]

SUMMARY

Common peritrochanteric space disorders include trochanteric bursitis, snapping hip syndrome, and gluteal tendinopathy or tearing. Gluteal tendon tears are more frequently being diagnosed in patients with lateral-sided hip pain and abduction weakness and might be accompanied by additional intra-articular hip pathology. Causes of gluteal tendon tears include chronic degeneration, postoperative complications from lateral approach to the hip, and traumatic tears. Degenerative tendinopathy is often an insidious onset of pain and progresses from bursitis, partial-thickness, full-thickness, to complete tendon tears. Fatty degeneration and atrophy of the gluteal muscles is associated with worse outcome following surgical therapy. Patients with more severe pathology are more likely to undergo open treatment, although open and endoscopic treatment have been reported to have decreased pain and increased abduction strength.

CLINICS CARE POINTS

- Although conservative measures might be adequate to address the symptoms of trochanteric bursitis, endoscopic bursectomy is the preferred surgical treatment in recalcitrant cases.

- Snapping hip syndrome must be suspected in dancers or other patients who present with audible click during hip motion and treatment should be guided based on the underlying anatomic abnormality.

- Gluteus medius tears are common in patients with lateral hip pain and hip abduction weakness. Open or endoscopic gluteus medius repair results in significant improvement in pain and function in patients with isolated gluteal tendinopathy or those who receive additional therapy to address intra-articular hip pathology.

ACKNOWLEDGMENTS

Authors acknowledge The Cappo Family Research Fund (no grant specific to this study)

DISCLOSURE

The authors have nothing to disclose.

REFERENCES

1. Voos JE, Rudzki JR, Shindle MK, et al. Arthroscopic anatomy and surgical techniques for peritrochanteric space disorders in the hip. Arthroscopy 2007;23(11): 1246.e1-5.
2. Byrd JWT. Disorders of the peritrochanteric and deep gluteal space: new frontiers for arthroscopy. Sports Med Arthrosc Rev 2015;23(4):221-31.
3. Chandrasekaran S, Lodhia P, Gui C, et al. Outcomes of open versus endoscopic repair of abductor muscle tears of the hip: a systematic review. Arthroscopy 2015;31(10):2057-67.e2.
4. Lall AC, Schwarzman GR, Battaglia MR, et al. Greater trochanteric pain syndrome: an intraoperative endoscopic classification system with pearls to surgical techniques and rehabilitation protocols. Arthrosc Tech 2019;8(8):e889-903.
5. Redmond JM, Chen AW, Domb BG. Greater trochanteric pain syndrome. J Am Acad Orthop Surg 2016;24(4):231-40.
6. Seidman AJ, Varacallo M. Trochanteric bursitis. StatPearls. Treasure Island (FL): StatPearls Publishing StatPearls Publishing LLC.; 2020.
7. Pozzi G, Lanza E, Parra CG, et al. Incidence of greater trochanteric pain syndrome in patients suspected for femoroacetabular impingement evaluated using magnetic resonance arthrography of the hip. Radiol Med 2017;122(3):208-14.
8. Speers CJ, Bhogal GS. Greater trochanteric pain syndrome: a review of diagnosis and management in general practice. Br J Gen Pract 2017;67(663):479-80.
9. Drummond J, Fary C, Tran P. The outcome of endoscopy for recalcitrant greater trochanteric pain syndrome. Arch Orthop Trauma Surg 2016;136(11):1547-54.
10. Ribeiro AG, Ricioli WJ, Silva AR, et al. PRP in the treatment of trochanteric syndrome: a pilot study. Acta Ortop Bras 2016;24(4):208-12.
11. Barratt PA, Brookes N, Newson A. Conservative treatments for greater trochanteric pain syndrome: a systematic review. Br J Sports Med 2017;51(2):97-104.
12. Maffulli N. Editorial commentary: hip trochanteric bursitis and femoroacetabular impingement: the arthroscope is only the tool. Arthroscopy 2018;34(5):1461-2.
13. Vap AR, Mitchell JJ, Briggs KK, et al. Outcomes of arthroscopic management of trochanteric bursitis in patients with femoroacetabular impingement: a comparison of two matched patient groups. Arthroscopy 2018;34(5):1455-60.

14. Ali M, Oderuth E, Atchia I, et al. The use of platelet-rich plasma in the treatment of greater trochanteric pain syndrome: a systematic literature review. J Hip Preserv Surg 2018;5(3):209–19.
15. Bolton WS, Kidanu D, Dube B, et al. Do ultrasound guided trochanteric bursa injections of corticosteroid for greater trochanteric pain syndrome provide sustained benefit and are imaging features associated with treatment response? Clin Radiol 2018;73(5):505.e9-15.
16. Mitchell WG, Kettwich SC, Sibbitt WL Jr, et al. Outcomes and cost-effectiveness of ultrasound-guided injection of the trochanteric bursa. Rheumatol Int 2018; 38(3):393–401.
17. Zibis AH, Mitrousias VD, Klontzas ME, et al. Great trochanter bursitis vs sciatica, a diagnostic-anatomic trap: differential diagnosis and brief review of the literature. Eur Spine J 2018;27(7):1509–16.
18. Mitchell JJ, Chahla J, Vap AR, et al. Endoscopic trochanteric bursectomy and iliotibial band release for persistent trochanteric bursitis. Arthrosc Tech 2016;5(5): e1185–9.
19. Musick SR, Varacallo M. Snapping hip syndrome. StatPearls. Treasure Island (FL): StatPearls Publishing LLC; 2020.
20. Lerch S, Stark D, Ruhmann O. [Extra-articular impingement of the hip: treatment of snapping hip by lengthening of the iliotibial band]. Oper Orthop Traumatol 2018;30(2):80–6.
21. Perets I, Mansor Y, Yuen LC, et al. Endoscopic gluteus medius repair with concomitant arthroscopy for labral tears: a case series with minimum 5-year outcomes. Arthroscopy 2017;33(12):2159–67.
22. Pierce TP, Kurowicki J, Issa K, et al. External snapping hip: a systematic review of outcomes following surgical intervention: external snapping hip systematic review. Hip Int 2018;28(5):468–72.
23. Winston P, Awan R, Cassidy JD, et al. Clinical examination and ultrasound of self-reported snapping hip syndrome in elite ballet dancers. Am J Sports Med 2007; 35(1):118–26.
24. Allen WC, Cope R. Coxa saltans: the snapping hip revisited. J Am Acad Orthop Surg 1995;3(5):303–8.
25. Wettstein M, Jung J, Dienst M. Arthroscopic psoas tenotomy. Arthroscopy 2006; 22(8):907.e1-4.
26. Della Valle CJ, Rafii M, Jaffe WL. Iliopsoas tendinitis after total hip arthroplasty. J Arthroplasty 2001;16(7):923–6.
27. Yamamoto Y, Hamada Y, Ide T, et al. Arthroscopic surgery to treat intra-articular type snapping hip. Arthroscopy 2005;21(9):1120–5.
28. Walsh MJ, Walton JR, Walsh NA. Surgical repair of the gluteal tendons: a report of 72 cases. J Arthroplasty 2011;26(8):1514–9.
29. Chandrasekaran S, Gui C, Hutchinson MR, et al. Outcomes of endoscopic gluteus medius repair: study of thirty-four patients with minimum two-year follow-up. J Bone Joint Surg Am 2015;97(16):1340–7.
30. Saltzman BM, Ukwuani G, Makhni EC, et al. The effect of platelet-rich fibrin matrix at the time of gluteus medius repair: a retrospective comparative study. Arthroscopy 2018;34(3):832–41.
31. Saltzman BM, Louie PK, Clapp IM, et al. Assessment of association between spino-pelvic parameters and outcomes following gluteus medius repair. Arthroscopy 2019;35(4):1092–8.
32. Ilizaliturri VM Jr, Camacho-Galindo J, Evia Ramirez AN, et al. Soft tissue pathology around the hip. Clin Sports Med 2011;30(2):391–415.

33. Lachiewicz PF. Abductor tendon tears of the hip: evaluation and management. J Am Acad Orthop Surg 2011;19(7):385–91.

34. Kong A, Van der Vliet A, Zadow S. MRI and US of gluteal tendinopathy in greater trochanteric pain syndrome. Eur Radiol 2007;17(7):1772–83.

35. Grimaldi A, Mellor R, Nicolson P, et al. Utility of clinical tests to diagnose MRI-confirmed gluteal tendinopathy in patients presenting with lateral hip pain. Br J Sports Med 2017;51(6):519–24.

36. Bogunovic L, Lee SX, Haro MS, et al. Application of the Goutallier/Fuchs rotator cuff classification to the evaluation of hip abductor tendon tears and the clinical correlation with outcome after repair. Arthroscopy 2015;31(11):2145–51.

37. Thaunat M, Chatellard R, Noel E, et al. Endoscopic repair of partial-thickness undersurface tears of the gluteus medius tendon. Orthop Traumatol Surg Res 2013; 99(7):853–7.

38. Maslaris A, Vail TP, Zhang A, et al. Equivalent mid term results of open versus endoscopic gluteal tendon tear repair using suture anchors in 45 patients. J Arthroplasty 2020;35(6S):S352–8.

39. Ebert JR, Bucher TA, Ball SV, et al. A review of surgical repair methods and patient outcomes for gluteal tendon tears. Hip Int 2015;25(1):15–23.

40. Davies H, Zhaeentan S, Tavakkolizadeh A, et al. Surgical repair of chronic tears of the hip abductor mechanism. Hip Int 2009;19(4):372–6.

41. Davies JF, Stiehl JB, Davies JA, et al. Surgical treatment of hip abductor tendon tears. J Bone Joint Surg Am 2013;95(15):1420–5.

42. Okoroha KR, Beck EC, Nwachukwu BU, et al. Defining minimal clinically important difference and patient acceptable symptom state after isolated endoscopic gluteus medius repair. Am J Sports Med 2019;47(13):3141–7.

43. Thaunat M, Clowez G, Desseaux A, et al. Influence of muscle fatty degeneration on functional outcomes after endoscopic gluteus medius repair. Arthroscopy 2018;34(6):1816–24.

44. Voos JE, Shindle MK, Pruett A, et al. Endoscopic repair of gluteus medius tendon tears of the hip. Am J Sports Med 2009;37(4):743–7.

45. McCormick F, Alpaugh K, Nwachukwu BU, et al. Endoscopic repair of full-thickness abductor tendon tears: surgical technique and outcome at minimum of 1-year follow-up. Arthroscopy 2013;29(12):1941–7.

46. Bucher TA, Darcy P, Ebert JR, et al. Gluteal tendon repair augmented with a synthetic ligament: surgical technique and a case series. Hip Int 2014;24(2):187–93.

Core Muscle and Adductor Injury

Timothy J. Mulry, DO[1], Paul E. Rodenhouse, DO[2], Brian D. Busconi, MD*

KEYWORDS

- Core muscle injury • Groin pain • Athletic pubalgia • Sports hernia
- Adductor longus strain

KEY POINTS

- Core muscle injury is a difficult problem to diagnose and treat with an expansive differential diagnosis.
- Core muscle injury is best treated with a multidisciplinary approach involving physical therapists, athletic trainers, radiologists, and both orthopedic and general surgeons.
- Nonoperative management, including rest, a core strengthening physical therapy regimen, nonsteroidal anti-inflammatories, and oral or injectable corticosteroids are the first line in management.
- Upon failure of conservative treatment, operative intervention to treat all pathology around the pubis using several techniques has been shown to be extremely successful.

INTRODUCTION

Groin pain can be a difficult problem for patients as well as practitioners. Lower abdominal and groin injuries are among the most common causes of both pain and lost playing time in sports.[1] These injuries affect athletes and nonathletes alike. Most lower abdominal and groin injuries are self-limited and only a small percentage cause symptoms for more than 3 weeks.[2] However, there are still many that do not improve despite conservative management. The majority of symptomatic core muscle injuries requiring surgical management occur in male athletes who play soccer, hockey, football, basketball, skiing, or rugby.[3] Core muscle injuries are also becoming increasingly recognized in the female athlete with women comprising about 5% to 15% of the injured population.[4] The differential diagnosis is expansive, including musculoskeletal, genitourinary, and intra-abdominal pathologies. We believe that a

Department of Orthopedics and Physical Rehabilitation, University of Massachusetts Medicine School, Worcester, MA, USA
[1] Present address: 65 Lake Avenue, Apartment #527, Worcester, MA 01604.
[2] Present address: 125 Franklin Street, Apartment #2228, Worcester, MA 01608.
* Corresponding author. 46 Proctor Street, Hopkinton, MA 01748.
E-mail address: Brian.Busconi@umassmemorial.org
Twitter: @PaulRodenhouse (P.E.R.)

Clin Sports Med 40 (2021) 323–338
https://doi.org/10.1016/j.csm.2020.12.001
0278-5919/21/© 2021 Elsevier Inc. All rights reserved.

multidisciplinary team approach to assess all patients with possible core muscle injury is important. This team involves athletic trainers, physical therapists, radiologists, operative and nonoperative sports medicine specialists, and a general surgeon with a special interest in abdominal wall disorders.[2]

TERMINOLOGY

Athletic pubalgia is an ill-defined term used in the literature. It is used to detail a constellation of symptoms that involve the inguinal region and core. Core muscle injury refers to damage to any skeletal muscle within the area between the chest and mid-thigh.[1] One of the difficulties with diagnosing athletic pubalgia is an inconclusive agreed upon nomenclature. Nonspecific terms including sports hernia, sportsman's hernia, sportsman's groin, athletic pubalgia, sports pubalgia, incipient hernia, Gilmore groin, hockey groin, and core muscle injury have been used, among others.[2] At our institution we have chosen to use the term core muscle injury. This terminology does not correlate with any anatomic structures, creating potential confusion for practitioners. Although none of these terms are perfect, they all seek to describe a poorly understood disease.[2] Historically, much of the literature on core muscle injury has been outside of the orthopedic arena. More recently, there has been an increasing awareness for core muscle injury among orthopedists owing to the growing number of diagnoses among high-profile athletes.[2]

HISTORY

Athletes presenting with a core muscle injury often report worsening groin pain located about the pubic symphysis, which may radiate into the lower abdomen or proximal adductors. Most patients describe an insidious onset of symptoms, but some recall a traumatic event involving a trunk hyperextension, hip hyperabduction mechanism.[5] Activities that involve repetitive cutting, pivoting, kicking, sprinting, or sudden acceleration–deceleration movements typically incite the pain.[6] Sports such as soccer, ice hockey, basketball, football, skiing, and rugby have been implicated as having a higher incidence of core muscle injury compared with other sports.[7] The cessation of rigorous activity may temporarily alleviate the pain, but symptoms often return once the athlete returns to sport without treatment. The pain may also be aggravated by coughing, sneezing, or sit-ups, and it is not uncommon for the pain to radiate into the perineum, inner thigh, or testicles.[6]

ANATOMY AND PATHOPHYSIOLOGY

A detailed understanding of inguinal anatomy is essential when evaluating the athlete presenting with a core muscle injury. Multiple musculotendinous, ligamentous, neurovascular, and bony structures converge in the inguinal region, which can make determining the specific underlying etiology a diagnostic challenge.

The rectus abdominis is a long, flat, paired muscle that spans the entire length of the anterior abdominal wall. It originates from the pubic symphysis, pubic crests, and pubic tubercles and it inserts onto the xiphoid process and costal cartilages of ribs V through VII.[8]

The lower abdomen is organized into several distinct layers on either side of the rectus muscle (**Fig. 1**). The most superficial layer beneath the skin and subcutaneous tissue is formed by the external oblique muscle and fascia. The external oblique muscle originates from the lower 8 ribs and inserts onto the iliac crest, anterior superior iliac spine, and pubic tubercle. Inferiorly, the external oblique aponeurosis is

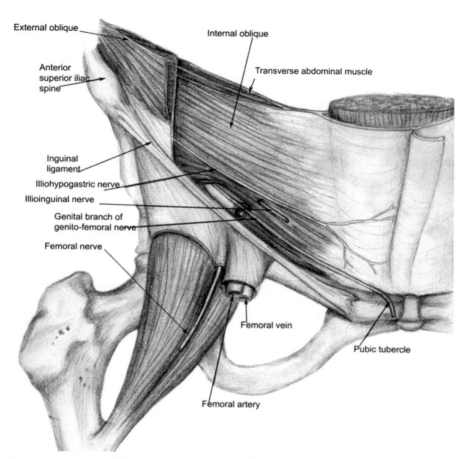

Fig. 1. Abdominal wall layers and their contributions to the inguinal canal. (*From* Firooza-badi R, Stafford P, Routt M. Inguinal abnormalities in male patients with acetabular fractures treated using an ilioinguinal exposure. Archives of Bone and Joint Surgery. 2015 Oct;3(4):274, with permission).

contiguous with the inguinal ligament. The inguinal ligament originates from the anterior superior iliac spine and inserts onto the pubic tubercle, forming the base of the inguinal canal. Together, the external oblique aponeurosis and inguinal ligament form the external inguinal ring that lies superficial and lateral to the pubic tubercle.[3]

The next layer deep to the external oblique muscle is formed by the internal oblique muscle and fascia. The internal oblique muscle originates from the iliac crest, thoracolumbar fascia, and lateral inguinal ligament. The internal oblique muscle forms the superior portion of the inguinal canal and envelopes the spermatic cord (or round ligament in females), the genital branch of the genitofemoral nerve, and the ilioinguinal nerve.[3]

The deepest structures of the abdominal wall are the transversus abdominis muscle and transversalis fascia. The transversus abdominis muscle originates from the thoracolumbar fascia, iliac crest, lateral inguinal ligament, and the costal cartilages of ribs VII through XII. The transversalis fascia forms the internal inguinal ring, which marks the entryway for the spermatic cord (or round ligament) into the inguinal canal.[3] Distally, the transversus abdominus and internal oblique muscles merge to form the conjoint tendon. The conjoint tendon blends with fibers of the rectus sheath and external oblique aponeurosis as they attach to the pubic tubercle. These fibers in turn coalesce with the origins of the adductor longus and gracilis tendons forming the "aponeurotic plate" anterior to the pubic symphysis (**Fig. 2**).[3,5]

Thus, the pubic symphysis is the focal point of the complex muscular anatomy of the lower abdomen.[9] A nonsynovial amphiarthroidal joint, the pubic symphysis marks the convergence of the 2 pubic bones at the center of the anterior pelvis. The pubic bones are separated by a fibrocartilaginous disk and are rigidly connected by anterior, posterior, superior, and inferior ligaments. The inferior ligament, or arcuate ligament, spans both inferior pubic rami and confers the greatest stability to the joint.[10] The rigidity of the pubic symphysis limits shear and tensile stresses, allowing it to act as a fulcrum for the muscular and ligamentous structures that attach to the aponeurotic plate.[5,9,10]

Given this complex anatomy, 3 prevailing theories exist with regard to the pathophysiologic causes of core muscle injury.[11,12] The first theory is that muscular imbalance between the rectus abdominis and the adductors leads to injury about the aponeurotic plate (**Fig. 3**).[13–15] A second theory suggests that pain related to core muscle injury stems from either a defect or weakness within the posterior inguinal canal.[2,16,17] Last, a third theory proposes that weakness of the posterior inguinal canal leads to dynamic compression of the genital branch of the genitofemoral nerve resulting in neuropathic pain.[12] Therefore, the management of core muscle injuries is aimed at identifying and treating the underlying anatomic etiology of the patient's pain.

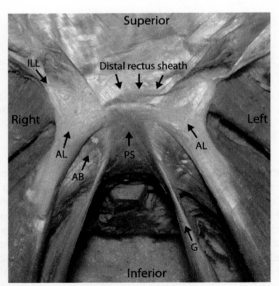

Fig. 2. Cadaveric dissection demonstrating the anatomic insertions at the aponeurotic plate. AB, adductor brevis tendon; AL, adductor longus tendon; G, gracilis; ILL, Ilioinguinal ligament; PS, pubic symphysis. (*From* Norton-old KJ, Schache AG, Barker PJ, Clark RA, Harrison SM, Briggs CA. Anatomic and mechanical relationship between the proximal attachment of adductor longus and the distal rectus sheath. Clinical Anatomy. 2013 May;26(4):522-30, with permission).

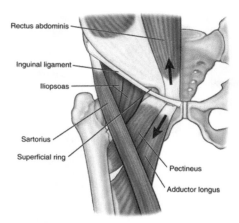

Fig. 3. The major force vectors acting at the aponeurotic plate. The *yellow arrows* indicate the opposing pull of the rectus abdominis and adductor longus. Note the proximity of the superficial (external) inguinal ring. (*From* DeLee, Drez and Miller's Orthopaedic Sports Medicine, 5th Edition, 2019, Elsevier; with permission.)

PHYSICAL EXAMINATION

Physical examination of an athlete presenting with a suspected core muscle injury should begin with direct visualization of the inguinal region. The patient's skin must be examined for any signs of ecchymosis or swelling that could indicate an acute injury, and any scars or previous surgical incisions should be documented.

After a careful visual inspection, palpation of several key anatomic landmarks should occur. The pubic symphysis, pubic tubercles, rectus abdominis tendon, conjoint tendons, and adductor longus tendons should all be palpated, and any localized tenderness or palpable defects should be noted. The external inguinal ring must also be assessed to rule out the possibility of an inguinal hernia (**Fig. 4**). According to the British Hernia Society's position statement from 2014, a diagnosis of a sports hernia can be made if 3 of the following 5 criteria are confirmed on clinical examination[18]:

1. Pinpoint tenderness over the pubic tubercle at the point of insertion of the conjoint tendon.
2. Palpable tenderness over the deep inguinal ring.
3. Pain and/or dilation of the external ring with no obvious hernia evident.
4. Pain at the origin of the adductor longus tendon.
5. Dull, diffuse pain in the groin, often radiating to the perineum and inner thigh or across the midline.

Further provocative testing is also helpful in determining the underlying etiology. Having the patient cough or perform a Valsalva maneuver classically reproduces groin pain in patients with a core muscle injury. Pain with resisted sit-ups can be indicative of rectus abdominis or conjoint tendon pathology (**Fig. 5**). Sit-ups can be performed with the patient's hips straight, at 45° flexion, and 90° of flexion to stress the rectus muscle in several different planes. The oblique muscles can be further isolated by asking the patient to perform a lateral bend against resistance toward the affected side. Pain with passive hip abduction or resisted hip adduction are suggestive of adductor longus tendon pathology.[19]

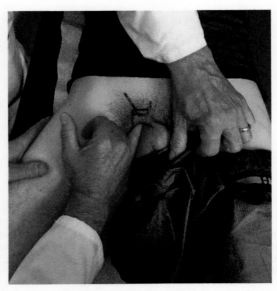

Fig. 4. Clinical photograph demonstrating the examiner palpating for an inguinal hernia at the external inguinal ring.

Last, careful consideration must be given to the patient's hip joint owing to the high association between core muscle injuries and femoroacetabular impingement (FAI).[20] Hip range of motion bilaterally should be evaluated in flexion/extension, abduction/adduction, and internal/external rotation. Provocative tests such as flexion, abduction, and external rotation; flexion, adduction, and internal rotation; and McCarthy's sign should also be performed to rule out a concomitant diagnosis of FAI.

In patients who exhibit a mixed clinical examination, injections can be used for both diagnostic and therapeutic purposes. The resolution of symptoms after the administration of a local anesthetic with or without a corticosteroid to either the rectus attachment, adductor longus origin, or pubic symphysis are more consistent with a

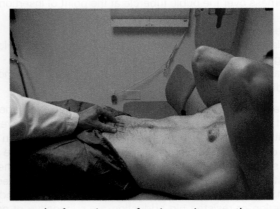

Fig. 5. Clinical photograph of a patient performing a sit-up as the examiner palpates the rectus insertion at the pubic tubercles.

diagnosis of core muscle injury. Pain relief with an intra-articular hip injection suggests a pathology related to FAI.[21]

IMAGING

Diagnostic imaging is valuable for both confirming the presence of a core muscle injury and excluding other causes from the differential. Radiographs of the pelvis and hip are the initial imaging modality of choice in all patients presenting with groin pain.

A standard anteroposterior view of the pelvis can be used to evaluate the pubic symphysis for any abnormal widening or erosive changes. Dedicated hip radiographs including an anteroposterior, frog-leg lateral, cross-table lateral, false profile view, and modified 45° Dunn view are all useful for evaluating FAI. Other pathologies that should always be considered include pelvic avulsion fractures, stress fractures, apophyseal injuries, apophysitis, degenerative joint disease, and hip dysplasia.[3,5]

Although radiographs are a useful screening tool, MRI is the imaging modality of choice for evaluating a core muscle injury. A dedicated sports hernia MRI protocol is recommended to enhance visualization of the affected area.[22] Standard coronal, sagittal, and axial sequences with a large field of view should be obtained first. These images are useful for evaluating the entire pelvis and ruling out other concomitant pathology such as osteitis pubis, osteonecrosis, stress fractures, tumors, myotendinous injuries, and intra-articular disorders.[5] A smaller field of view with a higher resolution is necessary to focus on the pubic symphysis and aponeurotic plate. Coronal oblique and axial oblique sequences through the rectus abdominis insertion and pubic symphysis give the most accurate representation of the anatomy.[22] Tears of the aponeurotic plate, fluid undermining the aponeurosis, and abnormal marrow signal in 1 or both pubic bones are best visualized on the axial oblique and sagittal sequences. Partial or complete tears of the adductor musculature are better appreciated on coronal oblique sequences. Overall, MRI has been found to be 68% sensitive and 100% specific for rectus abdominis pathology and 86% sensitive and 89% specific for adductor longus pathology. (**Figs. 6** and **7**)[23]

An estimated one-third of patients may not demonstrate any significant findings on MRI.[3] In this subset of patients computed tomography arthrography has been

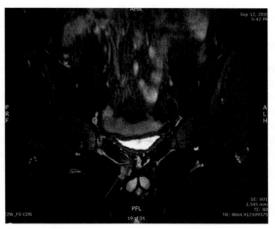

Fig. 6. Coronal fat-saturated T2-weighted MRI of a 17-year-old male with a right-sided adductor longus tendon strain (*red arrow*).

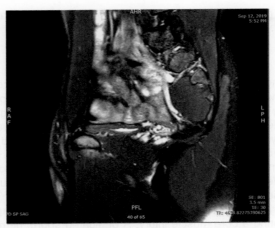

Fig. 7. Sagittal proton density-weighted MRI of a 17-year-old male with disruption of the rectus insertion at the right pubic tubercle with fluid undermining the pubic aponeurosis (*red arrow*). Also note the increased bone marrow edema in the pubis (*blue arrow*).

described as a useful adjunct that can identify tearing of the rectus or adductor insertions at the aponeurotic plate. Computed tomography arthrography is performed by injecting radiopaque dye into the pubic symphysis and can be used for diagnostic as well as therapeutic purposes.[24]

Dynamic ultrasound examination is another useful adjunct that can demonstrate posterior inguinal canal deficiency in real time. Ultrasound examination has several distinct advantages over MRI. It involves a direct patient interaction with flexible fields of view, and it allows observation of the patients' anatomy at both rest and under stress. It is also less expensive than MRI and, like computed tomography arthrography, can be used to guide diagnostic and therapeutic injections.[25] Dynamic ultrasound examination is performed by positioning the probe over the inguinal canal and then instructing the patient to perform a Valsalva maneuver. If an anterior bulge in the posterior wall of the inguinal canal is visualized, the test is considered positive. However, it is important to note that ultrasound techniques are highly operator dependent and should only be performed by an experienced technician.[2]

DIFFERENTIAL DIAGNOSIS

The differential diagnosis for groin pain is sizable (**Box 1**). Like with most conditions, a thorough history and physical examination can aid in the clinical diagnosis. Owing to the wide range of pathologies on the differential, there can be several that occur concomitantly. Further adding to the diagnostic difficulty is the fact that many of these pathologies fall under the umbrella of several different medical specialties. Imaging studies can also be beneficial in these cases once a history and physical examination have been completed. As mentioned elsewhere in this article, a thorough history, detailed physical examination, and evaluation of imaging studies can help to confirm the diagnosis.

NONOPERATIVE MANAGEMENT

Groin pain and abdominal wall injuries are frequently encountered among practitioners who care for athletes. In many instances, the injury goes on to heal and is self-limited.[2]

Box 1
Differential diagnosis of groin pain

Hernia
  Inguinal
    Direct
    Indirect
  Femoral

Visceral
  Inflammatory bowel disease
  Diverticulitis
  Crohn's disease

Genitourinary disease
  Testicular pathology
    Torsion
    Carcinoma
  Prostatitis
  Urethritis
  Epididymitis
  Orchitis
  Ovarian disease
  Pelvic inflammatory disease
  Endometriosis

Lumbar pathology
  Spinal stenosis
  Radiculopathy
  Herniated nucleus pulposus
  Degenerative joint disease
  Spondylolisthesis

Hip pathology
  Femoroacetabular impingement
  Labral tear
  Degenerative joint disease
  Avascular necrosis
  Snapping hip
  Iliotibial band syndrome
  Fracture/stress fracture
  Hip dysplasia
  Apophyseal injuries

Theoretic causes of core muscle injury
  Conjoint tendon tear
  Inguinal ligament tear
  Posterior canal weakness
  External oblique muscle strain/tear
  External ring tear
  Superficial ring dilation
  Rectus abdominis strain/tear
  Adductor longus tendon strain/tear
  Pubic joint instability

Despite the typical signs and symptoms, a trial of conservative therapy should be the first-line treatment.[2] There is some controversy in the literature about the efficacy of physical therapy versus surgery.[1] Some studies have reported that these injuries improve with rest but are reaggravated when activities are reinitiated. Although this may be the case in some, giving the body the opportunity to heal itself and potentially saving someone an unnecessary surgery is worth the risk. The literature has reported that nonoperative, exercise-based therapy has shown success ranging from 40% to 100%, the latter being closer to what we see in our patient population.[26] Surgery is only used for those who have failed conservative management. A minimum of 2 months of rehabilitation before any surgical intervention should be attempted first, whereas other studies have recommended waiting 3 to 6 months before surgical repair.[3] At our institution, it is unusual to perform surgery earlier than 3 months from the onset of symptoms.[2]

A 3- to 4-week trial of rest and oral nonsteroidal anti-inflammatory drugs is the mainstay in nonoperative treatment. Athletes should also be allowed to do closed chain lower extremity exercises during the rest period. Core strengthening and improving range of motion should also be emphasized during therapy. Specific exercises should include strengthening of the gluteus medius and maximus, transversus abdominis, erector spinae, lateral abdominis, hip flexors, and hamstrings.[3] This strengthening can help in the correction of the dynamic pathologic anterior pelvic tilt seen in core muscle injury and hamstring tightness.[27] The overall goal of therapy is to strengthen the stabilizers of functional motion and posture.[3] Sport-specific exercises should be introduced back into the routine later into the rest period.

Adjuncts to nonoperative therapy include a short course of oral corticosteroids with a taper or an injection of corticosteroid or platelet-rich plasma into the site of injury or inflammation.[1,2] Corticosteroid injections are used commonly in our practice. We tend to inject the site of most pain between the rectus abdominus attachment and/or adductor longus origin. If injecting one site, we use 4 mL of 0.25% bupivacaine hydrochloride and 1 mL of 80 mg methylprednisolone acetate (**Figs. 8** and **9**). When we

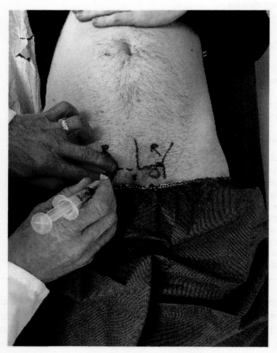

Fig. 8. Clinical photograph demonstrating a corticosteroid injection being administered to the rectus insertion at the right pubic tubercle.

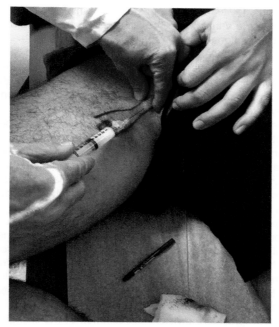

Fig. 9. Clinical photograph demonstrating a corticosteroid injection being administered to the right adductor longus tendon origin.

inject more than 1 site, we split the steroid between the sites so as to not go exceed 80 mg of corticosteroid. Although platelet-rich plasma has become more popular among physicians treating athletes, there have not been any prospective studies evaluating its efficacy in core muscle injury.[1] Thus, platelet-rich plasma does not have a role in our practice currently.

At the completion of the nonoperative rest period, a return-to-sport assessment is undertaken with the athlete. If successful, they are able to return to their sport. If pain persists, we leave it up to the athlete as to whether or not they believe that they can complete the season with the pain they have. Playing through the pain is not believed to worsen the tear or the surgical results of the repair.[2] Most athletes opt for surgical intervention in the off-season and once they have exhausted all of their nonoperative options.

OPERATIVE INTERVENTION

Given the variety of treatment options in the literature with similar results, the British Hernia Society recommends that the choice of surgery and operative approach be based on surgeon experience.[3] Many operative approaches have been described in the literature. The goal however remains the same despite the approach, that is, to relieve and minimize tension on the pubic joint while diminishing compression of the inguinal sensory nerves as well as repairing or reinforcing defects of the inguinal canal.[26] Treatment is aimed at restoring normal anatomy around the pubic bone. The 3 previously mentioned pathologic theories for the cause of core muscle injury are at the center of the treatment algorithm. This goal can be accomplished through open or laparoscopic techniques. Each of the techniques is a variation on an established operation for conventional groin hernia repairs.[2]

The most common open techniques include the mesh repair and sutured repair. The open mesh repairs are a variation on the Lichtenstein technique and have become very popular for conventional hernia repairs in the United States.[2] The thought is that the mesh will reinforce weakness in the abdominal wall and redistribute tension on the pubic joint.[26] Although mesh repairs are very common and recommended by many leading authors, there still is concern for mesh-related inguinodynia and persistent pain.[26] The success of the procedure has ranged in studies from 82% to 100% with return-to-play rates ranging from 93% to 100%.[26]

Open sutured repairs are probably the most common technique used for core muscle injury.[2] The sutured repairs satisfy the need to create stability of the anterior pelvis and can be performed in a number of different ways.[2] This stabilization is often done by broadening the attachment of the rectus abdominis insertion to the pubic bone and inguinal ligament.[2] Our preferred technique, a modified Bassini repair, reconstitutes the anterior column of the rectus muscle and secondarily reinforces the posterior inguinal wall (**Fig. 10**).[26]

The minimal repair of Muschaweck is done by opening the transversalis fascia and creating a plication repair by lateralizing the rectus abdominis.[26] In the Meyers repair, the rectus abdominis is reinforced to the pubic bone and lateralized to the inguinal ligament.[26] This technique also involves a complete epimysiotomy to free the adductor longus tendon. The epimysia is then sutured to the enthesial plate.[26] Treatment success for open sutured repairs in the literature has ranged from 79% to 100% with return-to-play rates of 64% to 100%.[26]

Performing a decompression, division, or resection of the ilioinguinal or genitofemoral nerves in the setting of an open core muscle injury repair remains controversial. It has been hypothesized that excessive scar tissue formation postoperatively can cause nerve irritation and chronic lower abdominal pain. Much of the reported literature demonstrates excellent or equivalent outcomes without neurectomy and, therefore, we do not routinely perform this procedure at our institution.[2]

The 2 most common laparoscopic techniques are the transabdominal preperitoneal approach and the totally extraperitoneal approach. Both are mesh repairs. With the transabdominal preperitoneal approach, the peritoneal cavity is entered, a flap of

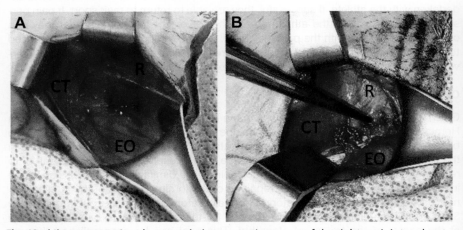

Fig. 10. (*A*) Intraoperative photograph demonstrating a tear of the right conjoint and rectus tendons (*B*) Photograph demonstrating the final repair of the defect. CT, conjoint tendon; EO, folded/shelving edge of the external oblique aponeurosis; R, rectus.

peritoneum is raised in the inguinal region, and a piece of mesh is placed in the pre-peritoneal space.[2] The peritoneum is not entered during the totally extraperitoneal approach. The dissection is maintained in the preperitoneal space where the mesh is appropriately placed in the inguinal region.[2]

Operative intervention for chronic adductor longus tendinopathy that is recalcitrant to conservative management is also associated with good outcomes. Several techniques have been described to address this pathology, including adductor repair, adductor longus tenotomy (**Fig. 11**), percutaneous partial tendon release, and, more recently, endoscopic tendon lengthening.[28,29]

Jørgensen and colleagues[30] recently performed a systematic review of the literature to evaluate the efficacy of surgical treatment options for core muscle injury. Eleven studies in this review evaluated the usefulness of adductor tenotomy alone in patients with chronic tendinopathy recalcitrant to conservative treatment. Nine of these 11 studies reported on the return to habitual activity. Of 323 patients, 287 (90%) were able to return to their daily activities at an average of 12 weeks postoperatively. Additionally, 6 of the 11 studies reviewed reported pain outcome measures. Of 70 patients, 63 (90%) reported no pain at final follow-up.[30]

Gill and colleagues[31] evaluated the outcomes of 32 professional and collegiate-level athletes who underwent open adductor longus tenotomy after failing conservative management. Twenty patients had concomitant core muscle injury pathology requiring repair and 12 patients underwent an isolated adductor tenotomy. Thirty-one athletes (97%) returned to their previous sport and 30 (94%) were able to return to their previous level of play. No patients reported any functional weakness or decreases in running speed or power. Furthermore, there were no statistical differences in the performance scores between the athletes who underwent isolated adductor tenotomy versus those who also underwent concomitant core muscle injury repair.[31]

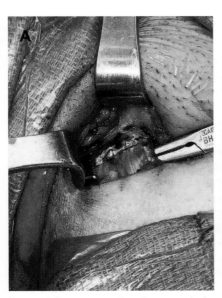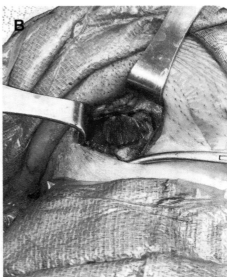

Fig. 11. (A) Intraoperative photograph demonstrating a left adductor longus origin on the pubic tubercle with planned level of resection. (B) Photograph of the same patient after complete tenotomy of the tendinous insertion of the adductor longus. The muscular origin beneath the tendon is now visible.

More recently, an endoscopic adductor longus tendon lengthening technique has been described. This technique allows for complete visualization of the adductor longus origin while mitigating the risk of wound healing complications observed in more open and invasive techniques. However, further investigation and long-term follow-up is still required to compare endoscopic release to more traditional surgical approaches.[28]

It is important to consider that groin injuries can involve more than just the rectus abdominis and the adductor longus. FAI can be a poor predictor of successful core muscle surgery.[3] FAI has been reported in as few as 12% but as many as 94% of patients with core muscle injuries.[32] In a systematic review of 72 articles on athletic groin pain, FAI was listed as the top cause for pain at 32%, followed by core muscle injury at 24%.[33] The treatment team should have a high suspicion for FAI given its prevalence in the athletic population. This finding again demonstrates the importance of a detailed history and physical examination on each patient with groin-related pain.

SUMMARY

Core muscle injuries are a significant cause of pain and lost playing time in sports, and they present a difficult problem for both athletes and health care practitioners alike. The complex anatomy of the inguinal region can make establishing the diagnosis quite challenging. A thorough history and clinical examination combined with the appropriate imaging studies will help to narrow down an extensive differential. A multidisciplinary team composed of athletic trainers, physical therapists, radiologists, sports medicine physicians, and general surgeons with extensive experience in treating abdominal wall disorders is beneficial in determining the best treatment approach. Core muscle injuries can respond well to conservative measures, yet there are still many athletes who will not improve with nonsurgical treatment. When operative intervention is indicated, surgical repair directed at the underlying anatomic defect is associated with excellent outcomes in returning athletes to their preinjury level of function.

CLINICS CARE POINTS

- Core muscle injury is one of many terms used to detail a constellation of symptoms that involve the core and inguinal region. It is also a nonanatomic, nondiagnostic term.[3]

- Most core muscle injuries are self-limited. Only a small percentage cause symptoms for more than 3 weeks.[2]

- Nonoperative, exercise-based therapy has shown success ranging from 40% to 100%.[26]

- There is a strong correlation between core muscle injury and FAI, as high as 94% that, when not appropriately diagnosed, can lead to unsuccessful outcomes.[32]

- Many of the operative techniques to treat core muscle injury are a variation on an established operation for conventional groin hernia repairs.[2]

- The literature on operative success rates for core muscle injury have ranged from 79% to 100% with return-to-play rates of 64% to 100%.[26]

- An open adductor tenotomy is associated with 97% rate of return to sport with minimal functional deficits in professional and collegiate-level athletes.[31]

DISCLOSURE

The authors have nothing to disclose.

REFERENCES

1. Poor AE, Roedl JB, Zoga AC, et al. Core muscle injuries in athletes. Curr Sports Med Rep 2018;17(2):54–8.
2. Litwin DE, Sneider EB, Mcenaney PM, et al. Athletic pubalgia (Sports Hernia). Clin Sports Med 2011;30(2):417–34.
3. Hopkins JN, Brown W, Lee CA. Sports hernia: definition, evaluation, and treatment. JBJS Rev 2017;5(9):e6.
4. Zoland MP, Iraci JC, Bharam S, et al. Sports hernia/athletic pubalgia among women. Orthop J Sports Med 2018;6(9). 2325967118796494.
5. Larson CM. Sports hernia/athletic pubalgia: evaluation and management. Sports Health 2014;6(2):139–44.
6. Choi HR, Elattar O, Dills VD, et al. Return to play after sports hernia surgery. Clin Sports Med 2016;35(4):621–36.
7. Farber AJ, Wilckens JH. Sports hernia: diagnosis and therapeutic approach. J Am Acad Orthop Surg 2007;15(8):507–14.
8. Drake RL, Vogl W, Mitchell AWM, et al. Grays anatomy for students. 2nd edition. Philadelphia (PA): Elsevier/Churchill Livingstone; 2005. p. 276–7.
9. Meyers WC, Yoo E, Devon ON, et al. Understanding "sports hernia" (athletic pubalgia): the anatomic and pathophysiologic basis for abdominal and groin pain in athletes. Oper Tech Sports Med 2012;20(1):33–45.
10. Gamble JG, Simmons SC, Freedman MA. The symphysis pubis. Anatomic and pathologic considerations. Clin Orthop Relat Res 1986;(203):261–72.
11. Miller MD, Thompson SR. 5th edition. DeLee, Drez, & Millers orthopaedic sports medicine: principles and practice, vol. 2. Philadelphia (PA): Elsevier; 2020. p. 1007–8.
12. Brunt LM. Hernia management in the athlete. Adv Surg 2016;50(1):187–202.
13. Norton-old KJ, Schache AG, Barker PJ, et al. Anatomical and mechanical relationship between the proximal attachment of adductor longus and the distal rectus sheath. Clin Anat 2013;26(4):522–30.
14. Riff AJ, Movassaghi K, Beck EC, et al. Surface mapping of the musculotendinous attachments at the pubic symphysis in cadaveric specimens: implications for the treatment of core muscle injury. Arthroscopy 2019;35(8):2358–64.
15. Ross JR, Stone RM, Larson CM. Core muscle injury/sports hernia/athletic pubalgia, and femoroacetabular impingement. Sports Med Arthrosc Rev 2015;23: 213–20.
16. Malycha P, Lovell G. Inguinal surgery in athletes with chronic groin pain: the "sportsman's" hernia. Aust N Z J Surg 1992;62(2):123–5.
17. Polglase AL, Frydman GM, Farmer KC. Inguinal surgery for debilitating chronic groin pain in athletes. Med J Aust 1991;155(10):674–7.
18. Sheen AJ, Stephenson BM, Lloyd DM, et al. 'Treatment of the sportsman's groin': British Hernia Society's 2014 position statement based on the Manchester Consensus Conference. Br J Sports Med 2014;48(14):1079–87.
19. Emblom BA, Mathis T, Aune K. Athletic pubalgia secondary to rectus abdominis–adductor longus aponeurotic plate injury: diagnosis, management, and operative treatment of 100 competitive athletes. Orthop J Sports Med 2018;6(9). 2325967118798333.
20. Economopoulos KJ, Milewski MD, Hanks JB, et al. Radiographic evidence of femoroacetabular impingement in athletes with athletic pubalgia. Sports Health 2014;6(2):171–7.

21. McCarthy E, Hegazi TM, Zoga AC, et al. Ultrasound-guided interventions for core and hip injuries in athletes. Radiol Clin 2016;54(5):875–92.
22. Lee SC, Endo Y, Potter HG. Imaging of groin pain: magnetic resonance and ultrasound imaging features. Sports Health 2017;9(5):428–35.
23. Omar IM, Zoga AC, Kavanagh EC, et al. Athletic pubalgia and "sports hernia": optimal MR imaging technique and findings. Radiographics 2008;28(5):1415–38.
24. McArthur TA, Narducci CA, Lopez-Ben RR. The role of pubic symphyseal CT arthrography in the imaging of athletic pubalgia. Am J Roentgenol 2014;203(5): 1063–8.
25. Morley N, Grant T, Blount K, et al. Sonographic evaluation of athletic pubalgia. Skeletal Radiol 2016;45(5):689–99.
26. Zuckerbraun BS, Cyr AR, Mauro CS. Groin pain syndrome known as sports hernia. JAMA Surg 2020;155(4):340–8.
27. Kuszewski MT, Gnat R, Gogola A. The impact of core muscles training on the range of anterior pelvic tilt in subjects with increased stiffness of the hamstrings. Hum Mov Sci 2018;57:32–9.
28. Bharam S, Bhagat PV, Spira MC, et al. Endoscopic proximal adductor lengthening for chronic adductor-related groin pain. Arthrosc Tech 2018;7(6):e675–8.
29. Rizio L, Salvo JP, Schürhoff MR, et al. Adductor longus rupture in professional football players: acute repair with suture anchors: a report of two cases. Am J Sports Med 2004;32(1):243–5.
30. Jørgensen SG, Öberg S, Rosenberg J. Treatment of longstanding groin pain: a systematic review. Hernia 2019;23. 1-0.
31. Gill TJ, Wall AJ, Gwathmey FW, et al. Surgical release of the adductor longus with or without sports hernia repair is a useful treatment for recalcitrant groin strains in the elite athlete. Orthop J Sports Med 2019;8(1). 2325967119896104.
32. Munegato D. Sports hernia and femoroacetabular impingement in athletes: a systematic review. World J Clin Cases 2015;3(9):823.
33. Sa DD, Hölmich P, Phillips M, et al. Athletic groin pain: a systematic review of surgical diagnoses, investigations, and treatment. Br J Sports Med 2016;50(19): 1181–6.

Proximal Hamstring Injuries

Amanda N. Fletcher, MD, MS[a], Jonathan W. Cheah, MD[b],
Shane J. Nho, MD, MS[c], Richard C. Mather III, MD, MBA[d],*

KEYWORDS

- Hamstring • Injury • Proximal hamstring injuries • Tendinosis • Tendinopathy
- Strain • Rupture • Chronic insertional tendinosis

KEY POINTS

- Proximal hamstring injuries can present as chronic tendinosis, acute strain, partial tendinous avulsions, or complete 3-tendon rupture. The mechanism of injury results from chronic repetitive or acute eccentric loading during hip flexion and knee extension.
- Patients often present with posterior hip pain located at the buttock/ischial tuberosity, posterior thigh ecchymosis, or a mass of retracted muscle if acutely injured, a stiff-leg gait, and exacerbation of pain with hip flexion and knee extension.
- Nonoperative management for chronic insertional tendinosis and low-grade, partial tears includes activity modification, oral anti-inflammatories, and physical therapy. Platelet-rich plasma injections, corticosteroid injections, dry needling, and shock wave therapy are newer treatment modalities being studied that may provide additional benefit.
- Surgical indications include complete, proximal avulsions; partial avulsions with least 2 tendons injured with greater than 2 cm of retraction in young and active patients; and partial avulsion injuries that have failed nonoperative management.
- Surgical management entails open primary repair, endoscopic primary repair, or augmentation/reconstruction.

INTRODUCTION

Hamstring injuries are one of the most frequently occurring injuries in sports, accounting for 12% to 29% of all injuries in athletes.[1–7] After an initial injury, athletes have increased rates of reinjury as high as 22% to 34%.[6–9] Injuries can occur at any level of the musculotendinous unit. Proximal hamstring injuries represent 12% of all hamstring injuries, whereas most injuries occur more commonly at the

[a] Department of Orthopaedic Surgery, Duke University Medical Center, 311 Trent Drive, Durham, NC 27710, USA; [b] Department of Orthopaedic Surgery, Santa Clara Valley Medical Center, 751 South Bascom Avenue, San Jose, CA 95128, USA; [c] Department of Orthopaedic Surgery, Midwest Orthopaedics at Rush, 1611 West Harrison Street, Orthopedic Building Suite 400, Chicago, IL 60612, USA; [d] Department of Orthopaedic Surgery, Duke University Medical Center, Duke Sports Science Institute, 3475 Erwin Road, Durham, NC 27705, USA
* Corresponding author.
E-mail address: mathe016@duke.edu

Clin Sports Med 40 (2021) 339–361
https://doi.org/10.1016/j.csm.2021.01.003
0278-5919/21/© 2021 Elsevier Inc. All rights reserved.

musculotendinous junction.[10] These injuries include a spectrum of disease from strain to complete rupture. Although proximal hamstring pathology has historically been recognized, proximal injuries were not reported on until 1988 when the first case series of complete proximal hamstring avulsions was published.[11] The management of these injuries continues to evolve depending on the severity of injury and patient-specific factors.

PERTINENT ANATOMY

There are 3 hamstring muscles: the semimembranosus, semitendinosus, and the long head of the biceps femoris. These muscles share a common origin at the ischial tuberosity; however, with 2 distinct footprints, as seen in **Fig. 1**. The semimembranosus originates from the superolateral ischial tuberosity. The semitendinosus and long head of the biceps femoris form the conjoint tendon, which originates medial to the semimembranosus at the superomedial ischial tuberosity. The hamstring muscles cross both the hip and knee joint, inserting distally below the knee on the proximal tibia. The hamstring muscles are innervated by the tibial branch of the sciatic nerve and receive their arterial supply from the perforating branches of profunda femoris artery, inferior gluteal artery, and the superior muscular branches of popliteal artery. Together the hamstring muscles extend the thigh, flex the knee, and internally rotate the tibia. They are active throughout the gait cycle, but primarily in terminal swing phase to slow knee extension.[1] The hamstrings also help initiate hip extension and continue to function during early stance phase to assist with hip extension.[1]

RISK FACTORS FOR HAMSTRING INJURY

Several risk factors for hamstring injuries have been proposed in the literature, including decreased flexibility,[12-14] strength deficits,[15] muscle fatigue,[16] poor core stability,[17] lack of proper warm-up,[18] poor lumbar posture,[14] and a prior hamstring injury.[19,20] Previous hamstring strain has been recognized as the strongest risk factor for recurrent strain among all the risk factors examined with an increased risk of recurrence by 2 to 6 times.[19-21] In addition, a 2015 epidemiologic study investigating hamstring injury in 25 National Collegiate Athletic Association sports demonstrated a higher rate of hamstring injury in male athletes than female athletes, specifically for soccer, baseball/softball, and indoor track.[22]

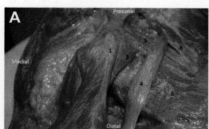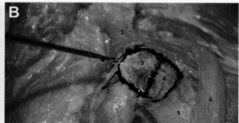

Fig. 1. (A) The gross anatomy of the proximal hamstring complex including the conjoint tendon. (A) is labeled as follows: (1) conjoint tendon, (2) semimembranosus, (3) superior gemellus, (4) sciatic nerve, (5) quadratus femoris, (6) piriformis. (B) is labeled as follows: (1) sacrotuberous ligament, (2) semitendinosus direct muscular attachment (3) conjoint tendon footprint, (4) semimembranosus footprint, (5) quadratus femoris, (6) sciatic nerve.

INJURY CLASSIFICATION

Hamstring injuries can occur at any level along the musculotendinous unit, but commonly occur at the myotendinous junction. Koulouris and Connell[10] demonstrated that only 12% of hamstring muscle injuries were proximal ruptures and 9% were complete. Understanding the location, severity, and acuity of proximal hamstring injuries is important when considering management options. When evaluating the injury severity and appropriate management options, classification considerations include the following:

Grade

- First described by the American Medical Association subcommittee in 1966, the 3-grade system for acute muscle injuries can help classify hamstring injuries.[23]
  - Grade 1 (tendinosis): Muscle soreness with no appreciable muscle tearing, less than 5% loss of function/strength
  - Grade 2 (partial): Partial damage to the musculotendinous unit, reduced strength, some residual function
  - Grade 3 (complete): Complete tear across the whole cross-section of the musculotendinous unit or discontinuity of the tendon-bone unit, loss of function, may have a palpable gap or mass from retraction

Location

- Insertional:
  - Bony involvement
    - Periosteal, bony, or apophyseal avulsion
      - This is typically seen in younger patients that are skeletally immature. Referred to as a "hurdler's fracture" or also commonly seen in water skiers.
  - Tendinous avulsion
- Musculotendinous junction
- Midsubstance muscle injury

Acuity

- Acute: less than 6 weeks of symptoms
  - There is no consensus on the definition of acute with studies ranging from less than 4 to 12 weeks
- Chronic: more than 6 weeks of symptoms

Mechanism

- Traumatic: Identifiable injury
- Atraumatic (attritional): No known injury or inciting event

Number of Tendon Involvement

- Hamstring injuries can involve 1, 2, or all 3 tendons. The most commonly injured tendons include the semitendinosus and biceps; the semimembranosus is the least commonly injured.[24]

Specific Terms

- Tendinopathy: Umbrella term for any tendon condition
  - The term proximal hamstring tendinopathy is used to describe an overuse injury that involves pain at the attachment of the hamstring tendons to the ischial tuberosity.

- Tendinosis: Noninflammatory degeneration of a tendon, often from strain injuries
- Tendinitis: Acute inflammation of the tendon due to small micro-tears

Broadly speaking, proximal hamstring pathology can be divided into 3 main categories: chronic insertional tendinopathy, partial-thickness hamstring tears, and full-thickness hamstring tears. Chronic insertional tendinopathy was first described as "hamstring syndrome" in 1988 and is common among long-distance runners and hurdlers.[25]

MECHANISM OF INJURY

The mechanism of injury is typically a result of an eccentric load during hip flexion and knee extension that results in excessive hamstring tension. This may occur as an acute injury or in the setting of chronic overuse. High-risk activities include sprinting, water skiing, or other sporting activities that require rapid acceleration and deceleration.

CLINICAL PRESENTATION

Injuries can occur in both young athletes or middle to older-aged individuals who sustain sudden or repetitive hip flexion and knee extension. It is important to obtain a thorough history of the patient's symptoms and baseline functional level. Patients with an acute proximal hamstring injury typically report a "popping" sensation with sudden severe pain about their ischium/buttock and startup pain with ambulation. They may recount a mechanism of injury with sudden concurrent hip flexion and knee extension such as a "split" type mechanism. They often present with ecchymosis in the posterior thigh and avoidance of painful simultaneous hip flexion and knee extension resulting in a stiff-leg gait pattern.

Chronic insertional tendinopathy is often more vague and difficult to diagnose. Chronic pathology is more commonly seen in endurance athletes, most notable when participating in running sports in which terminal hip flexion and knee extension elicits symptoms.[26] Patients present with insidious onset of symptoms including an ill-defined pain at the ischial tuberosity with radiation distally down the muscle belly to the popliteal fossa. Pain with prolonged sitting is common. Functional pain exacerbated with acceleration activities is a more specific finding. Occasionally, sciatic nerve irritation can occur due to the close proximity of the nerve to the hamstrings resulting in posterior thigh pain and radiation down the leg.[27]

PHYSICAL EXAMINATION

The physical examination should consist of a comprehensive examination of the involved lower extremity, contralateral side, and lumbar spine. Observe the patient's gait for a stiff-leg pattern and avoidance of hip and knee flexion. Inspection should include examining the posterior thigh for ecchymosis, swelling, a local mass of retracted muscle, or other evidence of trauma. Tenderness to palpation at the ischial tuberosity is common. Palpation over the mid-thigh can identify avulsed or retracted tendons. Hip range of motion and strength (flexion, extension, adduction, abduction, internal rotation, and external rotation) and knee range of motion (flexion, extension) should be evaluated. Patients with a proximal hamstring injury may guard with attempted hip flexion and exhibit weakness due to pain. A careful neurologic evaluation should be performed to assess for sciatic nerve irritation, including posterior thigh sensation and distal motor and sensory function of the tibial and peroneal nerves.

Any neurologic deficits not limited to the sciatic nerve should warrant a further spine workup.

There have been a few studies evaluating the diagnostic accuracy of orthopedic special tests for hamstring injuries to determine their clinical utility.[28–31] Suggested provocative tests are outlined in **Table 1** with their corresponding sensitivity, specificity, positive and negative predictive values, and positive and negative likelihood ratios. These tests can be especially important in the setting of chronic pathology or partial injuries in which the presentation is more equivocal.

DIFFERENTIAL DIAGNOSIS OF POSTERIOR HIP PAIN

The differential diagnosis for posterior hip and thigh pain includes hamstring injuries, piriformis syndrome (also known as deep gluteal syndrome), ischiofemoral impingement, lumbar sciatic pain, ischial stress fractures, apophysitis, and local infection or malignancy. A few diagnoses outlined in **Table 2** including common signs or symptoms help differentiate them from hamstring injuries. Special tests to consider, which may help ascertain other diagnoses, include the straight leg test; piriformis stretch test; and a combination of hip extension, adduction, and external rotation. Positive tests may suggest sciatica, piriformis syndrome, or iliofemoral impingement, respectively.

IMAGING

Diagnostic imaging modalities include radiographs, ultrasound, and MRI. Patients with a suspected acute proximal hamstring injury may undergo a workup with an anterior-posterior radiograph of the pelvis to evaluate for a bony avulsion off of the ischial tuberosity, enthesopathy suggesting chronic changes, or other local bony pathology. However, plain radiographs are largely inconclusive for this diagnosis, which typically requires an ultrasound or MRI evaluation.

Musculoskeletal ultrasound is being increasingly used when resources and trained personnel are available. It is especially useful in the acute setting when MRI may not be readily available. When available, dynamic ultrasound (sonography) provides several advantages over radiographs, computed tomography (CT), and MRI, including decreased cost, portability, lack of ionizing radiation, dynamic soft tissue imaging, color Doppler or power Doppler imaging, and determination of focal tenderness to sonopalpation.[34,35] In a longitudinal study comparing sonographic and MRI assessments of acute and healing hamstring injuries, Connell and colleagues[36] found that sonography has a similar sensitivity as MRI in depicting acute hamstring injuries, whereas MRI is more sensitive for follow-up imaging of healing injuries. **Fig. 2** depicts normal and pathologic hamstring ultrasound images.

MRI should be reserved for a high index of suspicion for complete rupture or patients being considered for surgical treatment after not responding to conservative management. An MRI can determine tendinopathy versus a partial or complete rupture, number of tendons involved, and extent of retraction. Representative MRIs are shown in **Fig. 3**. Specific findings associated with tendinopathy include increased tendon size, peri-tendinous T2 signal, and ischial tuberosity edema.[24] Thompson and colleagues[37] have cautioned for conservative use of MRI given that there is a high prevalence of hamstring pathology found in the asymptomatic population. In 235 consecutive patients with a median age of 51 years (range 13–88), Thompson and colleagues[37] concluded that 65% of patients had some abnormality on MRI, 5% of which of were bilateral partial tears and 2% were bilateral complete tears. This was described as the age-related natural history of degenerative change to the proximal

Table 1
Special orthopedic tests for evaluating proximal hamstring pathology

Test	How to Perform	Positive	Data
Chronic proximal hamstring tendinopathy			
Puraenen-Orava[25]	Patient standing Actively stretch the hamstring muscles with the hip flexed at about 90°, the knee fully extended, and the foot on a solid support surface.	Exacerbation of patient's symptoms	Sensitivity: 0.76 Specificity: 0.82 PPV: 0.81 NPV: 0.77 Positive likelihood ratio: 4.2 Negative likelihood ratio: 0.29 (Cacchio et al., 2012)[29]
Bent knee stretch[32]	Patient supine The hip and knee of the symptomatic leg are maximally flexed, and the examiner slowly straightens the knee while keeping the hip flexed.	Exacerbation of patient's symptoms	Sensitivity: 0.84 Specificity: 0.87 PPV: 0.86 NPV: 0.85 Positive likelihood ratio: 6.5 Negative likelihood ratio: 0.18 (Cacchio et al., 2012)[29]
Modified bent knee stretch[33]	Patient supine The lower extremities are fully extended. The examiner grasps the heel of the symptomatic limb with one hand and places the other hand on the knee. The examiner then maximally flexes the hip and knee of the symptomatic leg and rapidly extends/straightens the knee.	Exacerbation of patient's symptoms	Sensitivity: 0.89 Specificity: 0.91 PPV: 0.91 NPV: 0.89 Positive likelihood ratio: 10.2 Negative likelihood ratio: 0.12 (Cacchio et al., 2012)[29]

Hamstring strain

Taking-off-the-shoe test	Patient standing The patient attempts to take off the shoe on the affected side with the help of his or her other shoe. While performing this maneuver, the affected leg hindfoot must press the longitudinal arch of the noninvolved foot. The affected leg during the maneuver is in approximately 90° of external rotation at the hip and 20° to 25° of flexion at the knee.	The feeling of a sharp pain over the injured biceps femoris	Sensitivity: 1.0 Specificity: 1.0 PPV: 1.0 NPV: 1.0 Positive likelihood ratio: 208.0 Negative likelihood ratio: 0.0 (Zeren and Oztekin, 2006)[31]
Active range of motion test	Patient prone • Hip extension: The patient actively extends the hip with an extended knee. • Knee flexion: The patient flexes the knee as far as he or she can.	Reproduction of patient's pain with either test	Sensitivity: 0.55 Specificity: 1.0 PPV: 1.0 NPV: 0.70 Positive likelihood ratio: 154.6 Negative likelihood ratio: 0.5 (Zeren and Oztekin, 2006)[31]

(continued on next page)

Table 1
(continued)

Test	How to Perform	Positive	Data
Passive range of motion test	Passive hip flexion: The patient is supine with the pelvis stabilized by grasping the iliac crest. As the hip is flexed, the knee is allowed to flex from the tension placed on the hamstrings and gravity. With pressure applied proximal to the knee joint, the normal end feel for hip flexion is soft owing to the approximation of the quadriceps with the abdomen. Passive knee extension: The patient is supine with the hip flexed to 90° and with the knee flexed in a relaxed position. The lower leg (below the knee) is passively extended to a firm muscle tension end point.	Reproduction of patient's pain with either test	Sensitivity: 0.57 Specificity: 1.0 PPV: 1.0 NPV: 0.70 Positive likelihood ratio: 160.6 Negative likelihood ratio: 0.43 (Zeren and Oztekin, 2006)[31]
Resisted range of motion test	Hip extension with an extended knee: the patient is prone, with the knee extended and the pelvis stabilized with pressure on the iliac crest. An isometric break test is performed at end-range hip extension, with resistance applied to the popliteal fossa.	Reproduction of patient's pain with either test	Sensitivity: 0.61 Specificity: 1.0 PPV: 1.0 NPV: 0.72 Positive likelihood ratio: 170.6 Negative likelihood ratio: 0.4 (Zeren and Oztekin, 2006)[31]

Table 2
Differential diagnosis for posterior hip pain

Diagnosis	Pathology	Signs/Symptoms
Proximal hamstring injuries	Range of disease from sprains to complete avulsions	• Posterior thigh ecchymosis if acute or subacute • Pain with concomitant hip flexion and knee extension • Pain with acceleration • Stiff-leg gait pattern
Piriformis syndrome (deep gluteal syndrome)	Extra-pelvic sciatic nerve compression by the piriformis muscle	• Pain, tingling, or numbness in the buttocks • + piriformis stretch test (flexion, adduction, and internal rotation) • +/− sciatica symptoms with pain extending down the posterior leg
Ischiofemoral impingement	Impingement of soft tissues between the ischial tuberosity and lesser trochanter	• Risk factor: Femoral anteversion • Pain exacerbated by a combination of hip extension, adduction and external rotation • Shortened gait • Low back stiffness and pain
Lumbar radiculopathy	Sciatica due to compression on roots of the sciatic nerve by a herniated disc, spinal stenosis, etc	• Sciatica symptoms • + Straight leg test

hamstring complex that can be misinterpreted as pathologic in the asymptomatic population.

INDICATIONS

The management of hamstring injuries is directed by the severity of injury and patient-specific factors. A consensus agreement is lacking for the indications for surgical repair, along with the operative technique, and postoperative rehabilitation. Pasic and colleagues[38] recently surveyed 108 surgeon members of the American Orthopedic Society for Sports Medicine (AOSSM) and Arthroscopy Association of Canada (AAC) and described the disparity in practice patterns for the management of these injuries.

Nonoperative management of hamstring injuries is most commonly recommended in the setting of low-grade, partial tears and insertional tendinosis, which encompasses most proximal hamstring pathology. More specifically, conservative management is indicated for single-tendon injuries with retraction of less than 1 to 2 cm or rupture at the myotendinous juncture.[39] If the patient has inadequate improvement with conservative management, an ultrasound-guided corticosteroid injection has been shown to provide initial pain relief in up to 50% of patients at 1 month.[40]

Surgical indications include complete, proximal avulsions; partial avulsions with at least 2 tendons injured and more than 2 cm of retraction in young and active patients; and partial avulsion injuries that have failed nonoperative management with persistent symptoms after 6 months.[39] The top 3 considerations for surgery in the recent aforementioned survey of AOSSM and AAC surgeons were the following: number of tendons involved (most important factor = 42%, second most = 26%, third

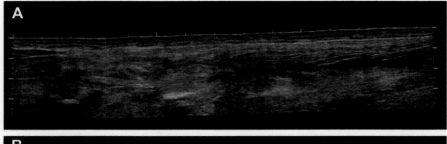

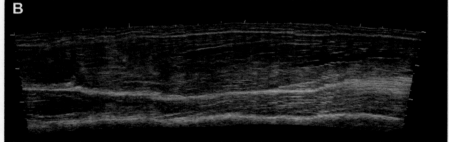

Fig. 2. (*A*) Ultrasound demonstration of a hamstring strain with disorganized, disrupted fibers. (*B*) Demonstration of an uninjured contralateral hamstring with normal organized and linear muscle patterns.

most = 13%), amount of tendon retraction (28%, 41%, 16%), and patient activity level (16%, 18%, 24%).[38] Surgical management has developed over the past couple of decades to include both open direct repair and endoscopic techniques. The generally recommended indications for management are outlined in **Table 3**.

NONOPERATIVE MANAGEMENT

Most patients with a hamstring injury are first treated with conservative management. Initial treatment consists of rest, ice, elevation, activity modification, oral nonsteroidal anti-inflammatory medications, and a graduated physical therapy program.[41] Physiotherapy focusing on eccentric exercises has been the mainstay of treatment for hamstring injury rehabilitation and prevention.[42] Lumbopelvic stabilization and

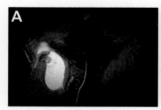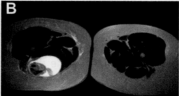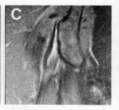

Fig. 3. Coronal (*A*) and axial (*B*) T2 MRI images of a complete, full-thickness proximal hamstring tear with a local fluid collection and retraction of the hamstring tendons. (*C*) Coronal T2 MRI image demonstrating a partial-thickness proximal hamstring tear. There is increased signal and attenuation in the semimembranosus tendon located superolateral on the ischial tuberosity. The conjoint tendon (semitendinosus and long head of biceps femoris) appears intact.

Table 3
Indications for the management of proximal hamstring injuries

| Nonoperative | Operative | | |
	Open Primary Repair[39]	Endoscopic Primary Repair	Augmentation or Reconstruction
Chronic insertional tendinosis	Complete injury with 3 hamstrings avulsed from ischial tuberosity	High-demand patient with an acute or chronic full-thickness tear with ~2–5-cm retraction of the tendon	Delayed cases of complete injuries where primary repair is not possible
Low-grade, partial tears	Two hamstring tendons that are retracted >2 cm from ischial tuberosity	Chronic tendinopathy with a partial or full-thickness tear after failure of conservative management	
Single tendon injuries regardless of retraction amount	Partial injuries with symptoms persistent after 6 mo		
Proximal ruptures of 1 to 3 tendons with minimal retraction (<2 cm)	Refractory cases of chronic insertional tendinosis		
Rupture at the myotendinous juncture			
Any hamstring injury in a low-demand patient, patients with multiple medical comorbidities at high risk for surgical intervention, or those unable to comply with postoperative restrictions			

improving the neuromuscular control of the hips and pelvis also help prepare patients for sports-specific movements. Depending on the severity of injury, programs typically include protected weightbearing followed by stretching and strengthening and gradual return to athletic activity over 4 to 6 weeks.[39,42]

If the patient fails to improve with initial conservative measures, additional nonsurgical options include platelet-rich plasma (PRP) injections,[43–49] corticosteroid injections,[40] dry needling,[50] and shock wave therapy.[33] These relatively new modalities have limited but positive results in the literature.

Two retrospective studies have demonstrated significant improvements in pain scores immediately following corticosteroid injections, with no reported short-term or long-term complications.[40,51] In a prospective level I randomized study of 40 patients, Cacchio and colleagues[33] described shockwave therapy as a viable methodology to treat proximal hamstring tendinitis, reporting 80% improvement in symptoms at 3 months. PRP injections have been studied in patients with chronic tendinopathy as well as acute hamstring injuries. In the 3 randomized controlled trials on acute hamstring injuries, one study reported that PRP injections following acute hamstring injury can decrease pain, increase ultrasonography regenerative indications, and decrease recovery time,[47] whereas the other 2 studies showed no difference between groups.[48,49] Given the inconsistent and limited quality evidence, PRP injections cannot be recommended as having value for hamstring injuries as compared with rehabilitative therapy alone (Grade B strength of recommendation).[52] However, the results of this same critically appraised topic suggested that PRP injections may be more beneficial in younger (high school and college aged), higher-level athletes who have sustained more severe acute hamstring injury, such as a grade IIa strain, or recurrent hamstring injuries.[52]

Hofmann and colleagues[53] reported on the largest series of 19 patients with complete proximal avulsion injuries managed nonoperatively. At an average follow-up duration of 31 months, the most notable finding was a persistent strength deficit, and 47% of patients wish they had undergone operative treatment at the time of injury. However, 71% of the patients were able to return to their previous sporting activities making nonoperative management worth consideration even in the setting of complete injuries.

SURGICAL TECHNIQUES
Open Primary Repair

When patients meet the operative indications, open debridement and primary repair with or without sciatic neurolysis remains the gold standard. However, endoscopic repair or open allograft reconstruction may be considered for select patients.

There have been many variants of open surgical repair. Most commonly, open surgical repair of the proximal hamstring is performed with the patient in the prone position with the knees slightly flexed to relieve tension at the hamstring insertion. The incision is most commonly oriented horizontally along the gluteal fold but can also be made longitudinally from the ischial tuberosity distally in cases of large retraction, chronic injuries with ample scar tissue suspected, and when careful neurolysis is warranted. These incisions are demonstrated in **Fig. 4** and can also be combined together for a T-type incision. The posterior hamstring fascia is exposed by elevating the inferior border of the gluteus maximus, taking care to avoid injuring the posterior femoral cutaneous nerve. In the acute setting, a large hematoma or seroma may be encountered and evacuated. The hamstring tendons are then identified and mobilized. Chronic injuries often require careful dissection of scar tissue around the retracted tendons and sciatic nerve. A sciatic neurolysis can be considered in the setting of chronic injuries and/or patients with preoperative neurologic symptoms.

The ischial tuberosity is then exposed and prepared for anchor placement. Anywhere from 2 to 5 anchors have been described, with the author's preferred technique being 4 anchors, 2 in the conjoint tendon footprint and 2 in the semimembranosus footprint. The repair is then completed with running, locking sutures or mattress sutures (**Fig. 5**).

Endoscopic Primary Repair

Endoscopic repair of proximal hamstring avulsion injuries was first described by Dierckman and Guanche[54] in 2012 with modified techniques outlined by others.[54–59] With

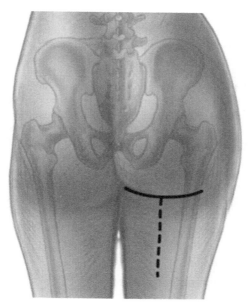

Fig. 4. Illustrative representation of the incision locations for open proximal hamstring repair. The incision can be oriented horizontally along the gluteal fold (*solid line*), longitudinally extending distal to the ischial tuberosity (*dotted line*), or combined in a T-type fashion.

the recent development of endoscopic techniques, the only reported patient outcomes specific to endoscopic hamstring repair was published in Germany in 2018; this study included 12 patients with good patient-reported outcomes (visual analog scale and subjective hip value) and no complications.[60] In general, the patient is

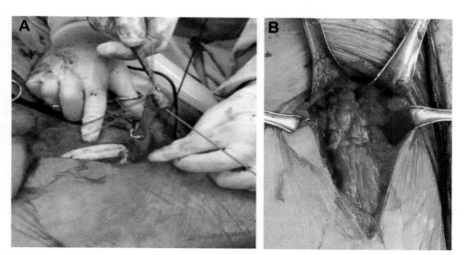

Fig. 5. Clinical photographs of an open proximal hamstring repair representing preparation of the proximal hamstring tendons (*A*) and the final completed repair (*B*) back to the ischial tuberosity footprint.

positioned prone with the feet at the head of the bed and table in reverse Trendelen-burg to level the spine in relation to the floor. The knees are flexed to 90°; this posi-tioning stabilizes the operative leg and takes tension off of the sciatic nerve. An unsterile assistant is positioned at the patient's feet with a hand on the operative foot to detect unintentional stimulation of the sciatic nerve throughout the case. Four portals are used, the first (accessory distal portal) within the gluteal fold overlying the palpable ischial tuberosity. A second portal (accessory proximal portal) is created directly superior, both within the interval between the hamstring tendon (medial) and sciatic nerve (lateral). Two portals are later created medial (posteromedial portal) and lateral (posterolateral portal) within the gluteal fold (**Fig. 6**). First, the sciatic nerve is identified, dissected, and mobilized away from the operative field for protection. Retraction sutures are used to help retract the gluteus maximus and further protect the sciatic nerve. Dissection is within the interval between the conjoint and semimem-branosus tendons. The tendons are freed and mobilized, the ischial tuberosity is decorticated, and an anatomic repair is carried out via 4 suture anchors, 2 at each tendon footprint. Endoscopic visualization of this technique is exhibited in **Fig. 7**.

Augmentation or Reconstruction

Augmented repairs have only been described in a total of 24 chronic complete avul-sions in the literature.[41] Most of these were performed with Achilles allograft[61,62]; how-ever fascia lata autograft and iliotibial band autograft have also been described.[41] Folsom and Larson[61] reported their new allograft technique using Achilles allograft for chronic reconstructions in 2008 and concluded that Achilles allograft appears to restore function and strength comparable to acute repairs.

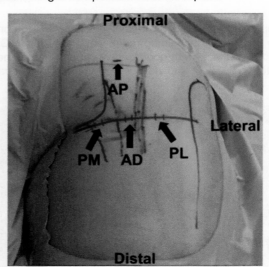

Fig. 6. Clinical photograph demonstrating landmarks and portal placement. The ischial tu-berosity and gluteal fold are palpated and drawn as well as the anticipated corresponding locations of the hamstring tendon and sciatic nerve. Four portals are used, 3 in horizontal alignment within the gluteal fold and 1 directly superior to the ischial tuberosity. The acces-sory distal (AD) portal is established first as the primary working portal and the accessory proximal portal second as the primary viewing portal. The posteromedial (PM) and postero-lateral (PL) portals are created in horizontal alignment with the AD portal at the level of the gluteal crease.

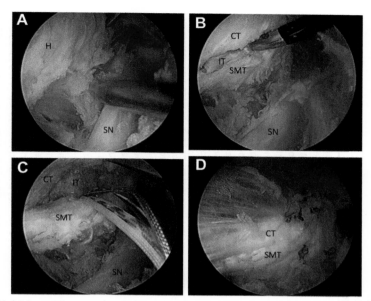

Fig. 7. Right hamstring repair: endoscopic visualization through the posterolateral portal with the patient positioned prone. (*A*) The hamstring insertion at the ischial tuberosity and sciatic nerve more laterally are identified. Soft tissue dissection is performed with a blunt switching stick to identify the sciatic nerve. The sciatic nerve is dissected and gently mobilized away from the operative field. (*B*) The proximal hamstring insertion is examined, and dissection is carried down to the ischial tuberosity in the interval between the conjoint and semimembranosus tendons. (*C*) Four suture anchors are placed, 2 at the footprint of the conjoint tendon and 2 at the footprint of the semimembranosus tendon.[4] (*D*) The final repair is visualized with anatomic restoration of both the conjoint and semimembranosus tendons to the ischial tuberosity. CT, conjoint tendon; H, hamstring; IT, ischial tuberosity; SMT, semimembranosus tendon; SN, sciatic nerve.

CLINICAL OUTCOMES

Within the past 2 decades, there have been multiple studies comparing the outcomes of operative and nonoperative management for proximal hamstring injuries. Many of these are retrospective, include small numbers of patients, and have conflicting conclusions. To date, there are 3 systematic reviews summarizing the current literature available for outcomes of proximal hamstring management.[41,63,64] The main conclusions from these systematic reviews are summarized in **Table 4**.

In general, it has been well established that open surgical repair for complete proximal ruptures has many benefits over nonoperative management, including significantly better subjective outcomes, greater rate of return to preinjury level of sport, and greater strength and endurance when compared with nonsurgical management.[41,63,64] In the review by Bodendorfer and colleagues,[41] these positive outcomes were quantified by significantly higher patient satisfaction (91% vs 53%), lower extremity function score (LEFS) (73 vs 70), and single-leg hop distance (119 cm vs 57 cm) in the operative group compared with the nonoperative group.

Agreement on the appropriate timing of surgery is less clear. This becomes important in deciding when conservative management should be trialed first versus early surgical intervention in the acute setting. Two of the aforementioned reviews

Table 4
Systematic reviews of proximal hamstring outcome studies, conclusions

Author (Publication Year)	Inclusion Criteria	N Studies Included	N Hamstring Repairs	Conclusions
Harris et al,[63] 2011	Proximal hamstring injury (partial and complete), >12-mo mean follow-up, operative or nonoperative treatment	18	300	• Acute surgical repair of proximal hamstring ruptures improves subjective clinical outcomes, strength, and endurance, with high rates of return to preinjury level of sport, and low risk of complications and rerupture. • Chronic surgical repair also improves outcomes, strength, and endurance, and return to sport, but not as well as acute repair. • Nonoperative treatment results in reduced patient satisfaction, with significantly lower rates of return to preinjury level of sport and reduced hamstring muscle strength.
Van der Made et al,[64] 2015	Proximal hamstring injury, >12-mo mean follow-up, operative treatment	13	387	• Surgical repair of proximal hamstring avulsions leads to a subjective highly satisfying outcome than nonoperative management. • However, it appears that both function and level of activity are not fully restored in all cases with a return to sports rate of 76%–100%, return to preinjury activity level rate of 55%–100%, and residual pain in 8%–61% of patients. • There are minimal to no differences in outcome of acute and delayed repairs with equivalent satisfaction, pain, functional scale scores, and strength/flexibility. • Achilles allograft reconstruction is a suitable alternative to primary repair in delayed cases in which primary repair is not possible.

| Bodendorfer et al,[41] 2018 | Proximal hamstring injury, >12-mo mean follow-up, operative or nonoperative treatment | 24 | 795 | • Operatively treated patients have higher patient satisfaction, return of strength, athletic capacity, and overall functional recovery.
• Patients undergoing acute repair have higher patient satisfaction, less pain, return of strength, and higher functional scores.
• Chronic repair was associated with a higher rate of sitting pain and neurologic complications.
• Compared with complete repairs, partial repairs demonstrated better strength and endurance testing and a lower complication rate, but worse patient satisfaction and pain scores. |

concluded that patients undergoing acute surgical repair had improved outcomes compared with chronic repair.[41,63] However, Van der Made and colleagues[64] reported minimal to no differences in outcome of acute and delayed repairs with equivalent satisfaction, pain, functional scale scores, and strength/flexibility. Collectively, results of these studies support that operative treatment provides good-to-excellent outcomes in terms of subjective function, objective strength evaluation, and patient-reported outcome measures, with acute repair favored over delayed/chronic repair.

COMPLICATIONS AND CONCERNS

Despite the positive clinical outcomes, open surgical repair results in a high complication rate of 23.17% and a return to sport of 79.75%.[8] Most commonly these complications include neurologic complications, peri-incisional numbness, infection/wound complications, reoperation, and rerupture. Thus, although open surgical repair of acute proximal hamstring injuries has significantly improved the functional prognosis of patients, preoperative counseling on potential complications is prudent. Advocates for advancing endoscopic repair techniques suggest a theoretic decreased rate of peri-incisional numbness and infection/wound complications.

DISCUSSION AND FUTURE DIRECTIONS

There is currently no widely accepted treatment protocol for hamstring injuries. In addition, outcomes after selected operative or nonoperative treatment pathways have not been well established. Evidence is limited to low-quality studies composed of case series and case-controls with conflicting data. There are no comparative, prospective, randomized trials comparing nonoperative with operative treatment or different surgical techniques. Thus, further high-level studies are needed to accurately assess outcomes after proximal hamstring injuries.

CASE STUDY/PRESENTATION

The patient is an active 36-year-old woman who presents to clinic with left buttock and posterior thigh pain 1 week after an injury. She has no significant past medical or surgical history. She notes the onset was sudden and occurred after she sustained a fall while water skiing. She denies any antecedent pain in the left lower extremity. She notes difficulty ambulating since her injury. On physical examination she has a stiff-legged gait pattern with avoidance of hip flexion. There is swelling and ecchymosis at her posterior thigh with no obvious mass. Her passive hip and knee range of motion is normal; however, she has decreased strength with hip extension and knee flexion. Her symptoms are reproduced with the resisted range of motion test. She is otherwise neurovascularly intact and the remainder of her examination is unrevealing.

Clinical Questions

- What is the next step in the workup?
  - Given her history and physical examination findings, the patient has presumably sustained a proximal hamstring injury. To further evaluate for a potential bony avulsion off of the ischial tuberosity or other bony pathology, an anterior-posterior pelvic radiograph can be considered. If readily available, an ultrasound will allow for examination of the soft tissues and comparison with the contralateral side.
- Should she get an MRI?

- ○ Given the patient's young age and active lifestyle, she is likely a surgical candidate if a high-grade injury is present. In addition, early surgical intervention may result in improved outcomes compared with nonoperative or delayed surgical intervention. An MRI will allow for characterization of the extent of tendon injury and preoperative planning.
  - If the patient was older with a low-demand lifestyle, it is appropriate to first discuss the suspected diagnosis and treatment options before advanced imaging. Initial conservative management is appropriate in this patient population. There is no need for advanced imaging if it will not change the treatment course at this time.
- Her MRI reveals an avulsion of the conjoint tendon with 3 cm of retraction. What is the best treatment option?
  - ○ This patient is young, healthy, and active. Given the 2-tendon involvement (long head of biceps femoris and semitendinosus) and greater than 2 cm retraction, she is indicated for primary operative fixation with either open or endoscopic techniques based on the patient preference and surgeon expertise.

SUMMARY

Proximal hamstring injuries can present as chronic tendinosis, acute strain, partial tendinous avulsions, or complete 3-tendon rupture. Nonoperative management for chronic insertional tendinosis and low-grade tears includes activity modification, anti-inflammatories, and physical therapy. Platelet-rich plasma injections, corticosteroid injections, dry needling, and shock wave therapy are newer therapies that also may provide benefit. Surgical indications include complete, proximal avulsions; partial avulsions with least 2 tendons injured with more than 2 cm of retraction in young, active patients; and partial avulsion injuries or chronic tendinosis that have failed nonoperative management. Surgical management entails open primary repair, endoscopic primary repair, or augmentation/reconstruction.

CLINICS CARE POINTS

- Proximal hamstring injuries represent 12% of all hamstring injuries.
- The proximal hamstring complex is composed of the semimembranosus, semitendinosus, and the long head of the biceps femoris.
- Proximal hamstring injuries include a spectrum of disease, including chronic tendinosis, acute strain, partial tendinous avulsions, and complete 3-tendon rupture.
- The mechanism of injury results from chronic repetitive or acute eccentric loading during hip flexion and knee extension. High-risk activities include sprinting, water skiing, or other sporting activities that require rapid acceleration and deceleration.
- Common physical examination findings include pain located at the buttock/ischial tuberosity, posterior thigh ecchymosis, or a mass of retracted muscle if acutely injured, a stiff-leg gait, and exacerbation of pain with hip flexion and knee extension.
- Ultrasound and MRI are most helpful in classifying the extent of soft tissue injury and are recommended in the setting of surgical consideration.
- Nonoperative management for chronic insertional tendinosis and low-grade, partial tears includes activity modification, oral anti-inflammatories, and physical therapy.

- Surgical indications include complete, proximal avulsions; partial avulsions with at least 2 tendons injured with greater than 2 cm of retraction in young and active patients; and partial avulsion injuries that have failed nonoperative management with persistent symptoms after 6 months.
- Surgical options include open primary repair, endoscopic primary repair, and augmentation/reconstruction.
- When indicated, operative treatment provides good-to-excellent outcomes in terms of subjective function, objective strength evaluation, and patient-reported outcome measures, with acute repair favored over delayed/chronic repair.

DISCLOSURE

A.N. Fletcher and J.W. Cheah: No conflicts to disclose. S.J. Nho receives research support from AlloSource, Arthrex, Athletico, DJ Orthopedics, Linvatec, Miomed, Smith and Nephew, and Stryker; is a board/committee member of American Orthopaedic Association, American Orthopaedic Society for Sports Medicine, and Arthroscopy Association of North America; receives intellectual property royalties from Ossur and Stryker; receives publishing royalties and financial/material support from Springer; and is a paid consultant for Stryker, outside the submitted work. R.C. Mather is a board or committee member of Arthroscopy Association of North America, North Carolina Orthopaedic Association, and International Society of Hip Arthroscopy; receives research support from Reflexion Health and Zimmer; receives intellectual property royalties from Stryker; and is a paid consultant for Stryker, outside the submitted work.

REFERENCES

1. Ahmad CS, Redler LH, Ciccotti MG, et al. Evaluation and management of hamstring injuries. Am J Sports Med 2013;41(12):2933–47.
2. Okoroha KR, Conte S, Makhni EC, et al. Hamstring injury trends in major and minor league baseball: epidemiological findings from the major league baseball health and injury tracking system. Orthop J Sports Med 2019;7(7). 2325967119861064.
3. Brooks JH, Fuller CW, Kemp SP, et al. Incidence, risk, and prevention of hamstring muscle injuries in professional rugby union. Am J Sports Med 2006; 34(8):1297–306.
4. Woods C, Hawkins RD, Maltby S, et al. The Football Association Medical Research Programme: an audit of injuries in professional football–analysis of hamstring injuries. Br J Sports Med 2004;38(1):36–41.
5. Ekstrand J, Hagglund M, Walden M. Epidemiology of muscle injuries in professional football (soccer). Am J Sports Med 2011;39(6):1226–32.
6. Elliott MC, Zarins B, Powell JW, et al. Hamstring muscle strains in professional football players: a 10-year review. Am J Sports Med 2011;39(4):843–50.
7. Orchard J, Seward H. Epidemiology of injuries in the Australian Football League, seasons 1997-2000. Br J Sports Med 2002;36(1):39–44.
8. Malliaropoulos N, Isinkaye T, Tsitas K, et al. Reinjury after acute posterior thigh muscle injuries in elite track and field athletes. Am J Sports Med 2011;39(2): 304–10.
9. Mendiguchia J, Alentorn-Geli E, Brughelli M. Hamstring strain injuries: are we heading in the right direction? Br J Sports Med 2012;46(2):81–5.
10. Koulouris G, Connell D. Evaluation of the hamstring muscle complex following acute injury. Skeletal Radiol 2003;32(10):582–9.

11. Ishikawa K, Kai K, Mizuta H. Avulsion of the hamstring muscles from the ischial tuberosity. A report of two cases. Clin Orthop Relat Res 1988;(232):153–5.

12. Watsford ML, Murphy AJ, McLachlan KA, et al. A prospective study of the relationship between lower body stiffness and hamstring injury in professional Australian rules footballers. Am J Sports Med 2010;38(10):2058–64.

13. Fousekis K, Tsepis E, Poulmedis P, et al. Intrinsic risk factors of non-contact quadriceps and hamstring strains in soccer: a prospective study of 100 professional players. Br J Sports Med 2011;45(9):709–14.

14. Hennessey L, Watson AW. Flexibility and posture assessment in relation to hamstring injury. Br J Sports Med 1993;27(4):243–6.

15. Orchard J, Marsden J, Lord S, et al. Preseason hamstring muscle weakness associated with hamstring muscle injury in Australian footballers. Am J Sports Med 1997;25(1):81–5.

16. Small K, McNaughton LR, Greig M, et al. Soccer fatigue, sprinting and hamstring injury risk. Int J Sports Med 2009;30(8):573–8.

17. Sherry MA, Best TM. A comparison of 2 rehabilitation programs in the treatment of acute hamstring strains. J Orthop Sports Phys Ther 2004;34(3):116–25.

18. Worrell TW. Factors associated with hamstring injuries. An approach to treatment and preventative measures. Sports Med 1994;17(5):338–45.

19. Engebretsen AH, Myklebust G, Holme I, et al. Intrinsic risk factors for hamstring injuries among male soccer players: a prospective cohort study. Am J Sports Med 2010;38(6):1147–53.

20. Hagglund M, Walden M, Ekstrand J. Previous injury as a risk factor for injury in elite football: a prospective study over two consecutive seasons. Br J Sports Med 2006;40(9):767–72.

21. Gabbe BJ, Bennell KL, Finch CF, et al. Predictors of hamstring injury at the elite level of Australian football. Scand J Med Sci Sports 2006;16(1):7–13.

22. Dalton SL, Kerr ZY, Dompier TP. Epidemiology of hamstring strains in 25 NCAA sports in the 2009-2010 to 2013-2014 academic years. Am J Sports Med 2015; 43(11):2671–9.

23. Rachun A. Standard nomenclature of athletic injuries. Chicago: American Medical Association; 1996.

24. De Smet AA, Blankenbaker DG, Alsheik NH, et al. MRI appearance of the proximal hamstring tendons in patients with and without symptomatic proximal hamstring tendinopathy. AJR Am J Roentgenol 2012;198(2):418–22.

25. Puranen J, Orava S. The hamstring syndrome. A new diagnosis of gluteal sciatic pain. Am J Sports Med 1988;16(5):517–21.

26. Chu SK, Rho ME. Hamstring injuries in the athlete: diagnosis, treatment, and return to play. Curr Sports Med Rep 2016;15(3):184–90.

27. Degen RM. Proximal hamstring injuries: management of tendinopathy and avulsion injuries. Curr Rev Musculoskelet Med 2019;12(2):138–46.

28. Reiman MP, Loudon JK, Goode AP. Diagnostic accuracy of clinical tests for assessment of hamstring injury: a systematic review. J Orthop Sports Phys Ther 2013;43(4):223–31.

29. Cacchio A, Borra F, Severini G, et al. Reliability and validity of three pain provocation tests used for the diagnosis of chronic proximal hamstring tendinopathy. Br J Sports Med 2012;46(12):883–7.

30. Schneider-Kolsky ME, Hoving JL, Warren P, et al. A comparison between clinical assessment and magnetic resonance imaging of acute hamstring injuries. Am J Sports Med 2006;34(6):1008–15.

31. Zeren B, Oztekin HH. A new self-diagnostic test for biceps femoris muscle strains. Clin J Sport Med 2006;16(2):166–9.

32. Fredericson M, Moore W, Guillet M, et al. High hamstring tendinopathy in runners: meeting the challenges of diagnosis, treatment, and rehabilitation. Phys Sportsmed 2005;33(5):32–43.

33. Cacchio A, Rompe JD, Furia JP, et al. Shockwave therapy for the treatment of chronic proximal hamstring tendinopathy in professional athletes. Am J Sports Med 2011;39(1):146–53.

34. Bengtzen RR, Ma OJ, Herzka A. Point-of-care ultrasound diagnosis of proximal hamstring rupture. J Emerg Med 2018;54(2):225–8.

35. Mariani C, Caldera FE, Kim W. Ultrasound versus magnetic resonance imaging in the diagnosis of an acute hamstring tear. PM R 2012;4(2):154–5.

36. Connell DA, Schneider-Kolsky ME, Hoving JL, et al. Longitudinal study comparing sonographic and MRI assessments of acute and healing hamstring injuries. AJR Am J Roentgenol 2004;183(4):975–84.

37. Thompson SM, Fung S, Wood DG. The prevalence of proximal hamstring pathology on MRI in the asymptomatic population. Knee Surg Sports Traumatol Arthrosc 2017;25(1):108–11.

38. Pasic N, Giffin JR, Degen RM. Practice patterns for the treatment of acute proximal hamstring ruptures. Phys Sportsmed 2020;48(1):116–22.

39. Cohen S, Bradley J. Acute proximal hamstring rupture. J Am Acad Orthop Surg 2007;15(6):350–5.

40. Zissen MH, Wallace G, Stevens KJ, et al. High hamstring tendinopathy: MRI and ultrasound imaging and therapeutic efficacy of percutaneous corticosteroid injection. AJR Am J Roentgenol 2010;195(4):993–8.

41. Bodendorfer BM, Curley AJ, Kotler JA, et al. Outcomes after operative and nonoperative treatment of proximal hamstring avulsions: a systematic review and meta-analysis. Am J Sports Med 2018;46(11):2798–808.

42. Schmitt B, Tim T, McHugh M. Hamstring injury rehabilitation and prevention of reinjury using lengthened state eccentric training: a new concept. Int J Sports Phys Ther 2012;7(3):333–41.

43. Wetzel RJ, Patel RM, Terry MA. Platelet-rich plasma as an effective treatment for proximal hamstring injuries. Orthopedics 2013;36(1):e64–70.

44. Park PYS, Cai C, Bawa P, et al. Platelet-rich plasma vs. steroid injections for hamstring injury-is there really a choice? Skeletal Radiol 2019;48(4):577–82.

45. Fader RR, Mitchell JJ, Traub S, et al. Platelet-rich plasma treatment improves outcomes for chronic proximal hamstring injuries in an athletic population. Muscles Ligaments Tendons J 2014;4(4):461–6.

46. Davenport KL, Campos JS, Nguyen J, et al. Ultrasound-guided intratendinous injections with platelet-rich plasma or autologous whole blood for treatment of proximal hamstring tendinopathy: a double-blind randomized controlled trial. J Ultrasound Med 2015;34(8):1455–63.

47. Hamid A, Mohamed Ali MR, Yusof A, et al. Platelet-rich plasma injections for the treatment of hamstring injuries: a randomized controlled trial. Am J Sports Med 2014;42(10):2410–8.

48. Reurink G, Goudswaard GJ, Moen MH, et al. Platelet-rich plasma injections in acute muscle injury. N Engl J Med 2014;370(26):2546–7.

49. Hamilton B, Tol JL, Almusa E, et al. Platelet-rich plasma does not enhance return to play in hamstring injuries: a randomised controlled trial. Br J Sports Med 2015;49(14):943–50.

50. Jayaseelan DJ, Moats N, Ricardo CR. Rehabilitation of proximal hamstring tendinopathy utilizing eccentric training, lumbopelvic stabilization, and trigger point dry needling: 2 case reports. J Orthop Sports Phys Ther 2014;44(3):198–205.

51. Nicholson LT, DiSegna S, Newman JS, et al. Fluoroscopically guided peritendinous corticosteroid injection for proximal hamstring tendinopathy: a retrospective review. Orthop J Sports Med 2014;2(3). 2325967114526135.

52. Manduca ML, Straub SJ. Effectiveness of PRP injection in reducing recovery time of acute hamstring injury: a critically appraised topic. J Sport Rehabil 2018;27(5):480–4.

53. Hofmann KJ, Paggi A, Connors D, et al. Complete avulsion of the proximal hamstring insertion: functional outcomes after nonsurgical treatment. J Bone Joint Surg Am 2014;96(12):1022–5.

54. Dierckman BD, Guanche CA. Endoscopic proximal hamstring repair and ischial bursectomy. Arthrosc Tech 2012;1(2):e201–7.

55. Laskovski JR, Kahn AJ, Urchek RJ, et al. Endoscopic proximal hamstring repair and ischial bursectomy using modified portal placement and patient positioning. Arthrosc Tech 2018;7(11):e1071–8.

56. Domb BG, Linder D, Sharp KG, et al. Endoscopic repair of proximal hamstring avulsion. Arthrosc Tech 2013;2(1):e35–9.

57. Jackson TJ, Trenga A, Lindner D, et al. Endoscopic transtendinous repair for partial-thickness proximal hamstring tendon tears. Arthrosc Tech 2014;3(1):e127–30.

58. Gomez-Hoyos J, Reddy M, Martin HD. Dry endoscopic-assisted mini-open approach with neuromonitoring for chronic hamstring avulsions and ischial tunnel syndrome. Arthrosc Tech 2015;4(3):e193–9.

59. Moatshe G, Chahla J, Vap AR, et al. Repair of proximal hamstring tears: a surgical technique. Arthrosc Tech 2017;6(2):e311–7.

60. Schroder JH, Gesslein M, Schutz M, et al. [Minimally invasive proximal hamstring insertion repair]. Oper Orthop Traumatol 2018;30(6):419–34.

61. Folsom GJ, Larson CM. Surgical treatment of acute versus chronic complete proximal hamstring ruptures: results of a new allograft technique for chronic reconstructions. Am J Sports Med 2008;36(1):104–9.

62. Rust DA, Giveans MR, Stone RM, et al. Functional outcomes and return to sports after acute repair, chronic repair, and allograft reconstruction for proximal hamstring ruptures. Am J Sports Med 2014;42(6):1377–83.

63. Harris JD, Griesser MJ, Best TM, et al. Treatment of proximal hamstring ruptures - a systematic review. Int J Sports Med 2011;32(7):490–5.

64. Van der Made AD, Reurink G, Gouttebarge V, et al. Outcome after surgical repair of proximal hamstring avulsions: a systematic review. Am J Sports Med 2015;43(11):2841–51.

Stress Fractures of the Hip and Pelvis

Rebecca A. Dutton, MD

KEYWORDS

- Stress fracture • Bone stress injury • Hip • Pelvis • Sacrum • Pubic ramus
- Femoral neck

KEY POINTS

- Stress fractures of the hip and pelvis have become increasingly recognized in the literature, and are observed more commonly in long-distance runners and military recruits.
- The diagnosis of stress fractures in the hip and pelvic region necessitates a high index of clinical suspicion, often combined with advanced imaging modalities such as MRI.
- The sacrum and pubic ramus reflect lower risk sites of injury and are typically managed with activity modification to a pain-free level.
- Stress fractures of the femoral neck necessitate more aggressive management to prevent complication, including at a minimum strict non-weightbearing, and in some cases, surgical fixation.

INTRODUCTION

Stress fractures refer to overuse injuries of bone resulting from repeated mechanical stress, none of which alone would be sufficient to produce structural demise. Such injuries are relatively common in athletes, especially those engaging in repetitive physical exercise including endurance athletes, dancers, gymnasts, and military recruits.[1,2] Injury rates as high as 20% to 31% annually have been reported in runners and military recruits respectively.[3,4] Stress fractures are overwhelmingly more common in the lower extremities. The tibia, fibula, and metatarsals appear to be the most vulnerable.[5] However, stress fractures of the hip and pelvis have become increasingly recognized in the literature.

Stress fracture development is multifactorial in nature, and various potentially contributing conditions have been identified. An excessively high volume or rapid escalation of training are some of the most consistently demonstrated contributors, especially in athletes.[6,7] Poor preparticipation fitness and a prior history of stress fracture are other common risk factors. Various anatomic influences have been identified including leg length discrepancy, genu valgum, pes planus or pes cavus deformities,

Department of Orthopaedics and Rehabilitation, University of New Mexico, MSC 10-5600, 1 University of New Mexico, Albuquerque, NM 87131, USA
E-mail address: radutton@salud.unm.edu

Clin Sports Med 40 (2021) 363–374
https://doi.org/10.1016/j.csm.2020.11.007
0278-5919/21/© 2020 Elsevier Inc. All rights reserved.
sportsmed.theclinics.com

and low bone mineral density and narrow bones in proportion to body size.[7] Finally, female gender is frequently cited, although it remains unclear whether gender reflects an independent risk factor or the influence of sex-associated conditions such as those embodied by the female athlete triad, namely menstrual irregularities and disordered eating, as well as biomechanical differences.[7]

Classically, a skeletal stress injury presents as localized mechanical pain that is not present at rest, but progresses with, or immediately following, activity.[8] On physical examination, the most sensitive finding is localized tenderness over the involved bone.[8] However, such assessment in the pelvic region is often challenged by the overlying soft tissues such that advanced imaging may be necessary to confirm diagnosis. MRI has generally become the imaging modality of choice in the diagnosis of bone stress injuries. Edema-sensitive sequences have utility to detect periosteal, muscle, or bone marrow edema, which may reflect the only finding in the initial stages of skeletal stress injury.[9] As the injury progresses, edema may become apparent on T1-weighted sequences, and ultimately in cases of a frank fracture, a band-like, low-signal fracture line will be evident.[9]

Early recognition of bone stress injuries is important to direct appropriate management, limit time lost from sport, and avoid potential complications. Management is largely dictated by the site of injury and associated risk of delayed union, nonunion, or progression to complete fracture. Injuries at high risk for these complications necessitate a more aggressive approach to management that includes at a minimum, a period of strict non-weight bearing, and in certain circumstances may require surgical fixation.[6,8] The femoral neck represents 1 such high-risk site. Lower-risk stress fractures, including the sacrum and the pubic ramus, may be managed less aggressively with activity modification to a pain-free level.[6,8] In all instances, it is critical to identify and address any modifiable risk factors to both promote recovery and prevent future injuries.[8] This article will review in greater detail the epidemiology, diagnosis, and management of bone stress injuries involving the hip and pelvic region.

STRESS FRACTURES OF THE SACRUM
Epidemiology

Located at the base of the spine, the sacrum is a triangular bone that articulates with the L5 vertebra superiorly, the coccyx inferiorly, and the ilium to either side by way of the sacroiliac joints. As the bridge between the spine and the iliac bones, the sacrum plays an important role in maintaining hip and pelvic stability.[10] The sacrum may be divided into zones based upon regional anatomy that, when injured, can influence clinical presentation. Zone I refers to the sacral ala, or the area medial to the sacroiliac joint and lateral to the neural foramen. Zone II is the region of the neural foramen. Zone III is the area medial to the neural foramen and includes the spinal canal.[11] Most sacral stress fractures are limited to Zone I.[12] Moreover, the fractures typically develop vertically, parallel to the sacroiliac joint, as a result of repetitive axial load transmitted downward through the spine to the sacrum.[12,13] It has also been suggested that instability of the pelvic ring, as can be seen in the context of osteitis pubis for example, may result in abnormal shear forces that further predispose to sacral stress fractures.[14]

Historically, stress fractures of the sacrum were considered relatively rare; however, it seems that these injuries may be more common than once thought.[12,15] Distance runners appear to reflect a particularly high-risk population.[15] Sacral bone stress injuries have also been reported in tennis, basketball, gymnastics, cycling, track and field, badminton, and weightlifting, as well as in military recruits.[16,17] In addition to the general risk factors for bone stress injury outlined previously, it has been suggested that increased pelvic anteversion may represent a more specific risk factor for the development of sacral stress fractures.[13]

Presentation and Evaluation

The clinical presentation of sacral bone stress injuries is notoriously vague. Patients may describe acute or insidious onset low back, buttock, pelvic or hip pain.[15] The pain tends to be exacerbated by weight-bearing activities and relieved by rest. Although the majority of sacral stress fractures are limited to the sacral ala, or Zone I, some patients may experience radicular symptoms because of involvement of the traversing lumbosacral nerve roots or fracture extension into Zone II.[17,18] On physical examination, reproducible tenderness to palpation in the sacral region is a common finding.[15,17,19] A single leg hop test may also reproduce pain.[15] Provocation maneuvers targeting the sacroiliac joint such as Gaenslen test and Patrick sign may be positive, but reflect a nonspecific finding.[12,17] It has been suggested that a prone fulcrum test, whereby the examiner applies an anteriorly directed force over the posterior sacrum, may have utility in diagnosis, although this has not been well validated.[17] Finally, neural tension signs (eg, slump test or straight leg raise) may be positive in the setting of accompanying nerve root involvement.[17]

Given the nonspecific nature of the history and physical examination, imaging studies are often necessary to confirm diagnosis. Plain radiographs are recommended initially to exclude potentially mimicking diagnoses. However, radiographs are poorly sensitive for the diagnosis of a sacral stress fracture.[20,21] MRI is currently considered the gold standard for diagnosis of sacral bone stress injuries.[17] MRI is notably more sensitive than computed tomography (CT), particularly in detecting earlier stages of bone stress injury.[20] Moreover, MRI can be useful to exclude alternative bone or soft tissue injuries.[15,17] Sacral bone stress injuries present with bone marrow edema limited to the sacrum, reflected by relatively high signal intensity on T2-weighted images, and often corresponding low signal intensity on T1-weighted images.[20] When present, a fracture line appears as a vertical, hypointense signal involving the superolateral anterior cortex and extending inferiorly through the first few sacral segments (**Fig. 1**).[15] As previously mentioned, sacral stress fractures almost exclusively involve the sacral ala, or Zone I of the sacrum. In select cases, perpetuated strain may lead to transverse extension into Zone II with consequent neural foraminal involvement.[12,18] CT or radionuclide bone scans may be considered in situations wherein MRI is contraindicated. Radionuclide bone scans, while less specific, are more sensitive than CT in the diagnosis of sacral bone stress injuries.[21]

Management

Relative rest, including cessation of offending and high-impact activities, is imperative in the management of sacral stress fractures. A brief, 1- to 2-week period of non-weightbearing or crutch-assisted ambulation is reasonable until the patient is able to walk without pain.[15] Thereafter, nonimpact cross-training such as stationary cycling, swimming, or deep water running may be introduced, using caution to maintain a pain-free level both during and after sessions.[22] Activity may be gradually advanced to include light-weighted exercise and sport-specific strengthening, followed by a progressive reintroduction of sport-specific activity.[22] Antigravity treadmills, which incorporate an air-filled, pressure-controlled compartment that permits body unweighting below the level of the waist, have become increasingly popular in the rehabilitation of running athletes. These devices allow an athlete to run at a high intensity but with reduced loading to the lower extremities.[23] One recent case report describes the successful return of a collegiate athlete with a pelvic stress fracture using this method.[24]

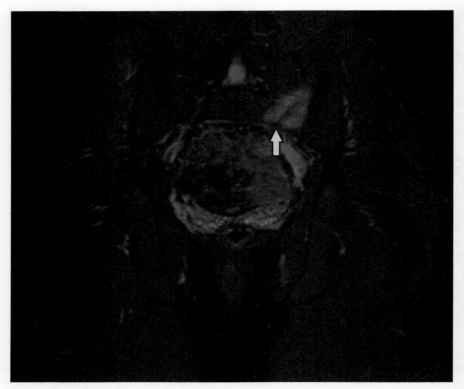

Fig. 1. Coronal, STIR MRI of the pelvis demonstrating a vertically oriented stress fracture (*arrow*) of the left sacral ala with extensive surrounding marrow edema.

During the initial recovery period, any underlying risk factors for bone stress injury should be identified and addressed, including education regarding training errors, reversal of energy imbalance, and correction of biomechanical deficits.[25] Calcium and vitamin D intake should be optimized to promote bone health.[25] Use of nonsteroidal anti-inflammatory drugs (NSAIDs) for pain control is somewhat controversial, although avoidance is generally recommended to limit any potential impairment of bone healing. Moreover, analgesic medications in general should be used with caution to avoid masking pain during rehabilitation and return to sport.[25]

Recovery and return to sport following sacral bone stress injuries are variable, but may require longer periods than some other low-risk stress fracture sites. Fredericson and colleagues[15] reported that return to preinjury training may take 3 to 6 months. Factors that can contribute to prolonged recovery include delay in diagnosis and the composition of the involved bone.[15,26] Bone stress injuries involving predominantly trabecular bone, such as the sacrum, appear to be associated with protracted recovery compared with those involving predominantly cortical bone.[26]

STRESS FRACTURES OF THE PUBIC RAMUS
Epidemiology

The literature regarding stress fractures of the pubis is relatively sparse, although like sacral stress fractures, it has been submitted that pubic stress fractures may be under-recognized.[27] One study involving military recruits over an 8-year period found that the pubic arch represented 8% of all diagnosed stress fractures.[27] Another study comprised of military recruits with stress-related hip, buttock, or groin pain identified a total of 174 bone stress injuries involving the pelvis or proximal femur, of which 37 (21%) involved the pubic arch.[28] Stress fractures of the pubic region most frequently occur within the inferior pubic ramus, near to the junction of the ischial ramus.[29] This has been attributed to repetitive tensile forces imparted by the adductor magnus resulting in an avulsion-type fatigue fracture.[30,31]

Stress fractures of the pubis have been reported most commonly in runners and military recruits.[29,32] Select cases have also been described in bowling, gymnastics, and swimming.[30,33] Excessive stride length, or overstriding, has been posited as a possible risk factor for such injuries, especially in female military recruits.[29,32]

Presentation and Evaluation

Stress fractures of the pubic ramus can present with pain involving the inguinal, perineal, sacral, and/or gluteal regions. The pain is generally associated with physical exercise and relieved with rest.[27] On physical examination, there may be tenderness to palpation over the anterior groin, inferior pubic ramus, or adductor muscle insertion.[27,32] The pain may be exacerbated by hip abduction and resisted hip adduction.[27,32] Thus, pubic stress fractures may be easily mistaken for groin or adductor strains.[32]

Plain radiographs represent the initial imaging modality of choice and may demonstrate a hypointense transverse fissure and/or surrounding cloud-like callus, most often within the inferior pubic ramus (**Fig. 2**A).[27] However, plain radiographs often fail to identify bone stress injuries of the pelvis including the pubic ramus, with a reported sensitivity of 47%.[28,31] Moreover, the symptoms of pelvic stress fractures often overlap with those of higher-risk sites, namely the femoral neck, such that advanced imaging is essential to attain an accurate diagnosis.[28] MRI is generally favored and should include the entire pelvis and both proximal femurs (**Fig. 2**B).[28]

Management

The management of pubic stress fractures should follow the principles of low-risk fracture sites, as previously described for the sacrum. This includes a period of relative rest and restricted activity to a pain-free level followed by a gradual rehabilitation and return-to-sport progression.[29] Underlying risk factors should be corrected

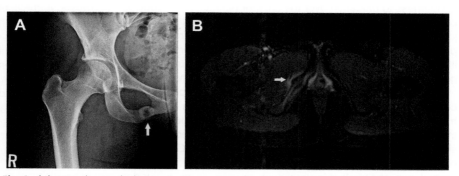

Fig. 2. (*A*) AP radiograph demonstrating a stress fracture (*arrow*) of the right inferior pubic ramus with surrounding cloud-like callus. (*B*) Axial, STIR MRI of the pelvis demonstrating a stress fracture (*arrow*) of the right inferior pubic ramus with surrounding marrow edema and periosteal fluid.

whenever possible, and calcium and vitamin D intake should be optimized. Like sacral stress fractures, those of the pubic ramus also often require a prolonged period of recovery, possibly related to the trabecular composition of the bone.[22,26] Delayed union[29] and nonunion[34] have been rarely reported. In at least 1 case of nonunion of an inferior pubic ramus stress fracture, successful treatment with percutaneous screw fixation has been described.[34]

STRESS FRACTURES OF THE FEMORAL NECK
Epidemiology

The femoral neck connects the femoral head to the femoral shaft. The junctional position of the femoral neck, and a relatively thin periosteum, subject it to higher risk of fracture. Stress fractures of the femoral neck are typically defined according to their location and corresponding distribution of forces across the bone.[35] Compression-sided fractures are overall more common and involve the inferomedial aspect of the neck, while tension-sided fractures involve the superolateral aspect of the neck.[35] Tension-sided fractures are more likely to displace if left untreated. Displaced fractures of the femoral neck, in particular, can disrupt the blood supply to the femoral head, increasing the risk of avascular necrosis and consequent joint destruction.[36]

Bone stress injuries of the femoral neck are fairly rare but are important to identify given the ominous nature of their location. Femoral neck stress fractures represent only about 2.5% to 5% of all bone stress injuries.[37,38] They are observed more commonly in runners than in other athlete groups.[39,40] Military recruits also appear to be at somewhat increased risk.[41] Other potential risk factors specific to the femoral neck may include decreased femoral bone mineral density,[42,43] gluteus medius weakness,[44] and femoroacetabular impingement (FAI).[44–46] Both cam- and pincer-type FAI have been associated with femoral neck stress fractures. It has been suggested that abnormal contact between the proximal femur and acetabular rim may lead to mechanical stress at the femoral neck that exceeds remodeling capacity and in turn results in bone stress injury.[45,46]

Presentation and Evaluation

Individuals with femoral neck stress fractures generally present with mechanical pain in the anterior hip, groin, or proximal thigh.[38,47] This may be accompanied with an antalgic gait.[38,47] On physical examination there can be pain-limited range of motion at the hip.[40] Tenderness to palpation over the anterior hip has been reported.[47] However, a precise palpatory examination is limited by the overlying soft tissues.[48] Manipulation of the hip joint including passive hip motion (especially internal rotation) and log roll, as well as hip provocation tests such as flexion, adduction, and internal rotation (FADIR) are often positive but nonspecific for stress fracture.[47] Heel percussion has been evaluated and is neither sensitive nor specific for the diagnosis of femoral neck stress fractures.[35,47]

Early diagnosis of femoral neck stress fractures is critical to minimize the potential for complication. Imaging evaluation should begin with plain radiographs, including at a minimum, an anteroposterior view of the pelvis and lateral view of the proximal femur. In the early stages, subtle ill definition of the affected cortex (known as a gray cortex sign) or a focal periosteal reaction may be present. Over time, a sclerotic linear region or cortical break may become apparent.[49] However, initial radiographs are frequently normal, and up to half of femoral neck stress fractures never demonstrate radiographic evidence of osseous injury.[49] Therefore, advanced imaging is often necessary to facilitate timely diagnosis and appropriate treatment. MRI has become the gold standard for the diagnosis of femoral neck stress fractures, and should be recommended in all individuals with suspected femoral neck stress fractures for whom initial radiographs are negative.[47,49] MRI exhibits exceptional sensitivity and specificity (approaching 100%) for femoral neck bone stress injuries and affords a comprehensive evaluation of the surrounding tissues to exclude alternative diagnoses.[50] Typical MRI findings include ill-defined bone marrow edema within the femoral neck. When present, a fracture line appears as a linear hypo-intense signal extending at right angles to the affected cortex (**Fig. 3**).[47,49] Radionuclide bone scans are a potential alternative to MRI, but are less specific, and have a high rate of false positives, exceeding 30%.[50]

MRI has also demonstrated a role in predicting outcomes related to bone stress injuries of the femoral neck. Steele and colleagues evaluated the risk of fracture progression in patients treated nonoperatively, and found that the initial presence of a hip joint effusion on MRI was a strong predictor for subsequent fracture progression requiring surgical fixation. Of note, no patients in their population with isolated edema without a fracture line (ie, stress reaction) had MRI progression necessitating surgical intervention.[51] The utility of MRI to predict return to activity has also been evaluated. Using the MRI grading scale proposed by Arendt and Griffiths[52] (**Table 1**), 1 study

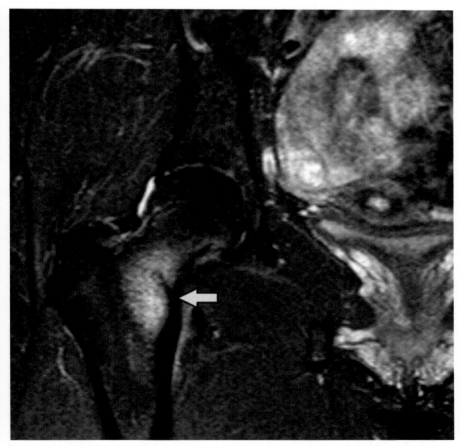

Fig. 3. Coronal, STIR MRI demonstrating a compression-sided stress fracture (*arrow*) of the femoral neck with surrounding marrow edema.

found that higher grade femoral neck stress injuries were associated with longer recovery periods and return to run.[53] Another study, using a modified grading scale (see **Table 1**), also found an association between higher grade injuries and military return to duty.[54] In this study, patients with high-grade femoral neck stress injuries had longer recovery times and higher rates of medical discharge, meaning an inability to complete basic training.[54]

Management

Given the higher risk of complication from femoral neck stress fractures, patients suspected of having such an injury should be made non-weightbearing pending definitive diagnosis. Long-term management is determined by the location, extent, and displacement of the fracture.[47] In general, compression-sided femoral neck stress fractures are more stable. Compression-sided stress reactions (ie, no fracture line present on MRI) or fractures involving less than 50% the width of the femoral neck are typically managed with a period of strict non-weightbearing.[50] Non-weightbearing status should be maintained until the patient is completely pain free, usually 6 to 8 weeks. During this time, patients must be followed closely, with serial radiographs every 1 to 2 weeks to evaluate for fracture progression.[50] Thereafter, progressive rehabilitation and weight-bearing activities may commence. A gradual return-to-sport progression is only permitted once there is clear clinical and radiographic evidence of fracture healing and union.

Surgical indications include compression-sided stress fractures involving greater than 50% of the width of the femoral neck or those with evidence of progression, malunion, or nonunion by follow-up imaging.[50] Initial management of tension-sided femoral neck stress fractures remains somewhat controversial, although most advocate for early percutaneous screw fixation.[47,50] Additionally, displaced fractures necessitate urgent surgical intervention to prevent avascular necrosis.[55,56] Although there is little evidence to guide implant selection for femoral neck stress fractures, it has been suggested that multiple cannulated screws are appropriate for compression-sided fractures, and a dynamic hip screw should be utilized for tension-sided fractures.[47] Postoperatively, 6 weeks of non-weightbearing, followed by an additional 6 weeks of partial weightbearing with crutches is recommended. It is reasonable to gradually resume lower-limb exercise once there is clinical and radiographic evidence of fracture union.[47]

Full return to sport following femoral neck stress fractures managed both conservatively and surgically often requires at least 3 to 6 months, but may exceed 1 year.[47] Moreover, many athletes may never achieve preinjury levels of activity. Johansson and colleagues[57] evaluated 23 elite and recreational athletes with femoral neck stress fractures (7 treated nonoperatively, 16 treated operatively) and found that 12 of 23

Table 1		
MRI grading scales for femoral neck bone stress injuries		
Grade	**Arendt & Griffiths,[52] 1997**	**Rohena-Quinquilla et al,[54] 2018**
Low	1	Signal change on STIR-image only	Endosteal marrow edema ≤6 mm
	2	Signal change on STIR- and T2-images	Endosteal marrow edema >6 mm and no macroscopic fracture
High	3	Signal change on T1- and T2-images; no fracture line	Macroscopic fracture <50% of femoral neck width
	4	Signal change on T1- and T2-images; fracture line present	Macroscopic fracture ≥50% of femoral neck width

(52%) were able to return to the same level of activity following treatment. Notably, the injury was career ending for all of the elite athletes in their cohort.[57] Similarly, Neubauer and colleagues[38] conducted a systematic review of elite and recreational runners with femoral neck stress fractures and reported that 58% were able to return to running; however, higher-performance runners were much less likely to resume running. In a recent study of military recruits with femoral neck stress fractures requiring surgical fixation, only 6 of 13 (46%) were able to return to full high-demand activity. Six of the 13 recruits were medically discharged, while the other remained on a permanent, no-run profile.[58] As previously stated, higher-grade femoral neck bone stress injuries have been correlated to prolonged recovery and lower likelihood of return to preinjury activity levels.[53,54] Correspondingly, displaced fractures have also been associated with worse outcomes and lower return-to-sport rates.[38,57]

SUMMARY

Bone stress injuries of the hip and pelvis are relatively rare, but have become increasingly recognized in certain populations, namely long-distance runners and military recruits. Sacral stress fractures are generally limited to the sacral ala, while stress fractures of the pubis most frequently involve the inferior pubic ramus near the junction of the ischial ramus. Stress fractures of the femoral neck may be compression-sided (inferomedial) or tension-sided (superolateral). In all cases, the diagnosis can be challenged by an often vague and nonspecific physical examination such that a high index of clinical suspicion is necessary to promote early detection and management. Advanced imaging is frequently required to confirm diagnosis, with MRI representing the current gold standard. Management is largely determined based upon the site of injury and its potential risk for complication. Lower-risk sites including the sacrum and the pubic ramus may be managed conservatively with activity modification to a pain-free level. Meanwhile, stress fractures of the femoral neck require, at a minimum, a period of strict non-weightbearing for at least 6 to 8 weeks. Surgical indications include compression-sided stress fractures involving greater than 50% of the width of the femoral neck, tension-sided fractures, and displaced fractures. In all instances of bone stress injury, it is critical to simultaneously identify and address any potentially modifiable risk factors including training errors, energy imbalance, poor bone health, and biomechanical deficits.

CLINICS CARE POINTS

- Stress fractures of the hip and pelvis require a high index of clinical suspicion for early diagnosis and to limit time lost from sport as well as to avoid potential complications.

- Specific risk factors for stress fractures of the hip and pelvis may include increased pelvic anteversion, excessive stride length, decreased femoral bone mineral density, gluteus medius weakness, and femoral acetabular impingement.

- The diagnostic yield of the physical examination and plain radiographs is often limited in the diagnosis of stress fractures involving the pelvic region, such that advanced imaging may be necessary to establish a diagnosis. MRI is currently the imaging modality of choice for the diagnosis of such injuries.

- MRI may have additional utility to predict fracture progression and return to play, particularly for stress fractures involving the femoral neck.

- Bone stress injuries of the sacrum and pubic ramus are typically managed with a period of relative rest, followed by progressive return-to-activity at a pain-free level; however, full return to preinjury training levels may require up to 3 to 6 months.

- Given a higher risk of potential complication with femoral neck stress fractures, a more aggressive treatment approach is warranted. A period of strict non-weightbearing for 6 to 8 weeks is recommended for compression-sided stress fractures involving less than 50% of the width of the femoral neck.

- Surgical indications for femoral neck stress fractures include compression-sided stress fractures involving greater than 50% of the width of the femoral neck, most tension-sided fractures, and displaced fractures.

ACKNOWLEDGMENTS

The author thanks Dr Jennifer Weaver and Dr Dustin Richter for their assistance procuring the radiographic figures included in the article.

DISCLOSURE

The author has nothing to disclose.

REFERENCES

1. Moreira CA, Bilezikian JP. Stress fractures: concepts and therapeutics. J Clin Endocrinol Metab 2016. https://doi.org/10.1210/jc.2016-2720.
2. Snyder RA, Koester MC, Dunn WR. Epidemiology of stress fractures. Clin Sports Med 2006;25(1):37–52.
3. Tenforde AS, Nattiv A, Barrack M, et al. Distribution of bone stress injuries in elite male and female collegiate runners: 3363 board #124 May 30, 9. Med Sci Sports Exerc 2015;47:905.
4. Milgrom C, Giladi M, Stein M, et al. Stress fractures in military recruits. A prospective study showing an unusually high incidence. J Bone Joint Surg Br 1985;67(5):732–5.
5. Bennell KL, Brukner PD. Epidemiology and site specificity of stress fractures. Clin Sports Med 1997;16(2):179–96.
6. Fredericson M, Jennings F, Beaulieu C, et al. Stress fractures in athletes. Top Magn Reson Imaging 2006;17(5):309–25.
7. Pepper M, Akuthota V, McCarty EC. The pathophysiology of stress fractures. Clin Sports Med 2006;25(1):1–16.
8. Warden SJ, Davis IS, Fredericson M. Management and prevention of bone stress injuries in long-distance runners. J Orthop Sports Phys Ther 2014;44(10):749–65.
9. Spitz DJ, Newberg AH. Imaging of stress fractures in the athlete. Radiol Clin North Am 2002;40(2):313–31.
10. Cheng JS, Song JK. Anatomy of the sacrum. Neurosurg Focus 2003;15(2):E3.
11. Denis F, Davis S, Comfort T. Sacral fractures: an important problem. Retrospective analysis of 236 cases. Clin Orthop Relat Res 1988;227:67–81.
12. Zaman FM, Frey M, Slipman CW. Sacral stress fractures. Curr Sports Med Rep 2006;5(1):37–43.
13. Leroux JL, Denat B, Thomas E, et al. Sacral insufficiency fractures presenting as acute low-back pain. Biomechanical aspects. Spine 1993;18(16):2502–6.
14. Major NM, Helms CA. Pelvic stress injuries: the relationship between osteitis pubis (symphysis pubis stress injury) and sacroiliac abnormalities in athletes. Skeletal Radiol 1997;26(12):711–7.

15. Fredericson M, Salamancha L, Beaulieu C. Sacral stress fractures: tracking down nonspecific pain in distance runners. Phys Sportsmed 2003;31(2):31–42.

16. Marchinkow A, Mallinson PI, Coupal T, et al. Sacral stress fractures in a sprint and throw athlete–a case report. Curr Sports Med Rep 2014;13(5):297–8.

17. Vajapey S, Matic G, Hartz C, et al. Sacral stress fractures: a rare but curable cause of back pain in athletes. Sports Health 2019;11(5):446–52.

18. Hameed F, McInnis KC. Sacral stress fracture causing radiculopathy in a female runner: a case report. PM R 2011;3(5):489–91.

19. Volpin G, Milgrom C, Goldsher D, et al. Stress fractures of the sacrum following strenuous activity. Clin Orthop Relat Res 1989;243:184–8.

20. Campbell S, Fajardo R. Imaging of stress injuries of the pelvis. Semin Musculoskelet Radiol 2008;12(1):062–71.

21. Spiegl U, Schnake K, Osterhoff G, et al. Imaging of sacral stress and insufficiency fractures. Z Orthop Unfall 2019;157(02):144–53.

22. Miller C, Major N, Toth A. Pelvic stress injuries in the athlete: management and prevention. Sports Med 2003;33(13):1003–12.

23. Liem BC, Truswell HJ, Harrast MA. Rehabilitation and return to running after lower limb stress fractures. Curr Sports Med Rep 2013;12(3):200–7.

24. Tenforde AS, Watanabe LM, Moreno TJ, et al. Use of an antigravity treadmill for rehabilitation of a pelvic stress injury. PM R 2012;4(8):629–31.

25. Raasch WG, Hergan DJ. Treatment of stress fractures: the fundamentals. Clin Sports Med 2006;25(1):29–36, vii.

26. Nattiv A, Kennedy G, Barrack MT, et al. Correlation of MRI grading of bone stress injuries with clinical risk factors and return to play: a 5-year prospective study in collegiate track and field athletes. Am J Sports Med 2013;41(8):1930–41.

27. Meurman KO. Stress fracture of the pubic arch in military recruits. Br J Radiol 1980;53(630):521–4.

28. Kiuru MJ, Pihlajamaki HK, Ahovuo JA. Fatigue stress injuries of the pelvic bones and proximal femur: evaluation with MR imaging. Eur Radiol 2003;13(3):605–11.

29. Pavlov H, Nelson TL, Warren RF, et al. Stress fractures of the pubic ramus. A report of twelve cases. J Bone Joint Surg Am 1982;64(7):1020–5.

30. Kim SM, Park CH, Gartland JJ. Stress fracture of the pubic ramus in a swimmer. Clin Nucl Med 1987;12(2):118–9.

31. Lee SW, Lee CH. Fatigue stress fractures of the pubic ramus in the army: imaging features with radiographic, scintigraphic and MR imaging findings. Korean J Radiol 2005;6(1):47–51.

32. Hill PF, Chatterji S, Chambers D, et al. Stress fracture of the pubic ramus in female recruits. J Bone Joint Surg Br 1996;78(3):383–6.

33. Schapira D, Militeanu D, Israel O, et al. Insufficiency fractures of the pubic ramus. Semin Arthritis Rheum 1996;25(6):373–82.

34. Okike K, Moritz BE. Minimally invasive screw fixation of inferior pubic ramus stress fracture nonunion in a runner: a case report. JBJS Case Connect 2016; 6(2):e261–6.

35. Fullerton LR, Snowdy HA. Femoral neck stress fractures. Am J Sports Med 1988; 16(4):365–77.

36. Boden BP, Osbahr DC. High-risk stress fractures: evaluation and treatment. J Am Acad Orthop Surg 2000;8(6):344–53.

37. Hulkko A, Orava S. Stress fractures in athletes. Int J Sports Med 1987;8(3):221–6.

38. Neubauer T, Brand J, Lidder S, et al. Stress fractures of the femoral neck in runners: a review. Res Sports Med 2016;24(3):283–97.

39. Taunton JE, Ryan MB, Clement DB, et al. A retrospective case-control analysis of 2002 running injuries. Br J Sports Med 2002;36(2):95–101.
40. Biz C, Berizzi A, Crimì A, et al. Management and treatment of femoral neck stress fractures in recreational runners: a report of four cases and review of the literature. Acta Biomed 2017;88(4S):96–106.
41. Waterman BR, Gun B, Bader JO, et al. Epidemiology of lower extremity stress fractures in the United States Military. Mil Med 2016;181(10):1308–13.
42. Pouilles JM, Bernard J, Tremollières F, et al. Femoral bone density in young male adults with stress fractures. Bone 1989;10(2):105–8.
43. Tenforde AS, Parziale AL, Popp KL, et al. Low bone mineral density in male athletes is associated with bone stress injuries at anatomic sites with greater trabecular composition. Am J Sports Med 2018;46(1):30–6.
44. Carpintero P, Leon F, Zafra M, et al. Stress fractures of the femoral neck and coxa vara. Arch Orthop Trauma Surg 2003;123(6):273–7.
45. Carey T, Key C, Oliver D, et al. Prevalence of radiographic findings consistent with femoroacetabular impingement in military personnel with femoral neck stress fractures. J Surg Orthop Adv 2013;22(1):54–8.
46. Goldin M, Anderson CN, Fredericson M, et al. Femoral neck stress fractures and imaging features of femoroacetabular impingement. PM R 2015;7(6):584–92.
47. Robertson GA, Wood AM. Femoral neck stress fractures in sport: a current concepts review. Sports Med Int Open 2017;1(2):E58–68.
48. McInnis KC, Ramey LN. High-risk stress fractures: diagnosis and management. PM R 2016;8(3S):S113–24.
49. Bencardino JT, Palmer WE. Imaging of hip disorders in athletes. Radiol Clin North Am 2002;40(2):267–87, vi-vii.
50. Shin AY, Morin WD, Gorman JD, et al. The superiority of magnetic resonance imaging in differentiating the cause of hip pain in endurance athletes. Am J Sports Med 1996;24(2):168–76.
51. Steele CE, Cochran G, Renninger C, et al. Femoral Neck Stress Fractures: MRI Risk Factors for Progression. J Bone Joint Surg Am 2018;100(17):1496–502.
52. Arendt EA, Griffiths HJ. The use of MR imaging in the assessment and clinical management of stress reactions of bone in high-performance athletes. Clin Sports Med 1997;16(2):291–306.
53. Ramey LN, McInnis KC, Palmer WE. Femoral neck stress fracture: can mri grade help predict return-to-running time? Am J Sports Med 2016;44(8):2122–9.
54. Rohena-Quinquilla IR, Rohena-Quinquilla FJ, Scully WF, et al. Femoral Neck Stress Injuries: Analysis of 156 Cases in a U.S. Military Population and Proposal of a New MRI classification system. AJR Am J Roentgenol 2018;210(3):601–7.
55. Lee C-H, Huang G-S, Chao K-H, et al. Surgical treatment of displaced stress fractures of the femoral neck in military recruits: a report of 42 cases. Arch Orthop Trauma Surg 2003;123(10):527–33.
56. Evans JT, Guyver PM, Kassam AM, et al. Displaced femoral neck stress fractures in Royal Marine recruits–management and results of operative treatment. J R Nav Med Serv 2012;98(2):3–5.
57. Johansson C, Ekenman I, Törnkvist H, et al. Stress fractures of the femoral neck in athletes. The consequence of a delay in diagnosis. Am J Sports Med 1990;18(5):524–8.
58. Kusnezov NA, Eisenstein ED, Dunn JC, et al. Functional Outcomes Following Surgical Management of Femoral Neck Stress Fractures. Orthopedics 2017;40(3):e395–9.

Pelvic Avulsion Injuries in the Adolescent Athlete

Kathryn C. Yeager, MD, Selina R. Silva, MD, Dustin L. Richter, MD*

KEYWORDS

- Pelvic avulsion • Adolescent hip avulsion • ASIS avulsion • AIIS avulsion
- Ischial avulsion • Iliac crest avulsion

KEY POINTS

- Apophyseal avulsion fractures are seen almost exclusively in the setting of pediatric sports participation. The apophysis is at risk during the time between the formation of the secondary ossification center and its closure.
- Older adolescents are more likely to sustain injuries to the iliac crest and anterior superior iliac spine (ASIS), and younger adolescents tend to sustain injuries at the anterior inferior iliac spine (AIIS) and ischium.
- The history and physical examination are excellent clues as to the diagnosis and usually confirmed with plain radiographs. Ischial avulsion fractures may require advanced imaging to evaluate the extent of hamstring tendon involvement.
- Pelvic avulsion fractures rely on the amount of fragment displacement to guide treatment. Conservative management is appropriate in most cases with recommendations of rest and avoiding use of the muscle(s) that attach to the avulsed piece. Operative treatment is typically reserved for widely displaced fractures or symptomatic nonunions.

INTRODUCTION

Growing numbers of children in the United States participate in sports each year. There are concerns that current trends placing higher demands on young athletes and a push toward earlier single sport specialization may contribute to greater risk of injury.[1,2] Physiologic differences in the pediatric skeletal system compared with that of an adult lead to differences in the types of injuries sustained during sporting activity.[3] One class of injuries unique to the pediatric population are apophyseal avulsion fractures, an entity almost exclusively seen in the setting of pediatric sports participation.

No outside research support or funding is pertinent to this review. The authors have no conflicts of interest to disclose.

Department of Orthopaedic Surgery, University of New Mexico, 1 University of New Mexico, MSC10 5600, Albuquerque, NM 87131, USA

* Corresponding author.

E-mail address: dustin.richter1818@gmail.com

Apophyseal avulsion injuries are rare injuries that occur in the setting of sudden, forceful, eccentric contraction of the lower extremity. Tensile force ultimately leads to avulsion of the musculotendinous attachment with fracture at the secondary apophysis. Apophyseal avulsions in the pediatric pelvis tend to occur with sudden eccentric forces, as seen in sprinting, jumping, swinging a bat, or kicking. In the pelvis, avulsion fractures are most commonly seen at the anterior superior iliac spine (ASIS), anterior inferior iliac spine (AIIS), and ischial tuberosity. Avulsions from the iliac crest and pubic symphysis also can be seen.

The pediatric pelvis is at risk of avulsion fractures due to tensile stress on the apophyseal growth plate. The cartilaginous growth plate tends to fail in tension before the musculotendinous unit, leading to avulsion fractures at the level of the apophysis. The apophysis is at risk of injury in the time between the formation of the secondary ossification center and its closure. Formation of the secondary ossification center typically begins in girls around age 10 at the AIIS, with closure ranging from age 11 to 16. The remainder of the iliac crest closes between 16 to 25 years of age.[4]

In a 2015 review of 228 pediatric pelvic avulsion fractures, it was determined that 49% were AIIS avulsions, 30% ASIS avulsions, 11% ischial tuberosity avulsions, and 10% iliac crest avulsions.[5] The most common mechanisms were running (39%) and kicking (29%), with the most common sports during which these injuries occurred being soccer (32%), track and field (24%), and football (14%).

Age, skeletal maturity, and sex have been found to be associated with specific types of avulsion fractures of the pelvis.[5,6] Older adolescents are more likely to sustain injuries to the iliac crest and ASIS, whereas younger adolescents tend to sustain injuries at the AIIS and ischium. Overall, boys are more likely than girls to sustain pelvic apophyseal avulsion fractures. Due to their earlier skeletal maturity and physeal closure, girls tend to sustain these injuries at a younger age than boys.

ANTERIOR SUPERIOR ILIAC SPINE AVULSION INJURY
Etiology

ASIS avulsions occur secondary to eccentric force at the hip with avulsion of the sartorius muscle. Although the tensor fascia lata also originates from the ASIS, these avulsions tend to cause iliac crest avulsion fractures instead of ASIS avulsions. ASIS avulsions are typically seen between age 11 and 16 in girls and 12 and 18 in boys. This injury is most commonly sustained in activities that involve running and kicking. ASIS avulsions are more likely to occur in the setting of a closed triradiate cartilage compared with AIIS avulsions.[5]

Presentation and Evaluation

Patients with ASIS avulsions will typically present with pain at the anterior pelvis and point tenderness over the ASIS. Patients will frequently report feeling or hearing a "pop" at the time of injury. Weight bearing may be limited secondary to pain. In acute injuries, swelling and ecchymosis also may be present over the ASIS. On physical examination, resisted hip flexion will likely be painful and weaker compared with the contralateral side.

Initial workup includes radiographs of the pelvis. Typically, an anterior-posterior (AP) and frog-leg lateral view of the pelvis will sufficiently demonstrate the avulsion from the ASIS while including the contralateral side for comparison (**Fig. 1**). Of note, ASIS avulsion injuries can be mistaken for AIIS avulsions due to lateral and inferior displacement of the avulsed fragment on radiographs. In children with delayed presentation, callus

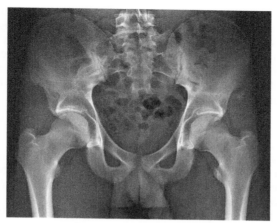

Fig. 1. AP radiograph of the pelvis in an adolescent athlete demonstrating a left-sided ASIS avulsion injury.

formation already may be present. Advanced imaging with computed tomography (CT) or MRI is rarely needed, but may assist in confirming the diagnosis.

Management

Nonoperative treatment with rest, protected weight bearing, and nonsteroidal anti-inflammatory drugs is the standard treatment for most ASIS avulsion injuries. Partial weight bearing with crutches is typically allowed at 0 to 3 weeks, with full weight bearing starting at 3 to 6 weeks. Return to sport is usually permitted approximately 3 months postinjury. Some studies report a longer delay in return to sport with conservative treatment when compared with surgical fixation.[7]

Surgical treatment for ASIS avulsions is typically reserved for fractures with more than 20 mm of displacement or in the setting of a chronic, painful nonunion. Some studies suggest a cutoff of 15 mm of fragment displacement for consideration of operative fixation.[8] Surgical fixation is most commonly performed with screws, with k-wires and plates less commonly used. The rate of nonunion for pelvic apophyseal avulsion fractures has been demonstrated to be lower with surgical fixation (0% vs 2.4%); however, there is a greater risk of heterotopic ossification reported after surgery in some studies (8.2% vs 2.4%).[8]

Postoperatively, patients are typically kept non–weight bearing for 7 to 10 days. Some literature suggests that it is safe to begin immediate partial weight bearing, with full weight bearing approximately 4 to 6 weeks after surgery. Return to sport is between 6 to 12 weeks based on patient recovery and radiographic healing.[7,8]

ANTERIOR INFERIOR ILIAC SPINE AVULSION INJURY
Etiology

AIIS avulsion fracture involves the direct head of the rectus femoris tendon. The direct head of the rectus femoris originates from the AIIS, whereas the indirect head originates from the anterior superior acetabular rim and is rarely affected by avulsion injuries. Avulsion injury of the AIIS typically occurs with eccentric force at the hip, such as seen in sprinting and kicking a ball.

AIIS injuries are more commonly seen in boys (82%) than girls, with greater gender disproportion than that seen in ASIS avulsions. AIIS avulsion fractures are also seen more commonly in sports played with a ball (70%) compared with ASIS avulsions, which are seen more equally between ball sports and other athletic activities.[8] Due to the earlier age at formation of the AIIS apophysis, these injuries are usually seen in younger patients who consequently have a greater rate of open triradiate cartilage at the time of injury.[5]

Presentation and Evaluation

Similar to ASIS avulsions, patients with AIIS injuries may describe feeling or hearing a "pop" at the time of injury. Swelling and ecchymosis may be present. Physical examination will demonstrate tenderness at the AIIS. Pain and weakness with hip flexion, knee extension, or a resisted straight leg raise also may be present.

Initial diagnostic workup includes plain radiographs with AP and frog-leg lateral of the pelvis and hip (**Fig. 2**). As with ASIS avulsions, CT or MRI are rarely needed for diagnosis but may assist if the diagnosis is unclear on initial radiographic evaluation.

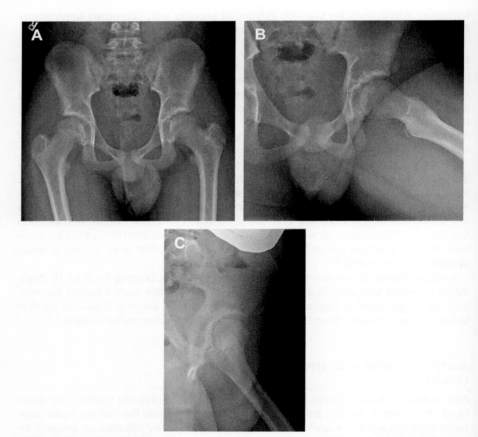

Fig. 2. (*A–C*) AP, frog-leg lateral, and false profile radiographs of the pelvis in an adolescent soccer player demonstrating a left-sided AIIS avulsion injury.

Management

Standard treatment for AIIS avulsion fractures is nonoperative with a period of protected weight bearing for 6 to 8 weeks. Traditionally, operative indications include displacement of greater than 20 mm, impingement with sitting, and painful nonunions. One meta-analysis of pelvic apophyseal avulsion fractures demonstrated that patients with more than 15 mm of fracture displacement had improved clinical outcomes with surgical intervention compared with nonoperative treatment.[8] In this review, overall clinical outcomes trended toward improvement in the operative group compared with nonoperative; however, failed to meet statistical significance.[8]

Although nonoperative treatment remains the standard of care for AIIS avulsions, some data have suggested greater rates of future hip pain with AIIS avulsions when compared with other avulsion fractures. Schuett and colleagues[5] reported the risk of future hip pain at 4.47 times more likely in AIIS avulsions. Furthermore, abnormal morphology of the AIIS after nonunion or malunion can lead to extra-articular femoroacetabular impingement[9] or subspine impingement. In this setting, patients may require surgery in later years to address symptomatic impingement due to the abnormal morphology of the AIIS (**Fig. 3**).

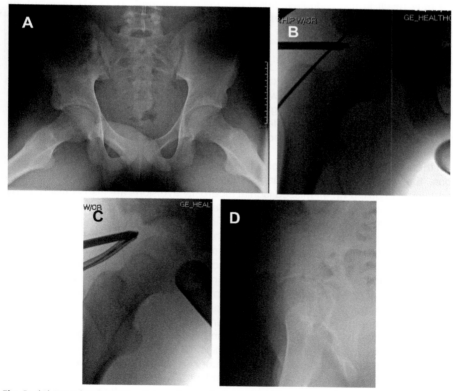

Fig. 3. (*A*) Frog-leg lateral pelvis radiograph demonstrating overgrowth of the right hip AIIS from prior healed avulsion injury, causing symptomatic subspine impingement. (*B, C*) Intraoperative fluoroscopic images of the right hip demonstrating localization of the AIIS and arthroscopic subspine decompression/acetabuloplasty. (*D*) Postoperative false profile radiograph showing final correction of the AIIS overgrowth.

ISCHIAL TUBEROSITY AVULSION INJURY
Etiology

The ischial tuberosity is the origin of the hamstring muscles (semitendinosus, semi-membranosus, and long head of the biceps femoris). The secondary ossification center of the ischial tuberosity appears between 12 and 14 years of age and closes at approximately 20 years of age.[4] Avulsion fractures off the ischial tuberosity occur from forceful flexion of the hip joint with concurrent knee extension. This specific leg position typically occurs during sprinting and kicking.[7] The incidence of ischial tuberosity avulsion is estimated to be 11% of all pediatric pelvic avulsion fractures.[5]

Presentation and Evaluation

Patients with ischial tuberosity avulsion fractures may experience a sudden "pop" at the time of injury. On physical examination, these patients will complain of pain with sitting, tenderness when palpating the ischium, and pain with bending forward, which puts the hamstrings on stretch. Swelling and ecchymosis is common along the posterior thigh.

Initial diagnostic workup includes plain radiographs with an AP of the pelvis. The extent of hamstring avulsion can be difficult to determine using plain radiographs and may result in misdiagnosis, which can delay treatment. Thus, CT or MRI may be required to ensure an accurate diagnosis in a timely manner and guide appropriate management.

Management

Conservative management is recommended for fragments displaced less than 15 mm, as shown in a small study with 13 patients.[10] Closed treatment should include decreasing the pull of the hamstrings on the avulsed fragment, which involves keeping the knee bent or preventing deep flexion of the hip joint. Bracing may be helpful to aid the patient in maintaining these precautions. In addition, we recommend avoiding athletic activities for 6 to 12 weeks.

In the setting of a delayed diagnosis or a patient having difficulty adhering to restrictions, the repetitive pull of the hamstrings on the avulsed fragment can lead to nonunion and pain (**Fig. 4**). Missed ischial tuberosity avulsions are also at risk of tardy sciatic nerve palsy in which the patient complains of pain radiating down the posterior thigh during prolonged periods of sitting. Sundar and Carty[11] observed 32 conservatively treated pelvic avulsion fractures over a 44-month time period and found that 31% went on to persistent pain and symptoms during sports. The cases that failed conservative treatment were primarily the ischial avulsion patients. Therefore, early recognition is important and surgical treatment is recommended for cases displaced more than 15 mm or in the setting of a symptomatic nonunion.[7] The most common surgical approach is a modified Kocher-Langenbeck for plate fixation of these injuries. Others have recommended a gluteal crease incision and fixation of the fracture fragment with screws, or excision of the piece and repair of the hamstrings back to the ischium through suture anchors or bone tunnels.[7] (**Fig. 5**).

Most investigators recommend a longer, conservative postoperative course with slow return to full weight bearing to avoid implant failure. Bracing can be used for 6 to 12 weeks to avoid excessive tension on the hamstrings insertion, with a full return to sports at 5 to 6 months. This is a much longer rehabilitation course when compared with the other pelvic avulsion injuries. Other treatment methods described in the literature, such as percutaneous fenestration of the avulsed fragment or the use of platelet-rich plasma, are not the standard of care and need further study.[7]

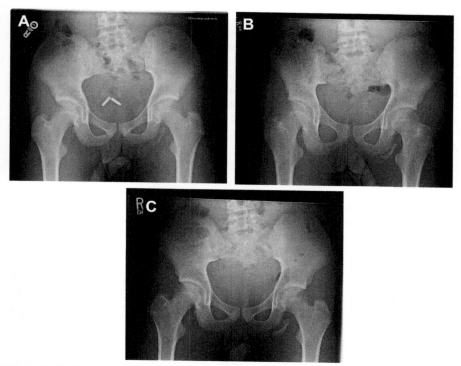

Fig. 4. (A–C) AP radiographs of the pelvis at time of injury (A), 6 weeks postinjury (B), and 12 weeks postinjury (C). Images demonstrate progression of the ischial tuberosity avulsion into a displaced and painful, symptomatic nonunion.

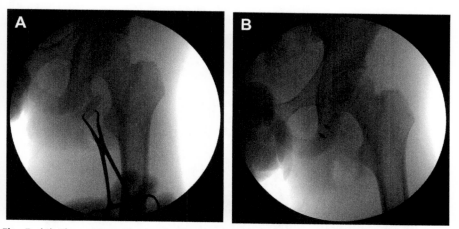

Fig. 5. (A) The patient previously described in **Fig. 4** with the painful ischial tuberosity nonunion underwent operative fixation. The avulsed fragment was not able to be mobilized adequately for fixation (A); thus, the fragment was excised and the hamstring tendon was advanced primarily repaired with suture anchors to the donor ischial tuberosity (B).

ILIAC CREST AVULSION INJURY
Etiology

The secondary ossification center of the iliac crest appears between 13 and 15 years of age and closes between 15 and 17 years of age.[7] Avulsion fractures of the iliac crest occur from forceful twisting or lateral flexion because of the strong abdominal muscles that attach along the crest. Eccentric contraction of the tensor fascia lata can also lead to avulsion of the iliac crest apophysis. This injury is rare and the incidence has been estimated to be 6% to 10% of all pediatric pelvic avulsion fractures.[5,7]

Presentation and Evaluation

Given the rarity of this injury, it can be more difficult to diagnose. Patients with iliac crest avulsions will demonstrate pain along the iliac crest and complain of pain with twisting motions or contraction of their tensor fascia lata or their abdominal external obliques. Initial diagnostic workup includes plain radiographs with an AP of the pelvis. CT or MRI may assist if the diagnosis is unclear on initial radiographic evaluation (**Fig. 6**). If these injuries are not identified and activity is not restricted, there is a risk of further displacement and the need for open reduction and internal fixation.

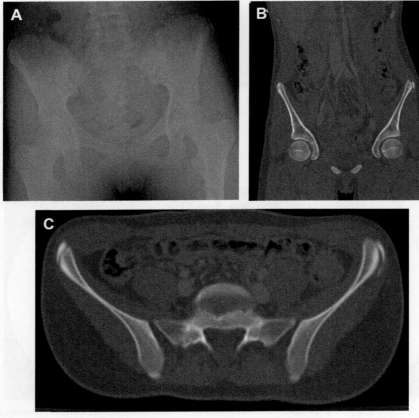

Fig. 6. (A) AP radiograph of the pelvis demonstrating a left-sided iliac crest avulsion injury. (B, C) Advanced CT imaging further demonstrates the size, location, and displacement of the iliac crest avulsion injury.

Management

When this type of avulsion fracture occurs, the apophyseal fragment is typically minimally displaced and can be treated conservatively with rest from athletic activities for 6 to 12 weeks.[5] It has been recommended that fragments more than 3 cm displaced should be reduced and fixed.[5] One technique described is open reduction of the fragment and use of 2 to 4 cannulated screws for internal fixation. Patients in one series did well with weight bearing at 2 weeks and return to sport at 4 weeks.[12]

PUBIC SYMPHYSIS AVULSION INJURY

Avulsion fractures of the pubic symphysis are extremely rare injuries. In the review by Schuett and colleagues[5] of 228 pelvic avulsion fractures, none of the injuries involved the pubic symphysis. The rectus abdominal sheath attaches to the superior pubic symphysis, whereas the hip adductors attach to the inferior pubic symphysis. Although adductor avulsion has been described during kicking,[13] core muscle injury (sports hernia) is a more likely diagnosis. Pubic symphysis avulsion injuries may be difficult to diagnose on plain radiographs, frequently requiring an MRI. Although fixation has rarely been described in adult patients, treatment in the youth population is almost universally nonoperative with activity modification and symptomatic management.[14]

SUMMARY

Pelvic avulsion fractures are common in young athletes, and many of these injuries can be treated conservatively. The history and physical examination are excellent clues to the diagnosis, which is usually confirmed with plain radiographs. Ischial avulsion fractures may require advanced imaging to evaluate the extent of hamstring tendon involvement. All of the adolescent pelvic avulsion fractures rely on the amount of displacement to guide treatment. Conservative management recommendations include rest and avoiding use of the muscle(s) that attach to the avulsed fragment. Operative treatment is typically reserved for widely displaced fractures or symptomatic nonunions. For operative ischial tuberosity avulsion cases, we advocate for excision of the ischial fragment and repair of the hamstrings back to the ischium. With appropriate treatment, young athletes can frequently return to their same level of sport.[5,6,8]

CLINICS CARE POINTS

- Apophyseal avulsion fractures of the pelvis are an uncommon entity almost exclusively seen in adolescent athletes due to eccentric forces on the secondary apophysis.

- Radiographs are generally sufficient to diagnose pelvic apophyseal avulsion fractures; advanced imaging with CT or MRI may be necessary in some cases for diagnosing ischial tuberosity and pubic symphysis avulsion fractures.

- Current literature lacks in large prospective studies on the management of pelvic apophyseal avulsion fractures.

- Standard of care is conservative treatment with protected weight bearing, activity restriction, and anti-inflammatory medications.

- Surgical intervention is reserved for painful nonunions and fractures with more than 20 mm displacement, although some studies suggest a cutoff of 15 mm for surgical intervention.

ACKNOWLEDGMENTS

The authors thank Zachary Hillman, MD, for his assistance in the identification and collection of radiographs and advanced imaging published in this article.

REFERENCES

1. Jayanthi NA, LaBella CR, Fischer D, et al. Sports-specialized intensive training and the risk of injury in young athletes: a clinical case-control study. Am J Sports Med 2015;43(4):794–801.
2. Myer GD, Jayanthi N, Difiori JP, et al. Sport specialization, part I: does early sports specialization increase negative outcomes and reduce the opportunity for success in young athletes? Sports Health 2015;7(5):437–42.
3. Adirim TA, Cheng TL. Overview of injuries in the young athlete. Sports Med 2003; 33(1):75–81.
4. Parvaresh KC, Upasani VV, Bomar JD, et al. Secondary ossification center appearance and closure in the pelvis and proximal femur. J Pediatr Orthop 2018;38(8):418–23.
5. Schuett DJ, Bomar JD, Pennock AT. Pelvic apophyseal avulsion fractures: a retrospective review of 228 cases. J Pediatr Orthop 2015;35(6):617–23.
6. Anduaga I, Seijas R, Pérez-Bellmunt A, et al. Anterior iliac spine avulsion fracture treatment options in young athletes. J Invest Surg 2020;33(2):159–63.
7. Schiller J, DeFroda S, Blood T. Lower extremity avulsion fractures in the pediatric and adolescent athlete. J Am Acad Orthop Surg 2017;25(4):251–9.
8. Eberbach H, Hohloch L, Feucht MJ, et al. Operative versus conservative treatment of apophyseal avulsion fractures of the pelvis in the adolescents: a systematical review with meta-analysis of clinical outcome and return to sports. BMC Musculoskelet Disord 2017;18. https://doi.org/10.1186/s12891-017-1527-z.
9. Novais EN, Riederer MF, Provance AJ. Anterior inferior iliac spine deformity as a cause for extra-articular hip impingement in young athletes after an avulsion fracture: a case report. Sports Health 2017;10(3):272–6.
10. Singer G, Eberl R, Wegmann H, et al. Diagnosis and treatment of apophyseal injuries of the pelvis in adolescents. Semin Musculoskelet Radiol 2014;18(5): 498–504.
11. Sundar M, Carty H. Avulsion fractures of the pelvis in children: a report of 32 fractures and their outcome. Skeletal Radiol 1994;23(2):85–90.
12. Li X, Xu S, Lin X, et al. Results of operative treatment of avulsion fractures of the iliac crest apophysis in adolescents. Injury 2014;45(4):721–4.
13. Rossi F, Dragoni S. Acute avulsion fractures of the pelvis in adolescent competitive athletes: Prevalence, location and sports distribution of 203 cases collected. Skeletal Radiol 2001;30(3):127–31.
14. Vogt S, Ansah P, Imhoff AB. Complete osseous avulsion of the adductor longus muscle: Acute repair with three fiberwire suture anchors. Arch Orthop Trauma Surg 2007;127(8):613–5.

Hip Injuries in the Adolescent Athlete

Paul B. Schroeder, MD[a], Marc A. Nicholes, BA[b], Matthew R. Schmitz, MD[a],*

KEYWORDS

- Adolescent athletic hip • Pediatric sports injuries • Legg-Calve-Perthes disease
- Femoroacetabular impingement • Apophyseal avulsion
- Developmental dysplasia of the hip • Coxa saltans
- Slipped capital femoral epiphysis

KEY POINTS

- Adolescents often have referred knee pain with hip pathology; therefore, a physical examination of the hip is necessary during initial evaluation of knee complaints.
- Radiographs are the diagnostic imaging modality of choice with advanced imaging being used when radiographs are equivocal, such as with suspected stress fractures and slipped capital femoral epiphysis (SCFE) (pre-slip).
- Learning radiographic measurements and relationships is necessary for diagnosing hip pathology.
- Early, proper diagnosis and treatment with conservative measures can avoid long-term complications and the need for surgery in many adolescent hip pathologies.
- Failure to diagnosis developmental dysplasia of the hip, femoral neck stress fractures, Legg-calve-Perthes disease, and SCFE can lead to detrimental osteoarthritis, completed fractures and avascular necrosis of the femoral head.

INTRODUCTION AND ETIOLOGY

Adolescent hip injuries encompass a wide range of disorders that are the result of not only acute trauma but also the manifestation of abnormal development. They commonly occur at a rate of approximately 53 per 100,000 athlete exposures based on National Collegiate Athletic Association reports.[1] It is important to note that sports involving explosive activities, as seen in soccer, ice hockey, and football, have a higher incidence of hip injuries. The temporal aspect of a person's hip pain also can provide insightful clues as to the underlying pathology. The acute onset of pain may represent

[a] Department of Orthopaedics, San Antonio Military Medical Center, 3851 Roger Brooke Drive, Fort Sam Houston, TX 78234, USA; [b] School of Osteopathic Medicine, University of the Incarnate Word, 7615 Kennedy Hill, Building 1, San Antonio, TX 78234, USA
* Corresponding author.
E-mail address: mattrschmitz@gmail.com
Twitter: @RugbyMD (M.R.S.)

Clin Sports Med 40 (2021) 385–398
https://doi.org/10.1016/j.csm.2020.12.003
0278-5919/21/Published by Elsevier Inc.

a fracture or soft tissue tear, whereas an insidious onset of pain may be related to developmental anatomy. The location of the athlete's pain can help determine the source, as groin pain is likely to represent intra-articular pathology. Lateral-based pain should raise concerns for anatomically pertinent pain generators, such as Iliotibial (IT) Band syndrome or abductor fatigue syndrome.[2] In younger patients, it is important to note that pain in the knee may be referred from the hip. Other important historical factors to assess for include the female athlete triad, family history of developmental disorders, or endocrinopathies.

PHYSICAL EXAMINATION

The physical examination of the hip consists of gait analysis, hip range of motion (ROM), muscular strength, and provocative testing to help elucidate a patient's potential pathology. The first assessment is to determine the ability to weight bear and abnormalities such as an antalgic gait and a Trendelenburg gait. A Trendelenburg gait occurs when there is associated hip abductor weakness and results in lateral trunk flexion to the affected side as the patient shifts their center of gravity to compensate for the associated abductor weakness.[3] Assessing hip ROM, specifically internal and external rotation, should be performed both prone to assess for femoral version, and supine with the hip flexed and extended. Dynamic testing of hip ROM can also be used to identify coxa saltans. Specialized examination maneuvers can be used to assist with differentiation between intra-articular and extra-articular pathologies. Flexion, adduction, and internal rotation (FADIR) is associated with femoroacetabular impingement, especially if there is a loss of associated internal rotation. Painful log roll test with the hip extended has been advocated to raise the suspicion for intra-articular pathology.[4] Flexion, abduction, and external rotation (FABER) can be used to diagnose posterior femoroacetabular impingement (FAI) or sacroiliac syndrome. It is considered positive for hip pathology when it produces groin pain or increased difference (>4 cm) between knee-to-table distance when compared with the contralateral side.[3] In addition, signs of hypermobility, including elevated Beighton Scores or anterior hip pain with the hip externally rotated in extension may help elucidate hip instability as the source of the problem.[2]

IMAGING

Imaging of the adolescent hip starts with the following radiographs: an anteroposterior (AP) pelvis, a false profile view, and a frog-leg or Dunn view. The decision to escalate to advanced imaging is mainly necessary for preoperative planning or to rule out injuries not seen on plain films. An MRI is used to visualize soft tissues, bony edema, and osteonecrosis. A computed tomography (CT) scan with 3-dimensional (3D) reconstructions provides improved bony anatomy visualization when compared with radiographs but should be completed with a low-dose protocol to limit radiation exposure.[5]

APOPHYSEAL AVULSIONS

Apophyseal avulsions are a noncontact injury resulting from rapid accelerations and decelerations during high-impact athletics. Repetitive stress on the musculoskeletal unit coupled with the intrinsic weakness of the epiphyseal plates explains why this fracture affects adolescents.[2] The same mechanism, in skeletally mature adults, usually results in a muscle or tendon injury.

This injury typically affects 14-year-old to 17-year-old athletes with a predilection for boys over girls.[6] The most common sports being soccer, football, gymnastics, and track. Acute symptoms include sudden, shooting pain and functional weakness. On examination, edema, ecchymosis, localized tenderness, and pain with passive ROM are often present.[7,8] Diagnosis is confirmed with radiographs with the most common locations in decreasing order being the anterior inferior iliac spine (AIIS), the ischial tuberosity, the anterior superior iliac spine (ASIS), the lesser trochanter, and the pubic symphysis (**Table 1**).[9] The degree of displacement is restricted by the surrounding periosteum and fascia.[3]

Conservative management is typically chosen for all avulsions with <2 cm of displacement. Rest, ice, and nonsteroidal anti-inflammatory drugs (NSAIDs) are used initially, followed by protection of weight bearing with crutches until symptom resolution. The athlete may return to sports after progressing through physical therapy involving isometric stretching and strengthening exercises.[2,3] Traditionally, surgical intervention is reserved for avulsions with >2 cm of displacement due to high risk of developing a symptomatic nonunion, chronic pain, or diminished function. Fixation is achieved by screws or suture anchors depending on surgeon preference and the size of the avulsed fragment.[7] However, a recent meta-analysis by Eberbach and colleagues[9] introduced some controversy to the historical treatment algorithm by showing an improved overall success rate in patients receiving surgery (88%) compared with those undergoing conservative treatment (79%) with a statistically significant return to sports rate of 92% and 80%, respectively. After stratifying using a cutoff of 1.5 cm versus 2.0 cm for operative intervention, their study showed an 84% success rate in operative patients versus 50% in the conservative group ($P = .04$).[9]

STRESS FRACTURES

Stress fractures occur in 2 generalized categories: fatigue fractures and insufficiency fractures. Fatigue fractures are the result of abnormal forces on normal bone, whereas insufficiency fractures result when normal forces act on abnormal bones. Typically, adolescents develop fatigue fractures due to repetitive microtrauma, whereas elderly patients develop insufficiency fractures.[6,10] The femoral neck encompasses 5% to 7% of all adolescent stress fractures, which is secondary only to the tibia.[11] Girls who participate in long-distance running are more likely to develop femoral neck stress fractures than their male counterparts. This higher prevalence in female individuals is also seen in military recruits.[11]

While assessing a female athlete with a femoral neck stress fracture, it is important to evaluate for the female athlete triad, consisting of amenorrhea, nutritional deficiencies or disordered eating, and osteopenia. Other risk factors include corticosteroid use, smoking, and hypermetabolic endocrinopathies. On examination, patients typically develop an insidious, progressive hip pain that may be localized to the groin

Table 1
Common adolescent avulsion fractures and their associated tendons and muscles

Apophysis	Common Muscle Avulsion
Anterior inferior iliac spine (AIIS)	Rectus femoris
Ischial tuberosity	Hamstrings
Anterior superior iliac spine (ASIS)	Tensor fascia lata, sartorius
Lesser trochanter	Iliopsoas
Pubic symphysis	Rectus abdominis

and is intensified with impact activity.[6] As symptoms worsen, pain will be elicited with hip internal rotation and with the hop test. Early in the disease process, radiographs have a low sensitivity of detecting an abnormality, and a rapid sequence MRI is a more sensitive imaging modality to assess for a stress fracture. Bony edema is what can be best visualized on T2-weighted images, but on T1-weighted sequences the presence and location of a fracture line largely determines the treatment (**Fig. 1**).

If the fracture remains confined to the compression side, which fortunately for adolescent athletes is more common as compared with tension-sided stress fractures, then conservative therapy can be attempted with toe-touch weight bearing for at least 4 weeks, NSAIDs, and physical therapy to increase core and hip strength.[6] If the adolescent fails conservative treatment or has a fracture line that involves any component of the tension side of the femoral neck, surgical intervention is necessary. Surgical options include either percutaneous screw fixation or other internal fixation devices to prevent propagation of the stress fracture into a complete femoral neck fracture. With either treatment, correcting underlying endocrinopathies, poor nutritional status, and osteoporosis is necessary to prevent future stress fractures and to promote adequate healing.

SLIPPED CAPITAL FEMORAL EPIPHYSIS

Slipped capital femoral epiphysis (SCFE) is one of the potentially devastating hip disorders that occurs in adolescent athletes. It has a higher prevalence in African American boys with elevated body mass indexes.[3] Frequently, it is a unilateral process, but it will be evident bilaterally in 20% to 50% of patients.[11] Those who suffer from bilateral disease often have an underlying endocrinopathy, most commonly being hypothyroidism, renal osteodystrophy, growth hormone deficiency, and panhypopituitarism. Younger age (<10 years old) and low height and/or weight (<10th percentile) warrants further workup for an endocrinopathy, as SCFE may be their initial presenting symptom[12–14]

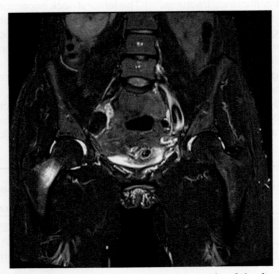

Fig. 1. MRI showing increased edema on the compression side of the femoral neck without discreet fracture line.

SCFE occurs most commonly with anterior displacement of the metaphysis relative to the epiphysis, with subsequent retrotorsion of the epiphysis. It has been associated with a pubertal growth spurt, trauma, and relative acetabular retroversion.[11,15] Adolescents typically present with an insidious onset of groin pain that is achy in nature and is exacerbated by physical activity. Like many hip disorders in adolescents, this pain can be referred to the knee. On examination, these patients ambulate with an external foot progression angle, have obligate hip external rotation with hip flexion, and have pain on any attempts of hip internal rotation. Per the Loder Classification, the ability to bear weight defines stability. This distinction is important because a stable SCFE has an osteonecrosis rate of less than 10% while an unstable SCFE has osteonecrosis rates reported up to 47%.[16,17]

Plain radiographs, including an AP pelvis and a lateral hip, will show that the Klein line does not intersect the epiphysis (**Fig. 2**). MRI is sometimes obtained if the radiographs are normal in the "pre-slip" condition. It will demonstrate edema around the physis as evidenced by hyperintensity on T2-weighted sequences and hypointensity on T1-weighted sequences (**Fig. 3**).

SCFE treatment involves surgical management to prevent continued displacement of the epiphysis relative to the metaphysis. The gold standard treatment is pinning in situ with the potential addition of a capsulotomy to theoretically decompress any intracapsular hematoma.[18,19] With more severe cases of displacement and deformities, more aggressive surgical techniques can be considered to attempt to restore joint biomechanics and theoretically delay hip degeneration. De Poorter and colleagues[19] assessed long-term outcomes averaging 18 years after patients underwent in situ pinning. In patients with mild to moderate slippage, approximately 5% developed early onset of osteoarthritis as compared with 75% in the severe group, showing

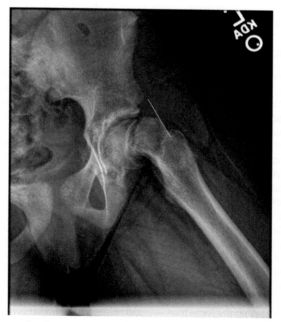

Fig. 2. Frog radiograph of a severe SCFE, which demonstrates a line along the anterior metaphysis (Klein line) not intersecting any of the epiphysis.

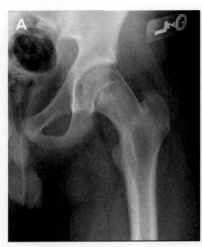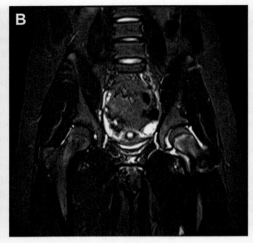

Fig. 3. Pre-slip. Plain radiographs (A) show that the Klein line still touches the epiphysis, but there is periphyseal lucency worrisome for a "pre-slip." MRI (B) shows increased edema around the physis indicative of pending SCFE.

that an increased level of deformity leads to premature degeneration of the hip.[19] Advanced treatment options including a surgical hip dislocation with sub-capital realignment (a modified Dunn procedure), open or arthroscopic osteochondroplasty, and intertrochanteric osteotomies can be used depending on the degree of deformity. Advanced procedures such as the modified Dunn should be performed by surgeons with specialized training because major complications such as avascular necrosis are not infrequent.[20]

FEMOROACETABULAR IMPINGEMENT

FAI is a common cause of hip pain among young athletes. Patients will often describe a sharp or achy pain deep within their groin or lateral hip in the shape of a C with an associated catching sensation.[2] Activities such as running, prolonged standing/sitting and pivoting exacerbate the pain. Common examination findings include pain with FADIR and decreased internal rotation with the hip in a flexed position.[8]

FAI has 2 major types: pincer and cam deformity, although a combination of the two is frequently found in patients. Pincer deformity refers to acetabular overcoverage with either focal or global acetabular retroversion, and cam deformity is an asphericity at the femoral head-neck junction.[2,6] Among adolescent populations, impingement may often be related to a preceding hip pathology such as SCFE, Legg-calve-Perthes Disease (LCPD), or trauma leading to the anatomic aberration. However, the role of intense sports among young patients is emerging as a potential causative factor. A study of 67 male collegiate football players showed that 95% had at least one hip with a cam or pincer morphology.[21] A separate study of male basketball players between the ages of 9 and 25 years showed a 10-fold increase in the probability of having a cam deformity when compared with age-controlled, nonathlete volunteers.[8,22]

Common radiographic findings that are associated with FAI morphology include an increased alpha angle of more than 55° on lateral hip radiographs, crossover sign, ischial spine sign, a posterior wall sign or an elevated posterior wall index (**Fig. 4**).

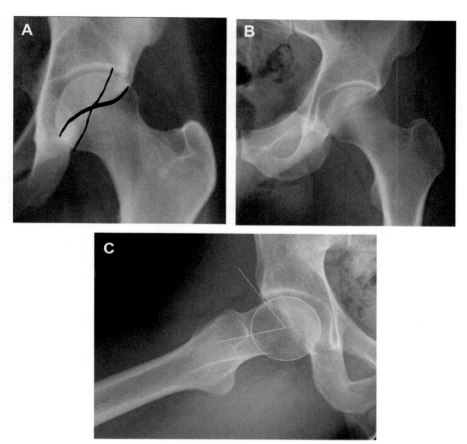

Fig. 4. Common radiographic findings in FAI. (*A*). Crossover sign indicated focal acetabular retroversion with the anterior wall crossing over the posterior wall caudally. (*B*). Ischial spine sign indicating relative acetabular retroversion with projection of the ischial spine medial to the iliopectineal line. (*C*). Alpha angle: increased alpha angle of more than 55° indicates asphericity at the femoral head/neck junction.

CT scans can be useful for 3D representation and preoperative planning. MRI/magnetic resonance angiography (MRA) will commonly demonstrate labral tears with a sensitivity of 76% to 91%.[2,8] However, a labral tear may be an incidental finding, as it is discovered in 81% to 86% of asymptomatic young adult volunteers with an increasing prevalence associated with age.[23,24] FAI and other abnormal bone morphologic conditions may predispose to the formation of acetabular labral tears, but studies have shown that the labral tear may not necessarily be the pain generator.[2,25,26]

Conservative treatment plays an important role in the management because many athletes have mild or quiescent FAI. Sports restriction with physical therapy, NSAIDs, and intra-articular cortisone injections may be considered.[8,27] Nevertheless, careful follow-up should be maintained, as significant injury to the labrum, articular cartilage, or osteoarthritis may result over time.[6] Pennock and colleagues[28] showed that 82% of nonoperatively treated patients could be managed successfully with improvement of outcomes scores at 2-year follow-up.[29] Surgical indications include failure of conservative management and limited functionality. A recent meta-analysis of adolescent and adult patients studied 600 open surgical hip dislocations and 1484 arthroscopies. The outcomes for both procedures were good, with arthroscopic surgery achieving higher general health-related quality of life scores.[27] A separate study of 218 hip arthroscopies in patients younger than 18 years showed a 1.8% complication rate with no cases of proximal femoral physeal separation, osteonecrosis, or growth disturbances.[2,30] Among adolescents, return to sports after surgery took an average of 7 months with a 95% return rate and 80% achieving presurgical level of function.[31]

DEVELOPMENTAL DYSPLASIA OF THE HIP

Developmental dysplasia of the hip (DDH) is a disorder that may present with increased symptomatology during adolescence. Risk factors include female sex, primiparity, a family history, and most importantly, intrauterine breech positioning. Like many other hip disorders in adolescents, patients typically present with an insidious onset of groin pain that may be referred to the knee. They may also present with laterally based pain and iliopsoas pain.[32] Trendelenburg gait can be seen with prolonged activity and hip abductor fatigue. Generalized laxity can be evaluated using the Beighton Criteria, whereas more specific examinations include anterior hip apprehension test and the prone external rotation test.[2,32] Frequently pain patterns vary, and instability is commonly represented by pain with the hip extended, as opposed to FAI, which commonly has pain with the hip flexed.

Radiographically, an AP pelvis, a lateral hip, and a false profile view should be obtained. The AP pelvis view is used to assess the lateral center edge angle and the Tonnis angle, which represents the slope of the sourcil (**Fig. 5**A, B). The anterior center edge angle is best assessed on the false profile view to assess for anterior acetabular coverage (**Fig. 5**C). Acetabular version is another key parameter that is typically assessed on the AP pelvis radiograph via the crossover sign but may be also assessed on axial CT scans.[32] MRI and MRA are also useful to evaluate for other common concomitant intra-articular pathologies.[32]

Currently, evidence to support nonoperative, conservative management of symptomatic DDH is greatly limited due to its known progression to cause premature osteoarthritis. Although when used, conservative management consists of activity modification, physical therapy focusing on core and abductor strengthening, and symptomatic relief with NSAIDs and corticosteroid injections.[32] A periacetabular osteotomy (PAO) is the mainstay of treatment for adolescents with symptomatic DDH. The overarching goal with a PAO is to reorient the dysplastic acetabulum to provide increased acetabular coverage. Fortunately, newer studies demonstrate survival rates of 92% at 15 years and 74% at 18 years when a PAO was performed by an experienced surgeon.[33,34] Arthroscopy can be used as an adjunct to treat the concomitant pathologies associated with dysplasia, but not as a stand-alone treatment as it does not address the underlying structural anatomic abnormality. Proximal femoral osteotomy can also help address the structural deformities associated with acetabular dysplasia.

LEGG-CALVE-PERTHES DISEASE

Legg-Calve-Perthes Disease (LCPD) is caused by avascular necrosis of the proximal femoral epiphysis resulting in coxa plana or coxa magna. The pathophysiology is largely idiopathic, but may be a result of trauma, coagulopathy, and steroid use.[35]

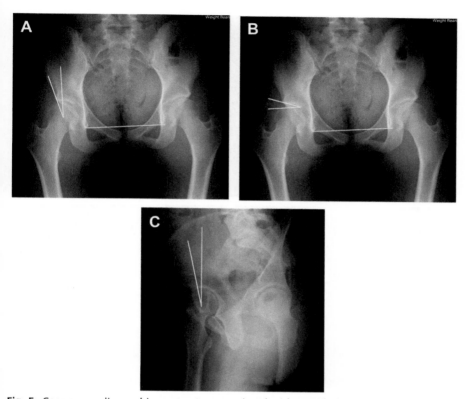

Fig. 5. Common radiographic parameters associated with acetabular dysplasia. (*A*). Lateral center edge angle: less than 20° indicates dysplasia with 20° to 25° being considered borderline dysplastic (*B*). Tonnis Angle: angle between horizontal and the sourcil with values over 10° indicating potential hip instability and dysplasia. (*C*). Anterior center edge angle: less than 25° indicates potential anterior undercoverage.

The best prognostic classification is the Lateral Pillar Classification, which assesses the maintenance of lateral height.[36,37]

Patients who have LCPD typically present from ages 4 to 12 years with a mean age of 7 years. There is a higher prevalence in boys, but when present bilaterally (10%–25%), it is more common in girls.[3,11] On examination, an insidious, painless limp typically precedes a painful limp by a few months. Like other pediatric hip disorders, this pain can be referred to the ipsilateral knee. Patients frequently develop decreases in hip ROM, especially internal rotation and abduction.[3] Radiographically, AP pelvis and frog-leg lateral views can be diagnostic. Early signs include a radiolucent subchondral zone in the anterolateral epiphysis (ie, the crescent sign). Advanced imaging such as MRI can be used to look at the potential amount of femoral head involvement.

Treatment for patients with LCPD is focused on retaining ROM during the early phases of the disease and treating deformities causing painful symptoms during adolescence after remodeling occurs (**Fig. 6**). Given the symbiotic relationship between femoral head growth and acetabular development, there is frequently head deformity with concomitant acetabular dysplasia and associated hip instability causing discomfort.[38] The structural deformities related to LCPD result in 50% of

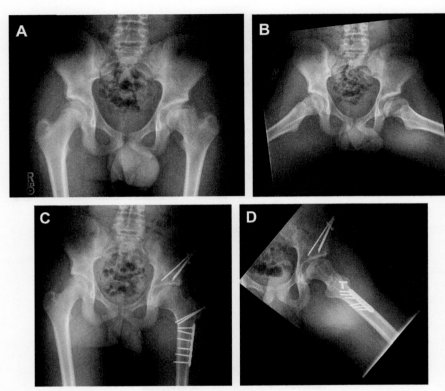

Fig. 6. Typical pathologic anatomic changes after Perthes disease with coxa magna, coxa plana, acetabular dysplasia both before (*A, B*) and after surgical treatment with surgical hip dislocation, femoroplasty, derotational osteotomy, relative femoral neck lengthening, and periacetabular osteotomy (*C, D*).

patients developing osteoarthritis in their fourth and fifth decade of life as evidenced in long-term studies.[11,39]

COXA SALTANS

Coxa saltans, or snapping hip syndrome (SHS), can be caused by several different potential pathologies. The main categories of SHS are coxa saltans interna and coxa saltans externa. Coxa saltans interna and externa frequently affect female athletes whose training or competition requires them to repetitively move into supraphysiological positions. For this reason, dancers are the most identified group with this pathology.[2,10]

Internal SHS results from a taught iliopsoas tendon as it moves from lateral to medial over the iliopectineal eminence or femoral head. Pain is typically localized to the anterior thigh with an associated ipsilateral low back pain. The snap can be elicited with extension, abduction, and external rotation. The Thomas test can also assist with clinical diagnosis.[40] Internal SHS and iliopsoas pain can also be seen in the setting of hip dysplasia, as the iliopsoas acts as a dynamic stabilizer of the under-covered hip.

External SHS occurs when the IT band or gluteus medius muscle snaps over the greater trochanter.[40] This most commonly arises when moving from flexion to extension.[2] Growth incongruity between soft tissue and bone is thought to be responsible for the tightness of the IT band; therefore, symptoms typically present during puberty. Pathology is often present bilaterally with pain worse on one side. Pain is felt near the greater trochanter with occasional radiation to the thigh or knee and is exacerbated by activity. The examiner can replicate the symptoms by palpating the greater trochanter while the athlete stands and circumducts the affected leg. The Ober examination, with the hip extended and knee flexed, is also useful for diagnosis when the leg cannot be adducted past neutral in this position.[40]

Dynamic ultrasound is helpful to show a sudden positional change in the IT band or the iliopsoas tendon as the snap occurs.[2,10] MRI may show thickening of the IT band, atrophy of the gluteus maximus, or intra-articular SHS pathology.[27,40]

Coxa saltans interna and externa always should be approached conservatively, as most vastly improve or resolve without surgical intervention. Sports restriction, NSAIDs, and physical therapy, with a focus on stretching of the affected structure paired with restoration of normal gait and movement patterns are the mainstays of treatment.[27] Corticosteroid injections may be considered to reduce symptoms for improved performance in physical therapy. Surgery is indicated when symptoms are severe, and after failing an extensive course of conservative therapy. Release or lengthening of the IT band can be performed open, endoscopically, or percutaneously with multiple methods, such as proximal or distal Z-lengthening or diamond-shaped resection. Scar-tethering and residual snapping are known complications. Release or fractional lengthening of the iliopsoas has been described arthroscopically at either the lesser trochanter or trans-capsular. Complications include hip flexor weakness and intra-abdominal fluid extravasation.[2,40] A recent study that assessed fractional lengthening of the iliopsoas at the musculotendinous junction had all adolescent patients return to their preoperative level of functioning; however, the number of lengthening procedures has decreased over the past decade secondary to reports of complications or failure to relieve symptoms.[11]

SUMMARY

Increased participation in sports, advances in imaging technology, and surgical innovation have led to more frequent diagnosis of adolescent athletic hip injuries. Although most hip injuries such as FAI and coxa saltans are given a trial of conservative therapy, more serious and potentially detrimental adolescent-specific pathology such as SCFE should be treated rapidly with surgical intervention to prevent devastating complications. This article reviews common adolescent sports-related hip injuries and provides concise, up-to-date pathophysiologic rationale, evaluation, and treatment options regarding the diagnosis. With advances in medicine, this information is ever-evolving to provide clinicians with information to properly care for our patients.

CLINICAL CARE POINTS

- Adolescent hip injuries include common adult pathologies such as FAI, snapping hip, and DDH, but also have unique pathologies to consider, such as SCFE, Perthes Disease, and avulsion fractures.
- Radiographic imaging can help with diagnosis in most hip disorders with advanced imaging needed for preoperative planning and in select cases of worry (femoral neck stress fracture, pre-slip in SCFE).
- Knee pain can often be the presenting symptoms for adolescents with hip pathology.

- When evaluating hip injuries in adolescents with atypical features, screening for endocrinopathies and the female athlete triad is necessary.
- Surgical intervention is based on severity of disease and symptomatology in most athletic hip conditions; however, certain conditions such as SCFE and femoral neck stress fractures warrant urgent workup and treatment.

DISCLOSURE

The authors have nothing to disclose.

REFERENCES

1. Kerbel Y, Smith C, Prodromo J, et al. Epidemiology of hip and groin injuries in collegiate athletes in the United States. Orthop J Sports Med 2018;6(5):1–8.
2. Frank J, Gambacorta P, Eisner E. Hip pathology in the adolescent athlete. J Am Acad Orthop Surg 2013;21(11):665–74.
3. Kocher M, Tucker R. Pediatric athlete hip disorders. Clin Sports Med 2006;25(2):241–53.
4. Byrd JWT. Evaluation of the hip: history and physical examination. N Am J Sports Phys Ther 2007;4(4):231–41.
5. Nepple J, Martel J, Kim Y, et al. Do plain radiographs correlate with CT for imaging of cam-type femoroacetabular impingement? Clin Orthop Relat Res 2012;470(12):3313–20.
6. Jacoby L, Yi-Meng Y, Kocher M. Hip problems and arthroscopy: adolescent hip as it relates to sports. Clin Sports Med 2011;30(2):435–51.
7. Roth J, Nepple JJ. Athletic injuries involving the hip. The Pediatric and Adolescent Hip 2019;841–53. https://doi.org/10.1007/978-3-030-12003-0_35.
8. Daley E, Zaltz I. Femoroacetabular impingement. The Pediatric and Adolescent Hip 2019;253–71. https://doi.org/10.1007/978-3-030-12003-0_9.
9. Eberbach H, Hohloch L, Feucht M, et al. Operative versus conservative treatment of apophyseal avulsion fractures of the pelvis in the adolescents: a systematical review with meta-analysis of clinical outcome and return to sports. BMC Musculoskelet Disord 2017;18(1). https://doi.org/10.1186/s12891-017-1527-z.
10. Paluska S. An overview of hip injuries in running. Sports Med 2005;35(11):991–1014.
11. Kovacevic D, Mariscalco M, Goodwin R. Injuries about the hip in the adolescent athlete. Sports Med Arthrosc Rev 2011;19(1):64–74.
12. Witbreuk M, van Kemenade F, van der Sluijs J, et al. Slipped capital femoral epiphysis and its association with endocrine, metabolic and chronic diseases: a systematic review of the literature. J Child Orthop 2013;7(3):213–23.
13. Burrow S, Alman B, Wright J. Short stature as a screening test for endocrinopathy in slipped capital femoral epiphysis. J Bone Joint Surg Br 2001;83-B(2):263–8.
14. Loder R, Starnes T, Dikos G. Atypical and typical (idiopathic) slipped capital femoral epiphysis. J Bone Joint Surg Am 2006;88(7):1574–81.
15. Hesper T, Bixby S, Kim Y, et al. Acetabular retroversion, but not increased acetabular depth or coverage, in slipped capital femoral epiphysis. J Bone Joint Surg Am 2017;99(12):1022–9.
16. Mahran M, Baraka M, Hefny H. Slipped capital femoral epiphysis: a review of management in the hip impingement era. SICOT J 2017;3:35.

17. Aprato A, Conti A, Bertolo F, et al. Slipped capital femoral epiphysis: current management strategies. Orthop Res Rev 2019;11:47–54.

18. Millis Michael, Novais EN. In situ fixation for slipped capital femoral epiphysis: perspectives in 2011. J Bone Joint Surg Am 2011;93:46–51.

19. De Poorter JJ, Beunder TJ, Gareb B, et al. Long-term outcomes of slipped capital femoral epiphysis treated with in situ pinning. J Child Orthop 2016;10(5):371–9.

20. Sankar W, Vanderhave K, Matheney T, et al. The modified Dunn procedure for unstable slipped capital femoral epiphysis. J Bone Joint Surg Am 2013;95(7): 585–91.

21. Kapron AL, Anderson AE, Aoki SK, et al. Radiographic prevalence of femoroacetabular impingement in collegiate football players. J Bone Joint Surg Am 2011; 93(19). https://doi.org/10.2106/jbjs.k.00544.

22. Giordano BD. Assessment and treatment of hip pain in the adolescent athlete. Pediatr Clin North Am 2014;61(6):1137–54.

23. Schmitz2 MR, Campbell SE, Fajardo RS, et al. Identification of acetabular labral pathological changes in asymptomatic volunteers using optimized, noncontrast 1.5-T magnetic resonance imaging. Am J Sports Med 2012;40(6):1337–41.

24. Kamath AF, Componovo R, Baldwin K, et al. Hip arthroscopy for labral tears. Am J Sports Med 2009;37(9):1721–7.

25. Martin RL, Irrgang JJ, Sekiya JK. The diagnostic accuracy of a clinical examination in determining intra-articular hip pain for potential hip arthroscopy candidates. Arthroscopy 2008;24(9):1013–8.

26. Santori N, Villar RN. Acetabular labral tears: result of arthroscopic partial limbectomy. Arthroscopy 2000;16(1):11–5.

27. Nwachukwu BU, Rebolledo BJ, Mccormick F, et al. Arthroscopic versus open treatment of femoroacetabular impingement. Am J Sports Med 2015;44(4): 1062–8.

28. Pennock AT, Bomar JD, Johnson KP, et al. Nonoperative management of femoroacetabular impingement: a prospective study. Am J Sports Med 2018;46(14): 3415–22.

29. Siebenrock KA, Ferner F, Noble PC, et al. Reply to letter to the editor: the cam-type deformity of the proximal femur arises in childhood in response to vigorous sporting activity. Clin Orthop Relat Res 2011;469(12):3508.

30. Nwachukwu BU, Mcfeely ED, Nasreddine AY, et al. Complications of hip arthroscopy in children and adolescents. J Pediatr Orthop 2011;31(3):227–31.

31. Reiman MP, Peters S, Sylvain J, et al. Femoroacetabular impingement surgery allows 74% of athletes to return to the same competitive level of sports participation but their level of performance remains unreported: a systematic review with meta-analysis. Br J Sports Med 2018;52(15):972–81.

32. Schmitz MR, Murtha AS, Clohisy JC. Developmental dysplasia of the hip in adolescents and young adults. J Am Acad Orthop Surg 2020;28(3):91–101.

33. Wells J, Schoenecker P, Duncan S, et al. Intermediate-term hip survivorship and patient-reported outcomes of periacetabular osteotomy. J Bone Joint Surg Am 2018;100(3):218–25.

34. Wells J, Millis M, Kim Y-J, et al. Survivorship of the Bernese periacetabular osteotomy: what factors are associated with long-term failure? Clin Orthop Relat Res 2016;475(2):396–405.

35. Mills S, Burroughs K. Legg calve perthes disease (calves disease). Stat pearls. Treasure Island (FL): National Institute of Health; 2019.

36. Herring JA, Ki HT, Browne R. Legg-Calve-Perthes disease. Part II: prospective multicenter study of the effect of treatment on outcome. J Bone Joint Surg Am 2004;86(10):2121–4.
37. Clohisy JC, Curry MC, Nunley RM, et al. Periacetabular osteotomy for the treatment of acetabular dysplasia associated with major aspherical femoral head deformities. J Bone Joint Surg Am 2007;89(7):1417–23.
38. Canavese F, Dimeglio A. Perthes' disease. J Bone Joint Surg Br 2008;90-B(7): 940–5.
39. Winston P, Awan R, Cassidy JD, et al. Clinical examination and ultrasound of self-reported snapping hip syndrome in elite ballet dancers. Am J Sports Med 2007; 35(1):118–26.
40. Lee LH, Gent E, Alshryda S. Snapping hip syndrome. The Pediatric and Adolescent Hip 2019;855–74. https://doi.org/10.1007/978-3-030-12003-0_36.

Sex-Related Differences in Hip Injury Rates and Strength and Conditioning

Arianna L. Gianakos, DO[a], John W. Yurek, DO[a],
Mary K. Mulcahey, MD[b],*

KEYWORDS

• Hip • Sex • Gender • Rehabilitation • Strength • Conditioning

KEY POINTS

• Although hip-related injuries are common in both the male and female populations, differences in anatomy, hip abductor strength and function, and landing biomechanics have been demonstrated within the literature.
• These differences can affect injury pattern, incidence, and outcomes.
• Both male and female athletes of all age groups benefit from injury prevention programs.
• Structured strength and conditioning programs are pivotal in developing an athlete's body both for on-field performance and to help prevent injury.

INTRODUCTION

Hip injuries are common in the athletic population, with a reported rate of approximately 1 per 2000 athletic exposures.[1,2] Of all collegiate sports, men's soccer (110.84 per 100,000 athletic exposures) and men's and women's ice hockey (104.9 and 76.88 per 100,000 athletic exposures, respectively) had the highest rates of hip injury.[2] Although previous epidemiologic studies have demonstrated that female athletes have a higher rate of hip injury in college athletics in sex-comparable sports, more recent studies dispute this by showing a higher rate of hip injury in male athletes both within the National Collegiate Athletic Association (NCAA) and in international athletic competition.[1–4] Hip injuries occur most commonly in sports that require impingement-type movements and can be a result of either contact or overuse. Higher rates of overuse hip injuries have been reported in female athletes compared with contact-related injuries in their male counterparts.[1,2] Although more than one-third

[a] Department of Orthopaedic Surgery, Robert Wood Johnson Barnabas Health – Jersey City Medical Center (Colony Plaza) Suite 14 Grand Street, Jersey City, NJ 07302, USA; [b] Department of Orthopaedic Surgery, Tulane University School of Medicine, 1430 Tulane Avenue #8632, New Orleans, LA 70112, USA
* Corresponding author.
E-mail address: mary.mulcahey.md@gmail.com

Clin Sports Med 40 (2021) 399–408
https://doi.org/10.1016/j.csm.2020.12.004
0278-5919/21/© 2021 Elsevier Inc. All rights reserved.

sportsmed.theclinics.com

of hip injuries in the NCAA led to time lost from competition, only approximately 1 in 100 injuries required surgery.[2] Therefore, in order to effectively diagnose and treat hip injuries in athletes, the differences in injury rates between male and female athletes, clinical presentation, treatment, and outcomes should be taken into consideration in order to expedite an athlete's return to play.

SEX-RELATED DIFFERENCES IN HIP ANATOMY AND BIOMECHANICS

Although hip-related injuries are common in both male and female athletes, differences in anatomy, hip abductor strength and function, and landing biomechanics have been demonstrated within the literature (**Table 1**). These differences can affect injury pattern, incidence, and outcomes. Anatomic-based differences have been described previously, with studies reporting that women have increased acetabular version, increased femoral anteversion, smaller alpha angles, and a decreased lateral center-edge angle.[5–7] Nguyen and colleagues[8] reported that women have greater anterior pelvic tilt, femoral internal rotation, knee hyperextension, and knee valgus compared with men. These described differences all may contribute to variations in injury patterns affecting male and female patients. Erector spinae and hip flexor tightness combined with abdominal and gluteal weakness has been found to contribute to greater anterior pelvic angles, which supports the findings that women tend to have decreased strength during hip range of motion as well as an increase in lumbar lordosis compared with men.[8–10]

Differences in abductor function and landing kinematics between men and women have also been demonstrated in the literature. Jacobs and colleagues[11] assessed landing kinematics of hopping from 2 legs onto 1 leg in 15 men (24.4 years ± 3 years) and 15 women (23.2 years ± 2.9 years). They evaluated for differences in peak torque, endurance capacity, and peak joint displacement and demonstrated that women have lower hip abductor peak torque values, increased knee valgus peak joint displacement, and a larger correlation between hip abductor strength and landing kinematics compared with their male counterparts (see **Table 1**). In addition, the investigators report a small positive correlation between strength and kinematics in men and a large negative correlation in women.[11] These differences suggest that hip abductor strength and lower extremity kinematics likely are dissimilar between men and women, with hip mechanics in women offering more protection around the hip joint during landing activities. Previous studies also have demonstrated that female athletes have a lower peak hip abduction torque related to body mass compared with their male counterparts. Brent and colleagues[12]

Table 1 Sex-related anatomic and kinematic differences		
Parameter	**Male**	**Female**
Acetabular version[6]	17.8° ± 6.5°	21.3° ± 7.6°
Acetabular inclination[6]	36° ± 3.6°	38.5° ± 4.5°
Femoral head diameter[6]	48.6 mm ± 2.3 mm	43 mm ± 2.4 mm
Femoral anteversion[6]	19.4° ± 10.4°	23.9° ± 9.8°
Alpha angle[7]	47.8°	63.6°
Lateral center-edge angle[7]	37.9° ± 5.3°	34.7° ± 6.1°
Hip abductor torque[11]	7.2% ± 1.5%	5.8% ± 1.2%
Knee valgus joint displacement[11]	7.26° ± 6.61°	3.29° ± 3.54°

conducted a biomechanical study evaluating the standing isokinetic hip-abduction torque in 79 male (13.65 years $\pm$ 1.6 years) and 272 female (14 years $\pm$ 2.2 years) adolescent soccer and basketball players using a dynamometer. They demonstrated that not only did male players have increased peak torque values compared with female players, but also they had greater increases in peak torque relative to body weight than did female players as they matured.[12] Therefore, hip-abductor strengthening exercises should be performed, especially in female athletes, as part of preventative and rehabilitative strengthening programs.[11]

SEX-RELATED DIFFERENCES IN HIP PATHOLOGY

A majority of injuries sustained during athletic competition typically are muscular in origin, comprising approximately 40% of all injuries.[13] Hamstring strains affect male athletes more commonly than female athletes in athletic competition.[13] When considering gender differences in hamstring injuries among all age groups, female athletes tend to be older and sustain injuries during everyday activities, whereas male athletes are younger and injured more commonly while playing sports.[14] Thigh muscle strains also are a common muscular injury, affecting both male and female athletes. Gender difference data are conflicting for these injuries. In high school soccer, thigh muscle strains were shown to occur more commonly in female athletes than in male athletes, with male athletes having a rate ratio of 0.66.[15] But, in adult international competition, thigh muscle strains occurred more often in male athletes, with an incidence of 52 per 1000 athletes compared with women, who had an incidence of 30 per 1000 athletes.[4] More research is required to determine whether gender differences in muscle injury truly are significant. Eckard and colleagues[16] evaluated hip flexor and adductor strains in collegiate athletes in 25 different NCAA sports and demonstrated that female collegiate athletes had higher rates of hip adductor muscle strains compared with male athletes in comparable sports, with an incidence rate ratio of 1.49, but the rates of hip flexor injury did not show significant statistical difference, at a rate ratio of 1.14. Regardless of potential differences between genders, it is clear that muscle injuries about the hip are common and should be included in the differential when evaluating an injured athlete.

A common cause of pain in athletes may be due to femoroacetabular impingement (FAI), and the sequelae created by this mechanical abnormality can cause significant disability and limit athletic performance. When treating athletes with this condition, gender may play a significant role in diagnosis, treatment, and eventual outcome. The clinical presentation of male athletes and female athletes with FAI is similar, with most patients having an insidious onset of groin pain made worse by activity, decreased hip range of motion, and a positive impingement test on physical examination.[17] In cadaver analysis, female acetabula demonstrate increased anteversion compared with male acetabula.[18] Increased anteversion can create over-coverage of the femoral head leading to pincer-type FAI. Therefore, female athletes may be expected to present with pincer-type FAIs more often than male athletes. Hooper and colleagues[19] conducted a retrospective review examining 177 adolescent patients aged 13 years to 18 years who underwent hip arthroscopy for treatment of FAI. They demonstrated that male patients had a smaller preoperative lateral center-edge angle than female patients. This supports the idea that female athletes are more likely to have pincer-type FAI because the lateral center-edge angle is a measure of coverage of the femoral head by the acetabulum. Previous studies have demonstrated that male athletes have a higher alpha angle, which is a measurement used to evaluate for a cam deformity, as well as increased chondral damage assessed intraoperatively.[19–21] This supports the concept that male athletes are more likely than female athletes to have cam-type FAI, which can lead to increased rates of chondral damage.

Hip arthroscopy is a common treatment of FAI and an extended recovery time can be expected after such a procedure. Among male patients, athletes have been shown to recover faster from hip arthroscopy than nonathletes.[22] In addition, high-level athletes who receive arthroscopic treatment of FAI are more likely to be male and younger, play a cutting sport, and have bilateral surgery compared with recreational athletes.[23] Therefore, participation in high-level athletics might cause clinical symptoms stemming from underlying structural abnormalities within the hip at an earlier age, especially in sports that require significant amounts of cutting. Joseph and colleagues[24] evaluated 156 female athletes and 73 male athletes with an average age of 31, who underwent arthroscopic treatment of FAI, and demonstrated that although female athletes had poorer preoperative function, both male and female patients reported continual functional improvement within their hip until 6 months postoperatively. The same study showed no significant differences between male athletes and female athletes in hip function 2 years after surgery.

Lastly, femoral neck stress fractures are a commonly reported injury within the athletic population and can be a major cause of disability. Studies have demonstrated higher rates of femoral neck stress fractures within the female international athletic population compared with their male counterparts.[4] Stress fractures around the hip are less common than other stress fractures in athletes with femoral neck stress fractures, accounting for only 3% of all sports-related stress fractures.[25] Femoral neck stress fractures are reported most commonly in sports involving long distance running; therefore, clinicians must have a high index of suspicion because early diagnosis has been shown to lead to improved outcomes. Reinking and colleagues[26] examined 64 female and 20 male collegiate athletes in several sports for lower extremity overuse bone injuries and found no association between risk of injury and gender. The investigators demonstrated that cross-country and track athletes are more likely to sustain these injuries than participants in other sports, with a relative risk of 2.26. They also found that athletes with lower bone mineral density within the calcaneus had a relative risk for developing an overuse injury of 2.1 compared with athletes with normal bone mineral density.

Within the current literature, gender differences in hip pathology have become increasingly recognized. Muscle injuries, FAI, and stress fractures are common injuries affecting both male and female athletes and understanding the differences between the sexes in their incidence, diagnosis, treatment, and outcomes is important in order to manage and treat patients more effectively (**Table 2**). Overall, more research is required to advance understanding of these topics in order to improve the care of both male and female athletic injuries.

SEX-RELATED DIFFERENCES IN THE REHABILITATION AND PREVENTION OF HIP INJURIES IN ATHLETES

After injury, athletes are motivated to return to their sport as soon as possible. Rehabilitation protocols are important to help guide athletes on their path to recovery. A vast majority of protocols are not gender-specific and, therefore, may lack individualization in order to maximize a male or female athlete's chance to return to play. In order to create gender-specific protocols, differences in muscle strength, injury recovery, strength and conditioning programs, and injury prevention strategies must be defined.

Male and female athletes have similarities and differences in individual muscle group strength as well as strength ratios between muscle groups. Male collegiate

Table 2
Sex-related differences in hip pathology

Pathology	Male	Female
Hamstring injury	Younger age, trauma-related	Older age, overuse-related
FAI	Cam-type, decreased anteversion, larger lateral center-edge angle, increased rates of associated chondral damage	Pincer-type, increased anteversion, over-coverage of femoral head, smaller lateral center-edge angle
Femoral neck stress fracture		Higher rates in female athletes, overuse related, low bone mineral density

athletes have greater hip abductor peak torque in isokinetic testing than female athletes, but hip adductor peak torques showed no significant difference.[27] Leetun and colleagues[28] evaluated core stability measurements in collegiate basketball and track athletes and reported that male athletes had increased strength compared with female athletes in hip abduction, external rotation, and quadratus lumborum strength when corrected for body weight. Athletes in this same group were less likely to sustain a lower extremity injury if they had increased hip abduction and external rotation strength. Lopes and colleagues[29] conducted a large cohort study of Navy cadets evaluating physical performance and showed that male athletes tested better than female athletes in muscle strength, power, and endurance. Female athletes were more flexible in sit and reach tests than male athletes, but there was no difference between genders in ankle dorsiflexion. In high school athletes, female athletes had greater hamstring flexibility than male athletes, but male athletes perceived hamstring stretching as more important to athletic performance.[30] This finding demonstrates that even with increased perceived importance of stretching, male athletes may be less flexible than female athletes at baseline. It also has been shown that despite having less peak torque with hip abduction than male athletes, female athletes had equivalent values in hip abduction endurance.[11] Therefore, female athletes are able to sustain muscle contraction for an equivalent amount of time compared with male athletes, even though their peak value of muscle contraction may not be as high. Nadler and colleagues[31] reported that female NCAA Division I collegiate athletes with weaker hip abduction were treated at a higher rate for low back pain, which indicates that hip strength may affect other areas of the body as well. In addition, previous studies have shown that there is greater disproportion in the velocity of contraction ratio between the quadriceps and hamstrings in female athletes compared with male athletes. These differences may create muscle imbalances, which could predispose a female athlete to injury.[32] Despite women having less muscle hypertrophy with strength improvement, it has been shown that women and men experience similar strength gain when training with the same routine.[33] Therefore, male and female athletes following the same workout routine can be expected to progress similarly, even though female athletes may not gain the same muscle mass as their male counterparts during this process.

Strength and conditioning programs have been shown to decrease risk of injury; therefore, both male and female athletes should be provided with equal opportunity to participate in such programs. In a survey of Idaho high school coaches of varsity soccer, basketball, softball, and baseball, 84% stated they provide strength and conditioning programs to their athletes, but only 37% required participation.[34] Coaches of female athletes were less likely to utilize certified strength coaches to plan and implement their training programs. This may place female athletes at a disadvantage by not having access to training programs that are equivalent to their male counterparts at the high school level. This same study reported that male athletes were more likely to have required training, have year-round strength training, and have more sessions per week.[34] This potentially could cause disproportionate strength increases among male and female athletes, which inherently may place female athletes at an increased risk of injury. Sommi and colleagues[35] conducted a meta-analysis examining female strength and conditioning programs and demonstrated a lack of programs offered to female adolescent athletes despite the benefits they provide in injury prevention. In youth athletes who have reached puberty, weight training has been shown to both prevent injury and decrease the risk of diabetes and metabolic syndrome.[36] In training prepubertal athletes, agility, balance, and coordination should be emphasized over strengthening in order to maximize the benefits of the plasticity of a developing child's brain. Therefore, more emphasis must be placed on providing both male and female athletes of all age groups access to training programs to maximize injury prevention.

Structured strength and conditioning programs are pivotal in developing an athlete's body both for on-field performance and to help prevent injury. Similarly, rehabilitation programs enable athletes to return their sport after an injury has occurred by increasing strength and proprioception within the injured extremity. After injury, muscle atrophy occurs from extended periods of immobilization, which can predispose an athlete to injury if significant strength is not regained before returning to play. Khayambashi and colleagues[37] showed that athletes were at high risk for sustaining a future anterior cruciate ligament injury when they had hip external rotation strength measures of less than 20% of their body weight or hip abduction strength of less than 35% of their body weight. Not only are athletes at increased risk for future injury with decreased hip strength, but also the lasting effects from a previous injury may be more severe. In athletes who sustained a lateral ankle sprain, those with decreased isometric hip strength were more likely to exhibit signs of chronic ankle instability after initial injury recovery.[38] This demonstrates that a well-rounded rehabilitation program that involves whole-body training is preferable in the treatment of isolated injuries. Decreased hip strength with abduction and external rotation also has been linked to an increase in symptoms of patellofemoral pain syndrome.[39] Therefore, physical therapy for this common diagnosis should target hip musculature as well as muscles surrounding the knee. Without proper rehabilitation after an injury, athletes' performance may decline after they return to their sport. In both male and female soccer players who sustained a previous hamstring injury, a shorter backswing and lower peak kicking velocity were observed, which may hinder their on-field performance.[40] Lastly, preventative proprioceptive training has been shown to decrease the rates of ankle sprains, knee injuries, and low back pain significantly in professional basketball players.[41] Therefore, proprioception as well as strength training should be included in training regimens for both injury prevention and rehabilitation.

Overall, strength and conditioning programs are important both for an athlete's performance on the field and to prevent future injury. There are discrepancies in the programs that are offered to male athletes and female athletes despite the clear benefits for all athletes. Proper rehabilitation of all lower extremity injures, not only those that involve the hip, should include hip strengthening to help prevent future injury. Athletes of all ages should be offered training programs tailored to their specific age group because prepubertal athletes benefit from training just as much as older athletes to help prevent injury. With proper implementation of preventative and rehabilitative strength, conditioning, and proprioceptive programs on a widespread scale, the rate of injuries in athletes of all genders and ages can be decreased significantly.

SUMMARY

Male and female athletes have both similarities and differences in hip anatomy, rates of hip injury, types of hip injury, and preventative and rehabilitative strength and conditioning programs that are provided to them. Although there has been increased recognition of sex-related differences with regard to injury patterns, anatomy, and biomechanics specific to hip injuries in athletes, future research is required to understand these differences adequately in order to better tailor treatment and rehabilitation protocols. It is important for physicians to take patient sex into consideration in order to better explain to patients how their anatomy may predispose them to certain conditions, educate them on which hip injuries they may be more likely to sustain, and discuss how a sex-specific strength and conditioning program can be beneficial in the prevention or rehabilitation of a hip injury.

CLINICS CARE POINTS

- Anatomic-based differences previously have been described, with studies reporting that women have greater pelvic tilt, increased acetabular version, increased femoral anteversion, smaller alpha angles, decreased lateral center-edge angle, greater knee hyperextension, and greater knee valgus compared with men.
- Studies also have demonstrated that women have lower hip abductor peak torque values, increased knee valgus peak joint displacement, and a larger correlation between hip abductor strength and landing kinematics compared with their male counterparts.
- Common causes of pain in athletes may be due to FAI, femoral neck stress fractures, and hamstring injuries.
- A vast majority of rehabilitation protocols are not gender-specific and, therefore, may lack individualization in order to maximize a male or female athlete's chance to return to play.
- With proper implementation of both preventative and rehabilitative strength, conditioning, and proprioceptive programs on a widespread scale, the rate of injuries in both male and female athletes can be decreased significantly.

DISCLOSURE

A.L. Gianakos and J.W. Yurek have nothing to disclose. M.K. Mulcahey disclosures: AAOS, board or committee member; ACSM Translational Journal of the American College of Sports Medicine, editorial or governing board; American Orthopaedic Society for Sports Medicine, board or committee member; Arthrex, Inc, paid presenter or speaker; Arthroscopy Association of North America, board or committee member; OrthoInfo, editorial or governing board; Ruth Jackson Orthopaedic Society, board or committee member; and The Forum, board or committee member.

REFERENCES

1. Cruz CA, Kerbel Y, Smith CM, et al. A sport-specific analysis of the epidemiology of hip injuries in national collegiate athletic association athletes from 2009 to 2014. Arthroscopy 2019;35(9):2724–32.
2. Kerbel YE, Smith CM, Prodromo JP, et al. Epidemiology of hip and groin injuries in collegiate athletes in the United States. Orthop J Sports Med 2018;6(5). 2325967118771676.

3. Sallis RE, Jones K, Sunshine S, et al. Comparing sports injuries in men and women. Int J Sports Med 2001;22(6):420–3.

4. Edouard P, Feddermann-Demont N, Alonso JM, et al. Sex differences in injury during top-level international athletics championships: surveillance data from 14 championships between 2007 and 2014. Br J Sports Med 2015;49(7):472–7.

5. Lindner D, El Bitar YF, Jackson TJ, et al. Sex-based differences in the clinical presentation of patients with symptomatic hip labral tears. Am J Sports Med 2014; 42(6):1365–9.

6. Nakahara I, Takao M, Sakai T, et al. Gender differences in 3D morphology and bony impingement of human hips. J Orthop Res 2011;29(3):333–9.

7. Hetsroni I, Dela Torre K, Duke G, et al. Sex differences of hip morphology in young adults with hip pain and labral tears. Arthroscopy 2013;29(1):54–63.

8. Nguyen A-D, Shultz SJ. Sex differences in clinical measures of lower extremity alignment. J Orthop Sports Phys Ther 2007;37(7):389–98.

9. Cahalan TD, Johnson ME, Liu S, et al. Quantitative measurements of hip strength in different age groups. Clin Orthop Relat Res 1989;246:136–45.

10. Day JW, Smidt GL, Lehmann T. Effect of pelvic tilt on standing posture. Phys Ther 1984;64(4):510–6.

11. Jacobs CA, Uhl TL, Mattacola CG, et al. Hip abductor function and lower extremity landing kinematics: sex differences. J Athl Train 2007;42(1):76–83.

12. Brent JL, Myer GD, Ford KR, et al. The effect of sex and age on isokinetic hip-abduction torques. J Sport Rehabil 2013;22(1):41–6.

13. Edouard P, Branco P, Alonso J-M. Muscle injury is the principal injury type and hamstring muscle injury is the first injury diagnosis during top-level international athletics championships between 2007 and 2015. Br J Sports Med 2016;50(10): 619–30.

14. Irger M, Willinger L, Lacheta L, et al. Proximal hamstring tendon avulsion injuries occur predominately in middle-aged patients with distinct gender differences: epidemiologic analysis of 263 surgically treated cases. Knee Surg Sports Traumatol Arthrosc 2019;28(4):1221–9.

15. Cross KM, Gurka KK, Saliba S, et al. Comparison of thigh muscle strain occurrence and injury patterns between male and female high school soccer athletes. J Sport Rehabil 2018;27(5):451–9.

16. Eckard TG, Padua DA, Dompier TP, et al. Epidemiology of hip flexor and hip adductor strains in national collegiate athletic association athletes, 2009/2010-2014/2015. Am J Sports Med 2017;45(12):2713–22.

17. Philippon MJ, Maxwell RB, Johnston TL, et al. Clinical presentation of femoroacetabular impingement. Knee Surg Sports Traumatol Arthrosc 2007;15(8):1041–7.

18. Tannenbaum E, Kopydlowski N, Smith M, et al. Gender and racial differences in focal and global acetabular version. J Arthroplasty 2014;29(2):373–6.

19. Hooper P, Oak SR, Lynch TS, et al. Adolescent femoroacetabular impingement: gender differences in hip morphology. Arthroscopy 2016;32(12):2495–502.

20. Gosvig KK, Jacobsen S, Sonne-Holm S, et al. Prevalence of malformations of the hip joint and their relationship to sex, groin pain, and risk of osteoarthritis: a population-based survey. J Bone Joint Surg Am 2010;92(5):1162–9.

21. Laborie LB, Lehmann TG, Engesæter IØ, et al. Prevalence of radiographic findings thought to be associated with femoroacetabular impingement in a population-based cohort of 2081 healthy young adults. Radiology 2011;260(2): 494–502.

22. Przybyl M, Walenczak K, Domzalski ME. Athletes do better after FAI arthroscopic treatment in male population. J Orthop Surg (Hong Kong) 2018;26(1). 2309499018760111.
23. Nawabi DH, Bedi A, Tibor LM, et al. The demographic characteristics of high-level and recreational athletes undergoing hip arthroscopy for femoroacetabular impingement: a sports-specific analysis. Arthroscopy 2014;30(3):398–405.
24. Joseph R, Pan X, Cenkus K, et al. Sex differences in self-reported hip function up to 2 years after arthroscopic surgery for femoroacetabular impingement. Am J Sports Med 2016;44(1):54–9.
25. Robertson GA, Wood AM. Femoral neck stress fractures in sport: a current concepts review. Sports Med Int Open 2017;1(2):E58–68.
26. Reinking MF, Austin TM, Bennett J, et al. Lower extremity overuse bone injury risk factors in collegiate athletes: a pilot study. Int J Sports Phys Ther 2015;10(2): 155–67.
27. Sugimoto D, Mattacola CG, Mullineaux DR, et al. Comparison of isokinetic hip abduction and adduction peak torques and ratio between sexes. Clin J Sport Med 2014;24(5):422–8.
28. Leetun DT, Ireland ML, Willson JD, et al. Core stability measures as risk factors for lower extremity injury in athletes. Med Sci Sports Exerc 2004;36(6):926–34.
29. Lopes TJA, Simic M, Alves D de S, et al. Physical performance measures of flexibility, hip strength, lower limb power and trunk endurance in healthy navy cadets: normative data and differences between sex and limb dominance. J Strength Cond Res 2018. https://doi.org/10.1519/JSC.0000000000002365.
30. Nyland J, Kocabey Y, Caborn DNM. Sex differences in perceived importance of hamstring stretching among high school athletes. Percept Mot Skills 2004; 99(1):3–11.
31. Nadler SF, Malanga GA, Bartoli LA, et al. Hip muscle imbalance and low back pain in athletes: influence of core strengthening. Med Sci Sports Exerc 2002; 34(1):9–16.
32. Martín-San Agustín R, Medina-Mirapeix F, Alakhdar Y, et al. Sex differences in the velocity of muscle contraction of the hamstring and quadriceps among recreationally active young adults. J Strength Cond Res 2019;33(5):1252–7.
33. Lewis DA, Kamon E, Hodgson JL. Physiological differences between genders. Implications for sports conditioning. Sports Med 1986;3(5):357–69.
34. Reynolds ML, Ransdell LB, Lucas SM, et al. An examination of current practices and gender differences in strength and conditioning in a sample of varsity high school athletic programs. J Strength Cond Res 2012;26(1):174–83.
35. Sommi C, Gill F, Trojan JD, et al. Strength and conditioning in adolescent female athletes. Phys Sportsmed 2018;46(4):420–6.
36. Walters BK, Read CR, Estes AR. The effects of resistance training, overtraining, and early specialization on youth athlete injury and development. J Sports Med Phys Fitness 2018;58(9):1339–48.
37. Khayambashi K, Ghoddosi N, Straub RK, et al. Hip muscle strength predicts noncontact anterior cruciate ligament injury in male and female athletes: a prospective study. Am J Sports Med 2016;44(2):355–61.
38. McCann RS, Bolding BA, Terada M, et al. Isometric hip strength and dynamic stability of individuals with chronic ankle instability. J Athl Train 2018;53(7):672–8.
39. Nakagawa TH, Moriya ETU, Maciel CD, et al. Trunk, pelvis, hip, and knee kinematics, hip strength, and gluteal muscle activation during a single-leg squat in males and females with and without patellofemoral pain syndrome. J Orthop Sports Phys Ther 2012;42(6):491–501.

40. Navandar A, Veiga S, Torres G, et al. A previous hamstring injury affects kicking mechanics in soccer players. J Sports Med Phys Fitness 2018; 58(12):1815–22.

41. Riva D, Bianchi R, Rocca F, et al. Proprioceptive training and injury prevention in a professional men's basketball team: a six-year prospective study. J Strength Cond Res 2016;30(2):461–75.

Rehabilitation of Soft Tissue Injuries of the Hip and Pelvis

Kyle E. Hammond, MD[a,*], Lee Kneer, MD[a], Pete Cicinelli, PT, DPT[b]

KEYWORDS

- Hip • Pelvis • Muscle strain • Gluteus • Iliopsoas • Rectus femoris • Adductor
- Proximal hamstring

KEY POINTS

- Understanding the prevalence of the more common soft tissue injuries around the hip and pelvis is essential to properly managing the athletes involved.
  - The more commonly injured muscle groups involve the adductors, abductors, hip flexors, and proximal hamstring attachment.
- Utilizing modern diagnostic skills and tools can drive an efficient work-up for soft tissue injuries around an athlete's hip.
  - Portable and bedside ultrasound techniques can provide real-time diagnostics in the training room setting for the high-level sports medicine provider.
- Implementing the proper rehabilitation phases and specific therapeutic techniques is crucial in succeeding with an athlete's recovery and return to sport.
  - Three phases apply to most injury rehabilitation, as the athlete moves from a recovery to a strengthening and ultimately a return-to-sport protocol.

 Video content accompanies this article at http://www.sportsmed.theclinics.com/.

INTRODUCTION

- There are 21 different muscles that cross the hip and pelvis.
- The complexity of these muscle groups and their differing functions aid in athletic function but also contribute to their predisposition to injury.
- Sprinting, cutting, and throwing sports all harness energy from the hip and pelvis, which makes these types of muscle injuries all too common across most sports.

[a] Emory University Sports Medicine Center, 1968 Hawks Lane, Atlanta, GA 30329, USA;
[b] Atlanta Braves, Truist Park, 755 Battery Avenue, Southeast, Atlanta, GA 30339, USA
* Corresponding author.
E-mail address: kehammond6@gmail.com
Twitter: @kylehammondmd (K.E.H.); @kneermd (L.K.)

Clin Sports Med 40 (2021) 409–428
https://doi.org/10.1016/j.csm.2021.01.002
0278-5919/21/© 2021 Elsevier Inc. All rights reserved.

- Professional baseball estimates have shown that approximately 5.5% of injuries are related to the hip or groin, which can place a player on the injured list for various amounts of lost time.[1]
- Strain and resultant injury sometimes can be complicated in an athlete's presentation, which requires diligent and accurate use of clinical skills and tools to arrive at the correct diagnosis and treatment protocol.
- The exact injury rate for hip and pelvic muscular strains is unknown because of the likelihood that milder injuries sometimes are unrecognized or under-reported.
- There are mixed opinions on the increased incidence of these injuries, because they sometimes are thought to be more common in the preseason time periods, due to lack of functional conditioning, but some report that later in the season injuries may increase, due to fatigue and/or overuse.
- Understanding a typical presentation for the most common muscular injuries and rehabilitation processes aids in a successful return to sport for the athlete.

HIP AND PELVIS BONY ANATOMY

- The pelvis consists of the fused os coxae (ilium, ischium, and pubis) and serves as the inferior connection between the axial and appendicular skeleton. This connection occurs at the diarthrodial synovial sacroiliac joints bilaterally, which serve both to transfer torque created in the lower extremities and to dampen the torso's vertical forces of ambulation.
  - Anteriorly, the pubic symphysis is a nonsynovial amphiarthrodial cartilaginous joint that sustains significant compressive forces with motion, attenuates the impulse of the forces of ambulation, and expands during childbirth.
  - Contributions from all 3 portions of the os coxae form the pelvic component of the femoroacetabular joint, the synovial ball-and-socket hip joint that serves as the structural foundation for locomotion.
  - In addition, the pelvis serves a protective function for the lower internal organs and neurovascular structures and is the attachment site of many muscles of locomotion.

MUSCLES OF THE PELVIS AND HIP

Table 1 depicts the various muscular anatomy and functional roles around the hip and pelvis.

ROLE OF THE HIPS AND PELVIS DURING DYNAMIC MOVEMENTS

- Absorption, transfer, and production of force (examples)
  - Trunk power is an independent predictor of pitching velocity in baseball.[2]
  - Energy transfer from pelvic torque force generation is a major contributor to rotational forces in the baseball pitching motion.[3]
  - Improving lumbosacral postural stabilization with as little as 6 weeks' training has been associated with improved baseball pitching accuracy and endurance.[4]
  - Sacroiliac extension torque is higher than any other joint during the block start in track events.[5]
  - A core stabilization training program has been associated with improved isometric shoulder strength in young female athletes.[6]
  - Lumbopelvic stability training improved performance on climbing-specific strength tasks in elite climbers.[7]

Table 1
Muscular anatomy and functional roles around the hip and pelvis

Muscle	Primary Function	Secondary Function(s)	Origin	Insertion	Innervation (Spinal Nerve)
Anterior compartment					
Iliacus	Hip flexion	Hip internal rotation	Iliac fossa	Femur–lesser trochanter	Femoral nerve (L1-3)
Psoas	Hip flexion	Hip external rotation; ipsilateral trunk lateral flexion	Transverse processes T4-12	Femur–lesser trochanter	Lumbar plexus (L1-3)
Rectus femoris	Knee extension	Hip flexion	Anterior-inferior iliac spine	Patella; tibial tuberosity	Femoral nerve (L2-4)
Sartorius	Hip flexion (weak)	Hip abduction, external rotation; knee flexion	Anterior-superior iliac spine	Anteromedial aspect of proximal tibia	Femoral nerve (L2-4)
Medial compartment					
Pectineus	Hip adduction	Hip flexion, internal rotation	Pubis-pectineal line	Femur–lesser trochanter; proximal linea aspera	Femoral nerve (L2, L3); obturator nerve in some patients (L2-4)
Adductor longus	Hip adduction	Hip flexion	Pubis—below pubic crest	Linea aspera	Obturator nerve, anterior branch (L2-4)
Adductor brevis	Hip adduction	Hip flexion	Pubis-body and inferior ramus	Femur–lesser trochanter; linea aspera	Obturator nerve (L2-4)
Adductor magnus	Hip adduction	Hip flexion, extension	Pubis-inferior ramus; ischial ramus and tuberosity	Gluteal tuberosity; linea aspera; femur–adductor tubercle	Obturator nerve (L2-4); small contribution from tibial nerve (L5-S1)

(continued on next page)

Table 1
(continued)

Muscle	Primary Function	Secondary Function(s)	Origin	Insertion	Innervation (Spinal Nerve)
Gracilis	Hip flexion	Hip external rotation; knee flexion	Pubis–body and inferior ramus; ischium–ramus	Anteromedial aspect of proximal tibia	Obturator nerve (L2-4)
Gluteals					
Gluteus maximus	Hip extension	Hip external rotation	Ilium–gluteal surface; sacrotuberous ligament; lumbar fascia; posterolateral sacrum	Femur–greater trochanter; iliotibial tract	Inferior gluteal nerve (L5, S1, S2)
Gluteus medius	Hip abduction	Hip internal rotation and flexion (anterior fibers); hip external rotation and extension (posterior fibers)	Ilium–gluteal surface	Femur–greater trochanter	Superior gluteal nerve (L4, L5, S1)
Gluteus minimus	Hip abduction	Hip internal rotation	Ilium–gluteal surface	Femur–greater trochanter	Superior gluteal nerve (L4, L5, S1)
Tensor fascia latae	Hip abduction	Hip flexion, internal rotation; knee external rotation	Outer lip of anterior iliac crest; anterior-superior iliac spine	Iliotibial tract	Superior gluteal nerve L4, L5, S1
Hamstrings					
Semimembranosus	Hip extension	Knee flexion; tibial internal rotation (flexed knee); hip internal rotation (extended hip)	Ischial tuberosity	Tibia–medial condyle	Tibial nerve (L5, S1, S2)
Semitendinosus	Hip extension	Knee flexion; Tibial internal rotation (flexed knee), external rotation (extended knee)	Ischial tuberosity	Anteromedial aspect of proximal tibia	Tibial nerve (L5, S1, S2) ura

Muscle	Action	Action	Origin	Insertion	Nerve
Biceps femoris (long head)	Hip extension	Knee flexion; hip external rotation	Ischial tuberosity; linea aspera	Fibular head	Tibial nerve (L5, S1, S2)
Deep hip external rotators					
Piriformis	Hip external rotation	Hip abduction (flexed hip)	Anterior sacrum	Femur–greater trochanter	Nerve to piriformis (L5, S1, S2)
Obturator externus	Hip external rotation	Hip adduction	Obturator foramen; obturator membrane	Femur–trochanteric fossa	Obturator nerve, posterior branch (L3, L4)
Obturator internus	Hip external rotation	Hip abduction	Ischiopubic ramus; greater sciatic notch; obturator membrane	Femur–greater trochanter	Nerve to obturator internus (L5, S1, S2)
Gemellus superior	Hip external rotation (extended thigh)	Hip abduction (flexed thigh)	Ischiopubic ramus; obturator membrane	Femur–greater trochanter	Nerve to obturator internus (L5, S1, S2)
Gemellus inferior	Hip external rotation (extended thigh)	Hip abduction (flexed thigh)	Ischiopubic ramus; obturator membrane	Femur–greater trochanter	Nerve to obturator internus (L5, S1, S2)
Quadratus femoris	Hip external rotation	Hip adduction	Ischial tuberosity	Femur–intertrochanteric crest	Nerve to quadratus femoris (L4, L5, S1)
Trunk stability					
Rectus abdominus	Knee extension	Hip flexion	Anterior-inferior iliac spine; superior aspect of iliac acetabulum	Patella; tibial tubercle	Femoral nerve (L2-4)
Internal oblique	Trunk rotation–ipsilateral	Abdominal flexion with bilateral activation	Anterior iliac crest; iliopectineal arch; thoracolumbar fascia	Inferior ribs 10–12; linea alba; pubic crest; conjoint tendon	Thoracoabdominal nerves T7-11; subcostal nerve (T12); iliohypogastric nerve (L1); ilioinguinal nerve (L1)

(continued on next page)

Table 1
(continued)

Muscle	Primary Function	Secondary Function(s)	Origin	Insertion	Innervation (Spinal Nerve)
External oblique	Trunk rotation–contralateral	Abdominal flexion with bilateral activation	Ribs 5–12	Anterior iliac crest; pubic crest and tubercle; linea alba; inguinal ligament; anterior-superior iliac spine	Thoracolumbar nerves (T7-11) Subcostal nerve (T12)
Pyramidalis	Linea alba tension		Pubic symphysis and crest	Linea alba	Subcostal nerve (T12)
Latissimus dorsi	Arm adduction	Arm internal rotation, extension; ipsilateral trunk rotation	T7-L5 spinous processes; thoracolumbar fascia; iliac crest; inferior ribs; inferior angle of scapula	Humerus–intertubercular sulcus	Thoracodorsal nerve (C6-8)
Multifidus	Back extension with bilateral activation	Contralateral trunk rotation and ipsilateral side bending with unilateral activation	Sacrum; posterior superior iliac spine; iliac crest	Spinous processes C2-L5	Medial branch nerve of the posterior ramus of spinal nerve at each level
Quadratus lumborum	Ipsilateral lumbar lateral flexion with unilateral activation	Trunk extension and rib cage depression with bilateral activation	Posterior iliac crest	Rib 12; transverse processes L1-5	T12 L1-4 ventral rami
Erector spinae—lumbar portion					
Iliocostalis	Ipsilateral lumbar lateral flexion with unilateral activation	Trunk extension with bilateral activation	Sacrum; posterior iliac crest; spinous processes of lumbar and lower thoracic vertebrae	Ribs 5–12; transverse processes L1-4	Lateral branch nerve of posterior ramus of spinal nerve at each level
Longissimus	Trunk extension with bilateral activation	Ipsilateral lumbar rotation with unilateral activation	Spinous and transverse processes of L1-5; lumbodorsal fascia; posterior iliac crest	Accessory and transverse processes L1-5	Lateral branch nerve of posterior ramus of spinal nerve at each level

Pelvic floor				
Ischiococcygeus	Coccyx flexion	Support of pelvic viscera	Sacrospinous ligament; ischial spine	Coccyx; sacrum	Pudendal nerve (S2-4) Spinal nerves S4, S5
Iliococcygeus	Support of pelvic viscera	None	Pubis–posterior body	Coccyx; anococcygeal ligament	Levator ani nerve (S4) Inferior rectal nerve (S3, S4) Coccygeal plexus
Pubococcygeus	Control of urinary flow	Support of pelvic viscera	Pubis–posterior body	Coccyx; anococcygeal ligament	Levator ani nerve (S4) Inferior rectal nerve (S3, S4) Coccygeal plexus
Puborectalis	Permission of defecation	Support of pelvic viscera	Ischial spine; obturator internus fascia	None (comprises puborectal sling)	Levator ani nerve (S4) S3, S4 spinal nerves

- Core endurance has been associated directly with superior isokinetic shoulder internal and external rotation and knee flexion strength in elite athletes of Olympic disciplines.[8]
- Core stability, balance, and resistance exercises have been shown to improve club head speed in golfers after an 8-week training program.[9,10]
- Superior trunk control has been associated with higher performance on rapid change-of-direction activities.[11]
- Horizontal arm swing velocity, critical in baseball, golf, and racquet sports, is directly dependent on trunk rotation of the arm and also indirectly by exerting interaction torque necessary for rapid elbow extension.[12]

- Helps to control body segments below the region
  - Increased knee valgus, a known risk factor for ACL injury, has been associated with decreased hip internal rotation, knee flexion, and trunk rotation strength.[13–16]
  - Altered trunk kinematics also are seen in patients with chronic ankle instability compared with controls, thought to be compensatory in nature. Those compensatory mechanisms have been associated with improvements in balance testing.[17,18]
- Relationship between trunk instability and inflexibility and injury risk
  - Overhead athletes with ulnar collateral ligament injuries of the elbow have been shown to have decreased trunk stability and balance but not hip range-of-motion (ROM) deficits.[19,20]
  - These balance deficits can be remedied, and a lower extremity neuromuscular control home exercise program has been shown to improve balance postoperatively in those with an ulnar collateral ligament tear.[21]
  - Increased hip, hamstring, and groin injury risk in professional baseball players with decreased hip internal rotation and total arc hip ROM.[22]
  - A training module, including leg and trunk stabilization, proprioceptive training with landing from a jump, postural stability, and lower extremity flexibility, led to a significant reduction of severe knee injury in elite soccer players.[23]
  - Core strength is an independent predictor of shoulder dysfunction in overhead athletes of all disciplines.[24,25]

CLASSIFICATIONS OF INJURIES

- Acute versus chronic onset
  - Acute injuries are more likely to occur during competition whereas those with an insidious onset are more likely to occur during training, where a vast majority of athletic exposures occur.[26,27]
  - Acute injuries are more likely to involve tendon avulsion whereas chronic-onset injuries are more likely to involve degenerative tendinopathy.

PRESENTATION

- Hip flexor injuries can involve the iliopsoas or rectus femoris, most commonly. These injuries typically are a product of an acute concentric or eccentric strain or a progressive overuse musculotendinous injury. The presentation usually involves a complaint of anterior hip pain that is located near the lesser trochanter and/or at the level of the anterior hip joint, whereas most of the anatomic makeup is musculotendinous structures. Less commonly, the pain can be more proximal in the lower abdomen involving more muscle belly fibers of the iliacus or psoas. Pain from rectus injuries usually is located at the joint or distal down the anterior thigh. Palpation is sensitive for rectus injuries, whereas the iliopsoas typically is deeper than allows for direct pressure to the injured structure. Pain is reproduced with concentric and eccentric resisted activity with hip flexion but also can be present with active or passive hip extension, which places the injured muscle on stretch.

- ○ Hip flexor strain key points
    - Acute or acute-on-chronic anterior hip pain after forced hip flexion
    - High rate of injury in competition, although higher overall incidence in training
    - Equal incidence in men and women
    - Most commonly noncontact
    - Typically results in less than 1 week's missed time from sport[28]
- Adductor injuries present with a similar mechanism but tend to be located anywhere from the pubic ramus down into the middle of the inner thigh. Pain is present more so with direct palpation, because the muscle groups are in more proximity to the superficial fascial layers. Sometimes, in higher-grade injuries, a palpable defect can be felt as well as the potential for ecchymosis and swelling with acute hemorrhage. With tendinous injuries, whether they are associated with a chronic tendinopathy or an acute avulsion, there typically is pain directly on the pubic bone. Pain and weakness can be present with adductor muscle testing and passive abduction of the hip.
    - ○ Adductor strain key points
        - Acute or acute-on-chronic medial proximal thigh (groin) pain or pain over ipsilateral pubis
        - High rate of injury in competition, although higher overall incidence in training
        - Higher incidence in men than women
        - Most commonly noncontact
        - Typically results in less than 1 week's missed time from sport[28]
- Gluteal tendon injuries tend to be more overuse or related to a chronic process rather than an acute injury, which may have resulted in a tendinopathy. Acute avulsions of the tendons from the greater trochanter and traumatic bursal or muscular injuries, however, also can occur with athletic injuries. The more commonly affected muscles are the gluteus medius and minimus. Both structures attach to the greater trochanter and function as hip abductors and stabilizers of the femoroacetabular joint as well as multiplanar pelvic control. Pain typically presents at the lateral aspect of the hip around the trochanter or proximal. Due to the more superficial location, just under the iliotibial fascia, there usually is pain to palpation and pain with active or resisted abduction and active or passive adduction. With acute, traumatic tendinous avulsions or bursal ruptures, there are swelling and ecchymosis at times.
    - ○ Gluteal tendon disorders key points
        - Typically, insidious onset and involves pain over the posterolateral hip
        - Can occur acutely after fall on the greater trochanter
        - Higher prevalence in older population[29]
- Proximal hamstring injuries also can involve acute injuries related to avulsions or strains but also can include more chronic processes like insertional tendinopathy. A common overlapping clinical presentation in this region may be a lumbar radicular or sciatic nerve issue, so the clinical awareness of both entities is crucial. Proximal muscle strains and chronic tendinopathy issues can resolve with nonsurgical treatment but do tend to require a lengthier treatment protocol

and sometimes time loss from their sport. With acute ruptures of the proximal hamstring attachment, there typically is a surgical reattachment performed for tears that involve at least 2 tendons and have a retraction of greater than 2 cm in high-level athletes. The recovery time from this surgery can take up to 9 months to return to sport.

- Proximal hamstring injury key points
  - Less common than midbelly hamstring injury[30]
  - Multifold increase in risk during competition compared with training[30]
  - More prevalent in older athletic populations
    - Incidence in male athletes associated with increased age (although younger than female athletes) and sport participation
    - Incidence in female athletes associated with increased age and occurrence during activities of daily living[31]
  - 5% co-incidence of sciatic nerve involvement[31]

CLINICAL ASSESSMENT

- General assessment of soft tissue injuries of the hip and pelvis
  - Subjective
    - Pain of muscular etiology typically most prominent with activation of the affected structure, especially in the stretched state (ie, activation of the hip flexor while supine in bed). Affected individuals typically can locate muscular pain with palpation.
    - Muscular pain is most pronounced more commonly after a period of rest, then abates before becoming more prevalent again with prolonged activity.
    - Patients with hip flexor (and its associated bursa) pathology may complain of snapping over the anterior hip, and this can present similarly over the lateral hip in external rotator/abductor tendinopathy or proximal iliotibial band friction syndrome, respectively.
    - Hip labral provocation with deep hip flexion, especially flexion and rotation movements, such as getting in and out of a vehicle
    - Pain not associated with motion or pain associated with urination/defecation suggests nonmusculoskeletal etiology
    - Diffuse discomfort or associated neurologic symptoms distally in the lower extremity should raise suspicion for a radiculopathic component as cause of the patient's symptoms.
  - Objective
    - Inspection
      - Evaluate for presence of ecchymosis/abrasions that may provide clues to the injured structure and mechanism of injury.
      - Muscle wasting
      - Pelvic tilt
      - Gait abnormalities
    - Palpation
      - Examine for area of maximal tenderness
      - Palpable tendinous defect in rupture/avulsion
      - Posterior-superior iliac spine for concomitant sacroiliac joint pathology
      - Firm pressure over gluteal musculature for reproduction of radicular pain in piriformis syndrome
      - Lateral femoral condyle in iliotibial band friction syndrome for distal component

- Knee joint for referred pain
- Passive testing
  - Important to evaluate hip ROM in the seated, supine, and prone positions
    - Evaluation of affected and unaffected sides is critical.
    - Special consideration to structures that cross 2 joints, such as the hamstring and iliotibial band (hip and knee)
- Special testing
  - Critical to assess bilaterally and serially to determine asymmetry and changes over time
  - Intra-articular pathology
    - Assess with log roll, scour, flexion-adduction-internal rotation testing
  - Extra-articular pathology
    - Thomas test/modified Thomas test
      - Hip flexor ROM restriction
      - Must control for pelvic tilt[32]
    - Ober test
      - Iliotibial band and/or tensor fascia latae ROM restriction
      - May be affected by tightness of gluteus medius/minimus[33]
    - Trendelenburg test
      - Ipsilateral hip abductor strength in single-leg stance
      - Assess after exercise to fatigue to tease out mild strength deficits
- Neurologic testing
  - Strength, sensation, and lower extremity reflexes are important to evaluate bilaterally for the presence of a neurologic component, such as with lower lumbosacral radiculopathies, which also provide motor input to hip girdle musculature.
  - Straight leg raise test to evaluate for radiculopathy
- Active testing
  - Strength testing
    - Stinchfield test
      - Resisted hip flexion past 30° to 45°
      - Aids in ruling out intra-articular pathology as a source of a patient's pain
    - Resisted internal rotation
      - More sensitive but less specific than Trendelenburg sign for detection of gluteus medius tears[34]
  - The evaluation of compound movements, such as the squat, lunge, and step-up/down, allows for the gross assessment of biomechanics but only when assessed by experienced practitioners.[35]
  - This evaluation also can help elucidate a possible femoroacetabular impingement component to the patient's symptoms.[36]
  - More ballistic, dynamic movement evaluation allows the practitioner to evaluate the interconnected kinematics between joints in the activities that most closely replicate the mechanism of injury. Although the most intensive of these require a laboratory setting with motion capture software, they also allow for evaluation of deficiencies that would not be detected with the typical office evaluation. Some examples of dynamic testing include the following:
    - Nine months post–anterior cruciate ligament (ACL) reconstruction, double-leg drop jump, single-leg drop jump, single-leg hop for distance, and hurdle hop all showed biomechanical deficiencies.[37]

- Also showed biomechanical alterations in change of direction activities
  - Knee valgus
  - Knee internal rotation and flexion angle
  - Knee extension and external rotation moment
  - Ankle external rotation moment[38]
- Single-leg triple hop
  - Increased anterior pelvic tilt, knee valgus, and contralateral pelvic drop in female athletes with patellofemoral pain[39]
- Single-leg hop
  - Simple in-office test to assist in evaluation of femoral neck and sacral stress injury. Avoid in patients experiencing pain with weight bearing.

Injury Rates

- Of all injuries sustained by Major League Baseball athletes, 5%
  - Of noncontact injuries during defensive fielding, 74%
  - Days missed for extra-articular injuries, on average: 12
  - Days of lost time for intra-articular injuries, on average: 123[1]
- There was an overall hip injury rate of 5.18 per 10,000 athlete exposures in National College Athletic Association football over a 10-year period. The most common were adductor strains (38.6%) and then hip flexor strains (28.5%), and these injuries were more common during the preseason.[40] A similar study investigated collegiate soccer players with similar results, and in addition they showed that they these injuries were noncontact injuries, 77.3%.[41]
- Hip and groin injuries led to lost time in one-fifth of professional soccer players.[42]
- In professional soccer players, 14% of all injuries [43]
- In professional dancers versus student dancers, 27.7% of all injuries versus 14.1% of injuries, respectively[44]
- Collegiate athlete exposures: 53.06 hip/groin injuries per 100,000
  - Most common in men's soccer (110.84) and men's (104.9) and women's (76.88) ice hockey
  - In sex-comparable sports, men with greater rate of hip/groin injury (59.53 vs 42.27)
  - Noncontact, 48.4%
  - Overuse/gradual, 20.4%
  - Resulted in missed time from sport, 39.3%
  - Resulted in surgery, 1.3% [45]

REHABILITATION PRINCIPLES

There is much overlap when considering the end goal of rehabilitation for hip flexor strains, adductor strains, proximal hamstring strains, and gluteal tendinopathy. Most sports involve various amounts of acceleration, deceleration, cutting, jumping, and sprinting at high speeds. All these components need to be trained during the rehabilitation process in order for an athlete to safely return to competitive sports. Phase 3 (return to competition) of the rehabilitation process might look similar for a soccer player who experienced an adductor strain and another soccer player who experienced gluteal tendinopathy. The reason for this is because phase 3 consists mostly of activities involving linear running, change of direction activities, sport-specific drills, and a graded return-to-game progression. Once athletes are physically able to perform phase 3 drills, they no longer are experiencing pain and should be either at normal or near normal in terms of their strength and coordinated movement strategies that once were affected by the injury.

On the other hand, the rehabilitation outlined for phase 1 and phase 2 of each of the 4 injuries in this article looks much different. The body needs to be put through specific movements and positions to properly strengthen and condition the injured tissue. Precise exercise prescription is required during these first 2 phases in order to overcome the specific deficits that an athlete presents to the clinician. **Fig. 1** provides a detailed overview of each phase (see **Fig. 1**).

Phase 1—Acute Management

The goal of phase 1 (acute management) is to protect the area of injury and initiate the rehabilitation program. The acronym POLICE (protection, optimal loading, ice, compression, and elevation) has been suggested as an early approach to treatment. It is similar to the classic recommendation of RICE (rest, ice, compression, and elevation), except that early optimal loading is encouraged instead of more extended rest.[46] Overall, pain management and swelling management are large components of the initial rehabilitation goals. Following the rules of POLICE helps achieve these goals.

Some research suggests that early initiation of a rehabilitation program after a soft tissue injury of the thigh and lower extremity might allow someone to return to their sport earlier after becoming injured.[47] In addition to this, allowing an athlete to participate in a graded rehabilitation program while still experiencing some pain might improve strength by the time they make a full return to their sport compared with undergoing a rehabilitation program that avoids pain. This has been shown in an randomized controlled trial for hamstring strains.[48]

In terms of exercises, the maintenance and restoration of strength, ROM, and stabilization strategies are large components of phase 1, along with the maintenance of cardiovascular fitness. The longer rehabilitation is delayed, the greater the chance that these characteristics can be impacted. Delays in the exercise component of rehabilitation might be needed due to the severity of the injury but should be initiated once tolerated in order to maximize function of the injured limb. Exercise for the injured tissue in this phase consists of isometric contractions, isotonic contractions, ROM activities, stabilization activities, and blood flow restriction (BFR) strengthening exercises. When the appropriate equipment is available, BFR exercises can be helpful because its application has been shown to enhance muscle protein synthesis, along with achieving similar muscle strength and muscle mass improvements when comparing the response of low-load BFR exercises to high-load exercises without using BFR.[49,50] The ROM component in the included rehabilitation programs is blended into all of the included categories of exercise. For example, performing a bodyweight squat with increasing depth is in the isotonic exercise category during phase 1 of a

Phases of Rehabilitation		
Phase Number: 1	**2**	**3**
Phase Name: Acute Management	Strengthening	Return to Competition
Goal: Protect area of injury and initiate rehabilitation program	Strengthen and recondition the injured tissue to the level required for full participation in the sporting activities	Return to full participation in sporting activities

Components: • POLICE
• Pain management
• Swelling management
• Maintenance/restoration of strength, ROM, and stabilization strategies
• Maintenance of cardiovascular fitness
• Assess and address movement qualities (ie, strength, ROM, stabilization) in neighboring body segments
	• Progress rehabilitations activities for
	  • Isometric strengthening
	  • Isotonic strengthening
	  • Stabilization/reactive strategies
	  • Cardiovascular fitness
	• Begin rehabilitation activities for
	  • Linear running
	  • Change of direction movements
	  • Plyometrics
	• Introduce sport-specific drills
	• Continue to address movement qualities away from the area of injury
		• Progress rehabilitation activities that were started in phase 2
		• Progress sport specific drills towards near competition intensity
		• Be able to run at maximal intensities and velocities
		• Initiate a gradual return to competition game/match plan so the athlete can safely return without any restrictions

Fig. 1. Phases of rehabilitation.

rectus femoris strain but should be considered an ROM activity just as much as a strengthening activity. In addition to exercise for the injured tissue, assessment and interventions for movement qualities (ie, strength, ROM, and stabilization) in neighboring body segments also should be included in this phase.

Therapeutic modalities and manual therapy (dry needling, joint mobilizations/manipulations, soft tissue manipulation, instrument-assisted soft tissue mobilization [IASTM], and so forth—targeted away from the site of injury) for pain management, swelling reduction, and increased circulation should be applied during phase 1. The application of manual therapy also can help maintain and improve ROM in this phase. Manual therapy initially should be applied away from the site of injury in order to not disrupt the innate healing mechanisms that are occurring. The role and application of various manual therapy techniques for acute muscle injuries are controversial somewhat due to much of the research being on animal models and not humans. When applied appropriately, human research has shown the following: dry needling techniques can improve blow flow[51] and reduce pain[52]; IASTM helps decrease pain[53]; and hands-on manual therapy techniques, such as joint mobilizations/manipulations and soft tissue treatment, often are included in rehabilitation programs that help decrease pain and increase function.[54]

A

Phases of Rehabilitation - Hip Flexor Strain (Rectus Femoris)

Phase Number:	1			2			3	
Phase Name:	Acute Management			Strengthening			Return to Competition	
Goal:	Protect area of injury and initiate rehabilitation program			Strengthen and recondition the injured tissue to the level required for full participation in the sporting activities			Return to full participation in sporting activities	
	Exercise - Tissue Specific	Isometrics	Low to medium intensity (Progress to increased ranges of knee flexion and hip extension) - Prone knee extension ISO (mid range knee flexion) - Supine hip flexion ISO (mid range hip flexion) - Split squat ISO (bottom position)	Exercise - Tissue Specific	Isometrics	Medium to high intensity (Progress to increased ROM and adding an external load KB, DB, or weight vest) - Prone knee extension ISO (from near max knee flexion) - Prone hip flexion ISO (from near max hip extension) - Split squat—ISO (bottom position) with weight - Rear foot elevated split squat ISO	Full-Strength Training Program	- Address any continued deficits through the previous used techniques in phase 2 - isometrics, isotonics, reactive/stabilization and BFR - Focus most of the athletes time in this phase on linear running, change of direction activities, sport-specific drills and a graded return to games and competitions - Strengthening and stabilization exercises are used to supplement the higher-demanding running and sporting activities
	Exercise - Tissue Specific	Isotonics	Partial ROM and bodyweight to start - Step-ups - Split squat - Reverse lunge - Lateral lunge - Squat - two-leg	Exercise - Tissue Specific	Isotonics	Add weight and increase ROM within the movement as tolerated by the athlete - Step ups - weighted and/or slow eccentric lowering - Split squat - Rear foot elevated split squat - Reverse lunge - Lateral lunge - Squat—two-leg and single-leg	Full-Strength Training Program	
	Exercise - Tissue Specific	ROM and Stabilization	- "A" marches in place→ "A" marches with forward progression - Sidestepping → side shuffle - Walking carioca → dynamic carioca - Half-kneeling medicine ball chest pass	Exercise - Tissue Specific	Stabilization and Reactive	- Split-stance medicine ball chest pass - Split-stance medicine ball diagonal chop - Scissor jumps in place - alternating - Scissor jumps with forward progression - lead with each leg separately	Additional Comments and Considerations	The dosage of an appropriate workload for each athlete is the key for a successful return to their sport and the completion of the rehabilitation process
	Exercise - Tissue Specific	BFR	If proper equipment is available - Perform at up to 80% LOP if tolerated - Standing hip flexion - Seated knee extension	Exercise - Tissue Specific	BFR	If proper equipment is available - Perform at up to 80% LOP if tolerated. Don't repeat isotonic movments from above. - Squats - Split squats - Step-ups		
	Additional Exercises (non-specific to injured tissue)		- Sidelying hip abduction - Sidelying clams - Glute bridges - Upper body/core training	Additional Exercises (non-specific to injured tissue)		- Additional exercises to target the posterior chain - RDLs, single-leg RDLs, Nordic hamstring curls - Upper Body/Core Training		
	Additional Comments and Considerations		- POLICE as needed - Modalties for pain management, swelling reduction and increased circulation (electrical stimulation, laser, hivamat, etc.) - Manual therapy away from the injured tissue - dry needling, soft tissue manipulation, IASTM	Additional Comments and Considerations		- Continuation of modalities for pain management, swelling reduction and increased circulation as needed - Manual therapy to the injured tissue - dry needling, soft tissue manipulation, IASTM		

B

Phases of Rehabilitation - Adductor Strain

Phase Number:	1			2			3	
Phase Name:	Acute Management			Strengthening			Return to Competition	
Goal:	Protect area of injury and initiate rehabilitation program			Strengthen and recondition the injured tissue to the level required for full participation in the sporting activities			Return to full participation in sporting activities	
	Exercise - Tissue Specific	Isometrics	Low to medium intensity (Progress to increased ROM) - Hooklying adductor ISO with posterior pelvic tilt - Sidelying supported adductor ISO - top leg in abduction on elevated surface - Half-kneeling adduction/IR ISO with band	Exercise - Tissue Specific	Isometrics	Medium to high intensity (Progress to increased ROM and adding an external load where appropriate - KB, DB, or weight vest) - Sidelying adductor hip lift ISO - Split-stance adduction/IR ISO with band - Split squat-ISO (bottom position)	Full-Strength Training Program	- Address any continued deficits through the previous used techniques in phase 2 - isometrics, isotonics, reactive/stabilization and BFR - Focus most of the athletes time in this phase on linear running, change of direction activities, sport specific drills and a graded return to games and competitions - Strengthening and stabilization exercises are used to supplement the higher demanding running and sporting activities
	Exercise - Tissue Specific	Isotonics	Partial ROM and bodyweight to start - Single-leg hip airplane - Lateral lunge - Crossover step up - Split squat –	Exercise - Tissue Specific	Isotonics	Add weight and increase ROM as tolerated for appropriate exercises - Sidelying adductor hip lift with eccentric lowering - Slide board lateral lunge - Crossover step up - Split squat–	Full-Strength Training Program	
	Exercise - Tissue Specific	ROM and Stabilization	- Half-kneeling medicine ball diagonal chop - "A" marches in place → "A" marches with forward progression - Sidestepping → side shuffle - Walking carioca → dynamic carioca	Exercise - Tissue Specific	Stabilization and Reactive	- Slide board - lateral slide intervals - Split-stance medicine ball diagonal chop - Split-stance medicine ball chest pass	Additional Comments and Considerations	The dosage of an appropriate workload for each athlete is the key for a successful return to their sport and the completion of the rehabilitation process
	Exercise - Tissue Specific	BFR	If proper equipment is available - Perform at up to 80% LOP if tolerated - Sidelying hip adduction raise - bottom leg - Squat	Exercise - Tissue Specific	BFR	If proper equipment is available - Perform at up to 80% LOP if tolerated. Don't repeat isotonic movments from above. - Lateral lunge - Step-up		
	Additional Exercises (non-specific to injured tissue)		- Sidelying hip abduction - Sidelying clams - Upper body/core training	Additional Exercises (non-specific to injured tissue)		- Additional exercises to target the posterior chain - RDLs, single-leg RDLs, Nordic hamstring curls - Upper Body/Core Training		
	Additional Comments and Considerations		- POLICE as needed - Modalties for pain management, swelling reduction and increased circulation (electrical stimulation, laser, hivamat, etc.) - Manual therapy away from the injured tissue - dry needling, soft tissue manipulation, IASTM	Additional Comments and Considerations		- Continuation of modalities for pain management, swelling reduction and increased circulation as needed - Manual therapy to the injured tissue - dry needling, soft tissue manipulation, IASTM		

Fig. 2. Four injury specifics. (*A*) Hip flexor (rectus femoris) strains. (*B*)Adductor strains. (*C*) Gluteal tendinopathy. (*D*) Proximal hamstring strains. AROM, active range of motion; DB, dumbbell; ER, external rotation; IR, internal rotation; ISO, isometric; KB, kettlebell; LOP, limb occlusion pressure; Max, maximal; RDL, romanian deadlift; SLR, straight leg raise.

C

		Phases of Rehabilitation - Gluteal Tendinopathy		
Phase Number:	1	2		3
Phase Name:	Acute Management	Strengthening		Return to Competition
Goal:	Protect area of injury and initiate rehabilitation program	Strengthen and recondition the injured tissue to the level required for full participation in the sporting activities		Return to full participation in sporting activities

D

		Phases of Rehabilitation - Proximal Hamstring Strain		
Phase Number:	1	2		3
Phase Name:	Acute Management	Strengthening		Return to Competition
Goal:	Protect area of injury and initiate rehabilitation program	Strengthen and recondition the injured tissue to the level required for full participation in the sporting activities		Return to full participation in sporting activities

Fig. 2. *Continued*

Phase 2—Strengthening

The goal of phase 2 (strengthening) is to strengthen and recondition the injured tissue to the level required for full participation in the sporting activities. Rehabilitation activities for strengthening (isometric and isotonic), stabilization/reactive strategies, and cardiovascular fitness are progressed. In addition to these, the athlete begins the following: linear running exercises, change of direction movements, plyometrics, and sport-specific drills.

This phase includes the continued utilization of both therapeutic modalities and manual therapy. Manual therapy can be applied to the injured tissue. Research is not clear on the exact timing for this to occur, but it is safe to do so in phase 2 because the tissue is well into the remodeling phase of tissue repair.

Phase 3—Return to Competition

The goal of phase 3 (return to competition) is for the athlete to return to full participation in their sporting activities. The athlete is pain-free and should have near-normal strength when entering this phase, but the dynamic movement ability is insufficient for a safe return. Most of the rehabilitation effort throughout this phase is spent on linear running, change of direction activities, sport-specific drills, and a graded return to games and competitions. The dosage of an appropriate workload for each athlete is key for a successful return to their sport and the completion of the rehabilitation process.

Running and Conditioning for Returning to Sport

Phase Number	1		
Phase Name:	Acute Management		
Goal:	Protect area of injury and initiate rehabilitation program		
	Cardiovascular Fitness		- Biking, elliptical, or walking in a pool if tolerated - Initially low intensity, but eventually higher heart rate when tolerated (heart rate goal of 120-150 BPM for 20-30 minutes) - The initial goal with these activities are to increase circulation to the area of injury. Eventually they will be done to achieve a cardiovascular effect

Phase Number	2		
Phase Name:	Strengthening		
Goal:	Strengthen and recondition the injured tissue to the level required for full participation in the sporting activities		
	Cardiovascular Fitness		- Continue longer duration, aerobic conditioning • Biking, elliptical, or any other cardio equipment - 20-30 minutes at a HR of 130-150 BPM - Initiate short duration, anaerobic conditioning • Bike intervals - Example: 10" on 20" off, repeated 6 times for two sets, 4 min rest between sets; HR will increase to >175 BPM
	Linear running progression	Drills	- "A" March - Various step heights to tolerance - "A" Skips - Various skip heights to tolerance - "A" Run - Various hip flexion ROM and cadence to tolerance
		Acceleration	- 10-yard accelerations (6–7 steps) - repeat in sets with short rest • Example: 10-yard accelerations @ 50%–70% intensity, repeated 5–10 times per set for 2–3 sets, resting 3 min between sets
		Jogging	Low intensity, increasing duration and distance to tolerance. This component is focused on less for sports where jogging long durations is not necessary (baseball, wrestling, volleyball, etc.)
		Tempo Runs	- 30–50+ yard runs at submaximal intensity (no more than 75%) • Example: 30-yard tempo runs at 75% intensity, repeated 5–10 times, with 30-60 s rest between reps
	Change of direction progression	Deceleration Drills	- Jump stop - Shuffle stop - Lateral jump stop - Lunge stop - forward and reverse
		Integrative Drills	- Lateral shuffle - quick change of direction - Carioca shuffle - quick change of direction - Forward/back jogging - quick change of direction
	Plyometrics	2 feet	- In place - Lateral over line - Forward/back over line - Forward for distance - Lateral for distance - each direction - Straddle jumps - Box
		1 foot	- In place - Lateral over line - Forward/back over line - Forward for distance - Lateral jump to two feet landing - Lateral jump to contralateral single leg landing - Box
	Sport specific drills		Start to integrate sporting drills with a graded increase in volume and intensity

Phase Number	3		
Phase Name:	Return to Competition		
Goal:	Return to full participation in sporting activities		
	Cardiovascular fitness		- Running, sport specific drills and game activity make up the majority of cardiovascular fitness in this phase - Use biking and cardio machines as needed for a non-impact option
	Linear running progression	Acceleration	- 10–15-yard accelerations at higher intensity than phase 2, along with increased rest time • Example: 5x10-yard and 5x15-yard accelerations @ 85%–100% intensity, resting 1–3 minutes between each rep and 5 minutes after the first set at 10-yards. Rest longer when running at higher intensities
		Jogging	Continue to increase distance and duration to meet the demands of the athletes sports they participate in
		Tempo Runs	- 80–100 yard runs at submaximal intensity (no more than 75%) • Example: 80-yard tempo runs at 75% intensity, repeated 5-10 times, with 2 minutes of rest between reps
		Maximal Velocity	- Maximal intensity sprinting at shorter distances (20–30 yds) • Example: 30 yard sprints at 95%-100% intensity, repeated 2–4 times with 5–6 minutes of rest between each rep (full recovery between reps)
	Change of direction progression	Integrative Drills	- Lateral run start - Shuttle runs (ie. 5–10–5) - T-Drill
	Sport Specific Drills		Progress volume and intensity of sporting drills
	Grade return to game activity		Create a graded return to unrestricted competition. Play part of a scrimmage, match or other component of the sport in a practice before going back to being in the regular competitive event. This should be done several times until the athlete feels comfortable to return and so they can achieve a high enough workload to return safely

Fig. 3. Running and conditioning for returning to sport. BPM, beats per minute; HR, heart rate; T-Drill, T-Drill.

Injury-Specific Rehabilitation Outlines

There are 4 separate figures with an example of a rehabilitation outline for each type of injury presented in this article: hip flexor (rectus femoris) strains, adductor strains, gluteal tendinopathy, and proximal hamstring strains. **Fig. 2** depicts specific rehabilitation details for each injury subgroup (see **Fig. 2**). They are broken down into suggested rehabilitation strategies for each type of injury. Videos are included for these 4 tables, demonstrating the exercises for each rehabilitation program (Videos 1–4).

In addition, **Fig. 3** includes rehabilitation guidelines for cardiovascular fitness, linear running, and change of direction movements and recommendations for returning to sporting activities. This table is a general framework that can be followed for each of the 4 different types of injuries.

These tables are not an exhaustive list of exercises and strategies to include for each injury. They provide a general framework to use when customizing a personalized rehabilitation plan for a patient experiencing one of these injuries.

SUMMARY

Hip and pelvis soft tissue injuries are common in all levels of athletics. The complex functional nature of the hip and pelvis anatomy is part of the reason why an organized approach to successfully treating and returning the athletes to their sport is prudent. The most common injuries involve the hip flexors, or adductors. Understanding the 3 phases of a rehabilitation process is crucial, and knowing that each athlete needs an individualized approach to a successful outcome helps hasten recovery. The authors break down these phases into acute management, strengthening, and return-to-competition phases. The acute phase should be implemented immediately and progression and/or overlap to the next phase is based on the injury severity and specific needs and goals of each athlete, in addition to but not limited to the athlete's physiologic makeup. High levels of successful return-to-sport rates are seen with the proper management of these soft tissue injuries around the hip and pelvis.

CLINICAL CARE POINTS

- Recognize the complexity of the multiple muscle groups connecting the hip and pelvis.
- Understand the coordinating function of the various muscle groups injured.
  - Hip flexors and adductors are the most commonly injured and sometimes can present with various overlap in their clinical presentation.
- Begin phase 1, acute-phase treatment, immediately.
- Individualize the treatment phases to each athlete.
- Return to sport should be highly successful in athletes with soft tissue injuries of the hip and pelvis, especially with adherence to the discussed previously principles.

DISCLOSURES

The authors have nothing to disclose.

SUPPLEMENTARY DATA

Supplementary video related to this article can be found at https://doi.org/10.1016/j.csm.2021.01.002.

REFERENCES

1. Coleman SH, Mayer SW, Tyson JJ, et al. The epidemiology of hip and groin injuries in professional baseball players. Am J Orthop (Belle Mead Nj) 2016; 45(3):168-175.
2. Aguinaldo A, Escamilla R. Segmental power analysis of sequential body motion and elbow valgus loading during baseball pitching: comparison between professional and high school baseball players. Orthop J Sports Med 2019;7(2). 2325967119827924.
3. Kimura A, Yoshioka S, Omura L, et al. Mechanical properties of upper torso rotation from the viewpoint of energetics during baseball pitching [published online ahead of print, 2019 Aug 6]. Eur J Sport Sci 2019;1-8. https://doi.org/10.1080/17461391.2019.1646810.
4. Lust KR, Sandrey MA, Bulger SM, et al. The effects of 6-week training programs on throwing accuracy, proprioception, and core endurance in baseball. J Sport Rehabil 2009;18(3):407-26.
5. Sado N, Yoshioka S, Fukashiro S. Three-dimensional kinetic function of the lumbo-pelvic-hip complex during block start. PLoS One 2020;15(3):e0230145.
6. Mısırlıoğlu TÖ, Eren İ, Canbulat N, et al. Does a core stabilization exercise program have a role on shoulder rehabilitation? A comparative study in young females. Turk J Phys Med Rehabil 2018;64(4):328-336.
7. Saeterbakken AH, Loken E, Scott S, et al. Effects of ten weeks dynamic or isometric core training on climbing performance among highly trained climbers. PLoS One 2018;13(10):e0203766.
8. Kocahan T, Akınoğlu B. Determination of the relationship between core endurance and isokinetic muscle strength of elite athletes. J Exerc Rehabil 2018; 14(3):413-418.
9. Thompson CJ, Cobb KM, Blackwell J. Functional training improves club head speed and functional fitness in older golfers. J Strength Cond Res 2007;21(1): 131-7.

10. Weston M, Coleman NJ, Spears IR. The effect of isolated core training on selected measures of golf swing performance. Med Sci Sports Exerc 2013; 45(12):2292–7.
11. Edwards S, Austin AP, Bird SP. The role of the trunk control in athletic performance of a reactive change-of-direction task. J Strength Cond Res 2017;31(1): 126–39.
12. Kim YK, Hinrichs RN, Dounskaia N. Multicomponent control strategy underlying production of maximal hand velocity during horizontal arm swing. J Neurophysiol 2009;102(5):2889–99.
13. Uebayashi K, Akasaka K, Tamura A, et al. Characteristics of trunk and lower limb alignment at maximum reach during the star excursion balance Test in subjects with increased knee valgus during jump landing. PLoS One 2019;14(1): e0211242.
14. Nguyen AD, Shultz SJ, Schmitz RJ. Landing biomechanics in participants with different static lower extremity alignment profiles. J Athl Train 2015;50(5): 498–507.
15. Krosshaug T, Nakamae A, Boden BP, et al. Mechanisms of anterior cruciate ligament injury in basketball: video analysis of 39 cases. Am J Sports Med 2007; 35(3):359–67.
16. Koga H, Nakamae A, Shima Y, et al. Mechanisms for noncontact anterior cruciate ligament injuries: knee joint kinematics in 10 injury situations from female team handball and basketball. Am J Sports Med 2010;38(11):2218–25.
17. Terada M, Morgan KD, Gribble PA. Altered movement strategy of chronic ankle instability individuals with postural instability classified based on Nyquist and Bode analyses. Clin Biomech (Bristol, Avon) 2019;69:39–43.
18. Hoch MC, Gaven SL, Weinhandl JT. Kinematic predictors of star excursion balance test performance in individuals with chronic ankle instability. Clin Biomech (Bristol, Avon) 2016;35:37–41.
19. Garrison JC, Arnold A, Macko MJ, et al. Baseball players diagnosed with ulnar collateral ligament tears demonstrate decreased balance compared to healthy controls. J Orthop Sports Phys Ther 2013;43(10):752–8.
20. Craig Garrison J, Hannon J, Conway J. No differences in hip range of motion exists between baseball players with an ulnar collateral ligament tear and healthy baseball players. Int J Sports Phys Ther 2019;14(6):920–6.
21. Hannon J, Garrison JC, Conway J. Lower extremity balance is improved at time of return to throwing in baseball players after an ulnar collateral ligament reconstruction when compared to pre-operative measurements. Int J Sports Phys Ther 2014;9(3):356–64.
22. Li X, Ma R, Zhou H, et al. Evaluation of Hip internal and external rotation range of motion as an injury risk factor for hip, abdominal and groin injuries in professional baseball players. Orthop Rev (Pavia) 2015;7(4):6142.
23. Krutsch W, Lehmann J, Jansen P, et al. Prevention of severe knee injuries in men's elite football by implementing specific training modules. Knee Surg Sports Traumatol Arthrosc 2020;28(2):519–27.
24. Radwan A, Francis J, Green A, et al. Is there a relation between shoulder dysfunction and core instability? Int J Sports Phys Ther 2014;9(1):8–13.
25. Reeser JC, Joy EA, Porucznik CA, et al. Risk factors for volleyball-related shoulder pain and dysfunction. PM R 2010;2(1):27–36.
26. Jones A, Jones G, Greig N, et al. Epidemiology of injury in English professional football players: a cohort study. Phys Ther Sport 2019;35:18–22.

27. Waldén M, Hägglund M, Ekstrand J. UEFA Champions League study: a prospective study of injuries in professional football during the 2001-2002 season. Br J Sports Med 2005;39(8):542–6.

28. Eckard TG, Padua DA, Dompier TP, et al. Epidemiology of hip flexor and hip adductor strains in national collegiate athletic association athletes, 2009/2010-2014/2015. Am J Sports Med 2017;45(12):2713–22.

29. Riel H, Lindstrøm CF, Rathleff MS, et al. Prevalence and incidence rate of lower-extremity tendinopathies in a Danish general practice: a registry-based study. BMC Musculoskelet Disord 2019;20(1):239.

30. Roe M, Murphy JC, Gissane C, et al. Hamstring injuries in elite Gaelic football: an 8-year investigation to identify injury rates, time-loss patterns and players at increased risk. Br J Sports Med 2018;52(15):982–8.

31. Irger M, Willinger L, Lacheta L, et al. Proximal hamstring tendon avulsion injuries occur predominately in middle-aged patients with distinct gender differences: epidemiologic analysis of 263 surgically treated cases. Knee Surg Sports Traumatol Arthrosc 2020;28(4):1221–9.

32. Vigotsky AD, Lehman GJ, Beardsley C, et al. The modified Thomas test is not a valid measure of hip extension unless pelvic tilt is controlled. PeerJ 2016;4:e2325.

33. Willett GM, Keim SA, Shostrom VK, et al. An anatomic investigation of the ober test. Am J Sports Med 2016;44(3):696–701.

34. Ortiz-Declet V, Chen AW, Maldonado DR, et al. Diagnostic accuracy of a new clinical test (resisted internal rotation) for detection of gluteus medius tears. J Hip Preserv Surg 2019;6(4):398–405.

35. Casartelli NC, Maffiuletti NA, Brunner R, et al. Clinical rating of movement-pattern quality in patients with femoroacetabular impingement syndrome: a methodological study. J Orthop Sports Phys Ther 2018;48(4):260–9.

36. Lewis CL, Loverro KL, Khuu A. Kinematic differences during single-leg step-down between individuals with femoroacetabular impingement syndrome and individuals without hip pain. J Orthop Sports Phys Ther 2018;48(4):270–9.

37. King E, Richter C, Franklyn-Miller A, et al. Whole-body biomechanical differences between limbs exist 9 months after ACL reconstruction across jump/landing tasks. Scand J Med Sci Sports 2018;28(12):2567–78.

38. King E, Richter C, Franklyn-Miller A, et al. Biomechanical but not timed performance asymmetries persist between limbs 9 months after ACL reconstruction during planned and unplanned change of direction. J Biomech 2018;81:93–103.

39. Alvim FC, Muniz AMS, Lucareli PRG, et al. Kinematics and muscle forces in women with patellofemoral pain during the propulsion phase of the single leg triple hop test. Gait Posture 2019;73:108–15.

40. Makovicka J, Chabbra A, Patel K, et al. A decade of hip injuries in national collegiate athletic association football players: an epidemiologic study using NCAA surveillance data. J Athl Train 2019;54(5):483–8.

41. Tummala S, Chhabra A, Makovicka J, et al. Hip and groin injuries among collegiate soccer players: the 10 year epidemiology, incidence and prevention. Orthopedics 2018;41(6):e831–6.

42. Mosler AB, Weir A, Eirale C, et al. Epidemiology of time loss groin injuries in a men's professional football league: a 2-year prospective study of 17 clubs and 606 players. Br J Sports Med 2018;52(5):292–7.

43. Werner J, Hägglund M, Ekstrand J, et al. Hip and groin time-loss injuries decreased slightly but injury burden remained constant in men's professional football: the 15-year prospective UEFA Elite Club Injury Study. Br J Sports Med 2019;53(9):539–46.

44. Trentacosta N, Sugimoto D, Micheli LJ. Hip and groin injuries in dancers: a systematic review. Sports Health 2017;9(5):422–7.
45. Kerbel YE, Smith CM, Prodromo JP, et al. Epidemiology of hip and groin injuries in collegiate athletes in the United States. Orthop J Sports Med 2018;6(5). 2325967118771676.
46. Bleakley CM, Glasgow P, MacAuley DC. PRICE needs updating, should we call the POLICE? Br J Sports Med 2012;46(4):220–1.
47. Bayer ML, Magnusson SP, Kjaer M, Tendon Research Group Bispebjerg. Early versus delayed rehabilitation after acute muscle injury. N Engl J Med 2017; 377(13):1300–1.
48. Hickey JT, Timmins RG, Maniar N, et al. Pain-free versus pain-threshold rehabilitation following acute hamstring strain injury: a randomized controlled trial. J Orthop Sports Phys Ther 2019;50(2):1–35.
49. Fry CS, Glynn EL, Drummond MJ, et al. Blood flow restriction exercise stimulates mTORC1 signaling and muscle protein synthesis in older men. J Appl Physiol (1985) 2010;108(5):1199–209.
50. Laurentino GC, Ugrinowitsch C, Roschel H, et al. Strength training with blood flow restriction diminishes myostatin gene expression. Med Sci Sports Exerc 2012; 44(3):406–12.
51. Cagnie B, Barbe T, De Ridder E, et al. The influence of dry needling of the trapezius muscle on muscle blood flow and oxygenation. J Manipulative Physiol Ther 2012;35(9):685–91.
52. Kaljić E, Trtak N, Avdić D, et al. The role of a dry needling technique in pain reduction. JHSCI 2018;8(3):128–39.
53. Karmali A, Walizada A, Stuber K. The efficacy of instrument-assisted soft tissue mobilization for musculoskeletal pain: a systematic review. J Contemporary Chiropr 2019;2:25–33.
54. Short S, Short G, Strack D, et al. A combined treatment approach emphasizing impairment-based manual therapy and exercise for hip-related compensatory injury in elite athletes: a case series. Int J Sports Phys Ther 2017;12(6):994–1010.

Printed and bound by CPI Group (UK) Ltd, Croydon, CR0 4YY

08/05/2025

01864694-0002